The Developmental Approach to Childhood Psychopathology

CLASSICAL PSYCHOANALYSIS AND ITS APPLICATIONS

A Series of Books
Edited by Robert Langs, M.D.

The Developmental Approach to Childhood Psychopathology

HUMBERTO NAGERA, M.D.

NEW YORK • JASON ARONSON • LONDON

ISBN: 0-87668-449-5

Library of Congress Catalog Number: 80-69668

Manufactured in the United States of America.

CONTENTS

PART III
ADOLESCENT DEVELOPMENT

PART IV
THE DEVELOPMENTAL APPROACH IN CLINICAL PRACTICE

PREFACE

The material in this volume is approached from a developmental point of view. I have always felt that it was necessary to pay attention to this particular approach which yields a great amount of understanding of and knowledge about human behavior in general and child psychopathology in particular.

There are many reasons for my interest. First, adults are the end product of a long developmental continuum of psychological processes that start at birth and possibly earlier. In other words, the child is always the father (and of course mother) of the adult he becomes. Just as during childhood one phase follows another and is influenced if not determined by the previous one, so adulthood is the outcome—the sum total—of all the developmental processes of childhood.

Second, without considering the developmental aspects of behavior, much of our knowledge would be one-dimensional and incomplete, frequently limited to a descriptive observation of a child or adult at a given moment in time. A developmental approach places these observations, along with the genetic givens and environmental influences that lead to normality and psychopathology, in their appropriate hierarchical and sequential order.

Thus, the developmental approach allows for a depth of genetic comprehensiveness that makes not only psychotherapy but also preventive work possible and rational, taking us well beyond a purely descriptive level of discourse. The developmental approach relates to the understanding of the child (and therefore the adult) as embryology does to anatomy, and in this way it is significant.

My years at the Hampstead Clinic in London and my contacts with Anna Freud and other members of the clinic stimulated my interest in the developmental aspects of normality and pathology. Indeed, a number of the chapters in this volume were written during that time and under their auspices. For what they taught me I am grateful.

Part I

GENERAL DEVELOPMENTAL CONSIDERATIONS

Chapter One

THE DEVELOPMENTAL PROFILE

The Developmental Profile can be considered a way of think-ing: more precisely, a metapsychological way of thinking and of organizing clinical material within the psychoanalytic frame of reference.[1] It collects from the mass of information available, clinical or otherwise, that which is relevant and necessary to gain a proper picture, as complete as possible, of a given personality at a given moment of development. It tends to discard the irrelevant, and at the same time highlights the areas in which the available information is incomplete though essential for the proper under-standing of a child's whole personality and conflicts.

This very point is one of the assets of the Profile. It largely solves the difficult question of how much and what kind of information

1. The following pages describe some aspects of the work of the Diagnostic Research Group at the Hampstead Clinic. In general our aims were to conduct an inquiry into the difficulties of diagnosing infantile disturbances, and to reevaluate initial diagnostic impressions and predictions recorded after the initial interviews and in the Diagnostic Conference. This initial material was compared with that gained from the same children after psychoanalytic treatment. It was hoped that as a result of this research, errors in assessment would be reduced and a more satisfactory and systematic technique for evaluat-ing the initial findings would be evolved. Several different approaches to the problem have been followed, but this paper is concerned with only one of these: the Developmental Profile as outlined by Anna Freud (1962).

During the course of the work of the Research Group, Anna Freud proposed a diagnostic scheme or, as she has called it, a *Developmental Profile*. This Profile was subsequently systematically applied to the cases being studied in the Diagnostic Research Group. Anna Freud made these suggestions after she had delivered her lectures "Four Contributions to the Psychoanalytic Study of the Child" (1960) in New York, lectures which contained the basic elements for the Developmental Profile.

is needed for a proper diagnostic evaluation of any specific case. By its very nature, the Profile is a metapsychological cross section of a personality structure at a given moment.

Attention should be paid to the fact that, in the Profile, *pathology is seen against the background of normal development and its possible variations.* This is, of course, of particular importance in child diagnosis, because the child, unlike the adult, is not yet a finished product.

The picture we may gain of a normal child and of his reactions will be different at different ages and stages of development. His capacity to react is different as he develops. Many phenomena seen in children represent aspects of development and are normal or nearly so at certain ages. Thus, for example, sleeping disturbances appear quite commonly in the second year of life. Similarly the child may deal with frustration or aggression by temper tantrums before more appropriate ways have been achieved developmentally. At a particular age, however, both symptoms lack the ominous quality they would have at a later age.

The developmental orientation of the Profile has a further advantage: by constantly forcing us to examine what is normal or pathological at different ages, it makes possible a clearer understanding and conceptualization of normal development.

As a concrete illustration of the Profile, I shall present the material of the diagnostic study of Arthur Z, eleven and a half years old. The information will be described and discussed under the main headings of the Profile. Examples will be given to illustrate some of the arguments and the many possibilities opened up by this approach. In addition, I hope to show the correlation existing among the various headings and I will attempt to convey something of our present experience in the use of the Profile.

DEVELOPMENTAL PICTURE AND GUIDE TO DIAGNOSIS
(PROFILE AT THE DIAGNOSTIC STAGE)

Material used:
Social History, June 11, 1954—Mrs. M

Psychiatric Interview, June 15, 1954—Dr. F
Intelligence Test Report, June 25, 1954—Miss W[2]

I. REASONS FOR REFFERAL

The mother felt that the child was retarded on account of persistent thumbsucking (which occurs only when he is at home and not when he is out). He has difficulties in school, where he does not cooperate and is not progressing properly. He is frequently absent from school due to slight rise in temperature, stomach pains, sickness, etc. His health has been checked several times and is fine.

II. DESCRIPTION OF THE CHILD

Arthur has a slight negroid appearance because of his crinkly hair and thick lips. He is a nice-looking lad, wears glasses, and is the size of a thirteen- or fourteen-year-old boy.

He can be quite independent (in spite of difficulties over separation) and will go anywhere alone. He will go skating or bicycling with his friends, though he is described as not making friends easily and being rather reserved.

Arthur tends to copy his little brother who is said to play with imagination. He likes his mother to read to him and prefers little-girl stories.

2. At Hampstead the diagnostic procedure varies according to the nature of the case involved. Broadly speaking, however, it consists of a social history, a psychiatric interview with the child, and psychological tests where indicated (but always, where possible, an intelligence test). Additional psychiatric interviews with parents and other relatives may be carried out as necessary.

A word needs to be said about our use of psychological test results. At the very beginning of the application of the Developmental Profile to our cases, we utilized mainly descriptions of the child's behavior in the test situation. The IQ was stated, but no special attention was paid to the content of the child's responses except where it gave information about the status of certain ego functions (relevant for this heading in the Profile). This procedure was followed because initially we wanted to base our assumptions as much as possible on purely clinical grounds. A much wider use of the test results (content) is of course perfectly valid and useful, and we are presently organizing a pilot study on this very aspect.

III. FAMILY BACKGROUND AND PERSONAL HISTORY

Arthur comes from a Jewish Nonorthodox background.

Mother: She has been in analytic treatment with Dr. W. She became increasingly depressed when the husband was away during the war. At that time, when Arthur was about two years old, she started working to cope with her misery. When she was pregnant with her second child, Arthur was three years nine months to four years six months old. She found him so irritating that she could not stand him. Arthur was then sent to a kindergarten.

It seems as if a certain amount of seduction goes on between Arthur and his mother. There are references to his making jokes about girls and laughing about nude pictures with his mother. He giggles, saying, "ooh," whenever he sees his mother not fully dressed.

Father: He is now established in business. He was away during the War when Arthur was between one year eight months to two years six months. At that time Mr. Z is said to have returned home after two months of convalescence following a nervous breakdown.

He was himself a difficult child, separating from his mother with difficulty. The father likes bathing the children on weekends (Arthur is now eleven and a half years) and has always cooperated a great deal in the care of Arthur.

Siblings: There is a seven-year-old brother. Arthur tends to copy this younger brother who is said to be imaginative. Arthur is now very jealous of him and constantly hits and teases him.

Friends: He is said not to make friends easily. While he did not refer to any special friend, he mentioned that he went out on his bike with a school friend and that he played with others in the street.

Personal History: The mother was well during the pregnancy. Arthur was born three weeks premature, but the birth is said to have been easy. The mother described him as a beautiful and happy baby. He was breast-fed for six months; was fed to the hour; and was weaned to the bottle at six months, refusing it at first.

He walked at a year; talked between two to two and a half years with slight setbacks when he went to the nursery. He has sucked his thumb since birth.

His toilet training is described as having been difficult. Arthur used to retain his bowel movements and still does so. He had bowel movements only at home. Frequently his pants were slightly soiled and still are nowadays. He achieved urinary control at the age of two years, though there were occasional accidents later.

IV. POSSIBLY SIGNIFICANT ENVIRONMENTAL INFLUENCES

1. Mother's and father's seductive attitude toward the children.

2. There have been a number of enforced early and later separations (and withdrawal on the mother's side due to her depression) that may have played a role in Arthur's difficulties. He tended to react to these experiences with extreme distress and regression.

For example, when during the War Arthur's mother became depressed due to the absence of her husband, Arthur (then aged two and a half) was sent to a nursery. There he never settled in; he stood in a corner, sucked his thumb, and bit and scratched the other children. There was a setback in talking as well. He was kept at this place for three months.

At the end of this third year he was sent to kindergarten. The mother, who was then pregnant again, referred to her not being able to stand the child at the time. He had always to be dragged screaming to the kindergarten.

At the age of five he went to a progressive school, where he was again not able to settle. He started soiling, wetting, and developed a tic in one eye.

V. ASSESSMENT OF DEVELOPMENT

GENERAL COMMENTS

This section has three main subsections: the development of (a) drives (libido and aggression), (b) Ego and Superego, and (c) Total Personality.

In regard to libido development, the essential point is the determination of whether a child has ever reached the phallic (oedipal) phase, at about the age of three or four. The type of object relationship is included here; attention should be paid to the way in which libido and aggression are used in relation to the objects and the self, and how objects are used in general.

In a similar way, we can ask at a later age whether the child has ever entered latency or puberty; whether this is a normal latency or puberty or one disturbed by neurotic conflicts or in some other way.

It is important in this context to distinguish the phallic phase from isolated phallic manifestations which may occur even though the bulk of the libido is still at an earlier stage. For example, a two-year-old girl may have penis envy for purely narcissistic reasons. We speak here of phallic dominance as a phase, and not as isolated phallic manifestations while another phase is dominant.

Has regression from the phallic phase taken place and, if so, to where? Of course, a relationship exists between this heading and that of Section VI, Regression and Fixation Points, since one of the prerequisites for regression is the existence of previous developmental points at which the libido has remained fixated.

It is not always easy to determine clearly how much of the libido one sees at a particular pregenital fixation point is present there as the result of regression and how much has always remained fixated at that point and has never moved forward. In brief, how much can be attributed to regression and how much to fixation? We have gained the impression that in many cases it is possible to have a relative, quantitative, idea of how much of the libido seen at a particular point may be attributed to fixation and how much to regression as a consequence of conflicts at later stages. A thorough developmental history of the child is necessary here.

In this connection, several possibilities may exist. Take, for instance, a child who was able to pass through the pregenital phases without too many difficulties and who shows what may be called the usual and normal fixation points at the oral and anal level. Further, let us suppose that as a result of the conflicts of the oedipal situation and because of castration fear the child regresses from the phallic level to the anal and oral levels.

The developmental history may show the picture of a child with no more than slight signs, if any, of fixations at the earlier levels. These may not be very outstanding, but at a certain point in development, for example, at the age of five years, as a consequence of the regression mentioned above, we can begin to observe the appearance of libidinal manifestations appropriate to the oral and anal phases, either as symptoms or as pieces of behavior which were previously absent.

If one pays proper attention to the details of the social history and in particular the developmental history, it will be seen that this picture differs markedly from that of another child in whom thumb-sucking (or some other oral manifestation. e.g., excessive clinging and demandingness) had been present throughout his development, far beyond the age at which such behavior corresponds to a specific stage of development and is therefore accepted as normal. The picture also differs from that of a child who shows in some way that his character bears the imprint of difficulties in one particular phase of development. The latter child may have moved through to the phallic phase, but the manifest signs of fixation to the early levels will at no point have disappeared from his developmental picture. If at a later stage conflict induces a regression of libido from the phallic phase, reinforcing the libido already present at earlier levels, one may be able to assess how much is attributable to this reinforcement through regression and how much to the ever-present fixations (though only in relative terms).

The outcome of further regression is an intensification of such manifestations as thumbsucking, clinging, and demandingness, or indeed of whatever signs of the anal or oral phases are present. What we observe is a reinforcement and intensification of the manifestation previously present.

Such a distinction is naturally of prognostic importance. It is no doubt easier to help the forward movement of libido which has regressed than of libido which has always been arrested at earlier stages. In assessing the total personality it is of value to have a relative estimate of how much of the libido was able to move forward to the phallic phase, even though it may at present be seen in a regressed state. It is important to know that at some time most or part of the libido had moved forward and had made its contribution at the proper time to the development of the ego and to the personality as a whole. This is in contrast to those cases in whom, through excessive fixation, large amounts of libido have remained arrested and were unable to contribute to normal development at the time when that contribution was required.

We believe that through collecting the material of a sufficient number of cases, light will be thrown on how, when, where, and why the libido makes its contribution to proper development. The same argument applies to the aggressive drive which will be dealt with below.

Finally, an examination of the libido is required in regard to its distribution in the self, objects, etc. Similarly, whenever relevant and possible, statements as to the mechanisms of self-esteem regulation and well-being can be included.

I return now to the assessment of development in the case of Arthur Z.

CASE ILLUSTRATION

A. *Drive Development*

1. Libido

(a) *With regard to phase development*

Arthur has reached the phallic-oedipal phase. (He giggles and says, "ooh," whenever he sees his mother not fully dressed; he makes jokes about girls and laughs about nude pictures with his mother; used to write "like love letters" to mother when away from her at nine years, etc.) There is evidence that he has very strong fixation points at the oral and anal levels to which large amounts of his libido are now regressed.

The latency period is being interfered with by the lack of a proper solution of the oedipal conflict and the regression that has followed. It can be said that latency is further complicated by a certain amount of seduction and stimulation exerted particularly, though not exclusively, by the mother. This factor makes it all the more difficult for him to renounce the pleasure he experiences when he succeeds in inducing his mother to care for him and look after him physically as if he were younger than he is (being dressed, bathed, etc.).

(b) *With regard to libido distribution*

(i) *Cathexis of self:* The cathexis of the self in Arthur's case seems to be interfered with in certain circumstances. In the test situation he showed an unusual degree of diffidence and self-criticism. He would present perfectly correct solutions, saying he was sure they were wrong, "I am not very good at this. . . ."

Similarly, the excessive use of turning aggression against the self may point either to a low narcissistic cathexis of the self (in relative terms) that allows and accounts for the choice and excessive use of this mechanism of defense or at least to a secondary interference with that cathexis when pressure on the side of the aggressive drive rises and defense has to be enforced.

(ii) *Cathexis of objects:* Arthur has, of course, reached the stage of object constancy, but that stage is constantly interfered with due to very strong and early fixations at the oral level.

2. Aggression

GENERAL COMMENTS

Here we look for the presence or absence of aggression on the surface, since we still know little about the vicissitudes of the different phases.

Quantitative, qualitative, and directional considerations are appropriate here.

The types of defense utilized to deal with aggressive drives should be noted and included here if relevant, or under the heading Ego, Defenses.

We hope that in time the systematic collection of information under this heading, and the correlation of that information with other aspects covered by the Profile, coming as it does from children of all ages and from all sorts of pathology, will ultimately make a contribution to our knowledge of the vicissitudes and development of the aggressive drive.

In Arthur's case the following material is recorded under the subheading of aggression.

CASE ILLUSTRATION

Arthur has not achieved adequate control of his aggressive impulses. Arthur's aggression breaks through frequently, particularly in the relationship with his mother. Whenever he is frustrated by her in any way, he attacks her and screams and yells with temper. On the other hand, at school he finds it difficult to read in a loud voice.

There is constant teasing and hitting of the brother.

He deals with aggression partly by turning it against himself (hurting himself frequently) and by means of his passivity.

B. *Ego and Superego Development*

GENERAL COMMENTS

This is the second main subheading in Section V, Assessment of Development. Under this heading are four main subdivisions: (1) ego apparatuses; (2) ego functions; (3) defenses; and (4) secondary interference of defenses with ego functions.

Ego development, like drive development, must be viewed against the background of normal development. One must constantly make allowances for the fact there are many variations or deviations in the normal development of ego function, and that, developmentally speaking, the child is not yet a finished product. Because of this, temporary regressions in ego functions or in libidinal development must under certain conditions be considered as normal.

Further allowance must be made for the processes of interaction between the child's endowment or innate capacity and the function of the environment as the releasing agent for the development of these innate capacities and as the stimulating agent for further ego development. For every infant and every environment (mainly represented by the mother at this early stage), the types of interaction will vary greatly.

The releasing and stimulating role of the mother depends of course on her interests and the possibilities for cathexis she provides. This factor plays a large role in the many variations of development which occur within normal limits.

It has previously been mentioned that there exists a link between the stage of libidinal development and the contribution made by it to further ego development.

(1) Under the subheading Ego Apparatuses, the intactness or defects of the ego apparatus are examined.

(2) Under the subheading Ego Functions, we look for the intactness of the various functions, always bearing it mind the age and stage of development of the particular child. We assess these functions against the background of our picture of normal development.

Particular attention should be paid to the existence of primary or developmental deficiencies.

When this point in the Profile has been reached we are able to categorize a very large number of cases diagnostically, i.e., those with an arrested libidinal or ego development. The value of the information recorded under this subheading for differential diagnosis and for prognosis cannot be overemphasized.

A good developmental history allows us to follow when certain functions appear, what their character is, and how they have developed since early in life. This is most useful for clarifying whether there is a "primary disturbance" based on an ego defect (organic damage being the possible substrate in many cases), or whether there is a "developmental disturbance" of the particular function or functions under consideration. In the latter case the cause might well be the lack of proper and adequate mothering. In this case the environment has failed in its releasing and stimulating function necessary for the proper development of the ego functions and apparatus (the extreme cases being those described by Spitz (1945) as "hospitalism").

The final picture presented by both types of cases may be similar, particularly if in the brain-damaged or deficient cases the neurological examination happens to be negative. Yet in one case there is an organic substrate, while in the other case there is a more functional defect (which nevertheless might be as irreversible as the first).

Both types of cases have a poor prognosis. The outcome depends on both the extent of the damage and the particular functions affected. In these cases analytic treatment will be limited since we cannot undo the organic defect, nor can we provide at a later date the stimulation and care which was required earlier.

A careful developmental history within the social history will help us here, and will at times allow us to make a differential diagnosis. For this purpose we should at the same time consider heading E in Section VII, Dynamic and Structural Assessment (Conflicts): External Conflicts, as well as the heading Background in Section III. There we will find descriptions of the sort of mothering the child has had in early life. Such details as normal siblings, coupled with the absence of information which might make us suspect the early mother-child relationship, and so on, will assist us. In other cases, the typical picture of the institutionalized child will complete our diagnosis.

On the other hand, in many cases of arrested ego development (of whatever nature), it is not possible to show or to point to conflicts of an internalized character (conflicts between superego, ego, and id), but only to conflicts of an internal nature (between opposites in the id) and to those of an external character. At a given age the absence of or incomplete picture of internalized conflicts can be a strong indicator of this type of problem, as shown by the lack of development in the structural sense. Furthermore, some of our cases used and needed their objects as auxiliary egos, to deal with fear and anxiety. They showed "an obsessionallike" organization. Any small change in the daily routine aroused extreme distress and anxiety. These cases are not obsessionals in the true meaning of the word but resemble them due to the incapacity of their egos to deal with any new situation or any change. These children were not withdrawn or autistic, but were quite able to cathect objects as long as they were approached at the level to which they had been able to develop. This latter point is important for the differential diagnosis of withdrawn or autistic children.

Some of these children showed phallic manifestations and reactions, but the ego development that should go with it and the rich fantasy life (oedipal) that should accompany these phallic reactions in normal children were never present. This is of great significance for the purpose of differential diagnosis. These cases represent the more or less extreme end of a scale which comprises all sorts of grades. The diagnostic procedure, and especially the prognostic evaluation, becomes more difficult as we approach the other end of the scale.

(3) Our third subheading under Ego and Superego Development deals with defenses, which we scrutinize in terms of their age adequacy.

Denial, identification, and projection are primitive defenses. Complete denial is adequate for a two-year-old but very abnormal later on. By the time of latency most of the primitive defenses should be in the background; one would then expect to see repression, reaction formation, sublimation, identification with the aggressor, turning passivity into activity, etc.

In adolescence all the primitive defenses seem to reappear for a time. Personal problems are now looked at impersonally, expressed in racial, social struggles, etc. (externalization). Attention should be paid to the excessive and untimely use of specific defenses, the availability of a variety of defenses, and the ego's effectiveness to deal with the drives in an adequate form. We should examine the type of defense not only in relation to its age adequacy but also in regard to the economic factor involved; whether, for example, the types of defense used require permanent and large expenditure of energy in the form of countercathexis. It should be borne in mind that the ego can use functions and mechanisms not normally meant for the purpose in a defensive fashion at a given time.

(4) Secondary Interference of Defenses with Ego Functions is the fourth subheading in the section Ego and Superego Development. Here we try to describe how the type of defense used by the ego interfere with certain ego functions. If the defenses can be removed

during the course of treatment the functions will reappear intact, in contrast with the case of primary defective functions.

It is easy to see, for example, that excessive use of withdrawal into fantasy will to a greater or lesser degree affect such functions as attention, perception, apperception, concentration, memory, and thought processes. At a given age this implies a severe interference with schooling and the process of learning. Other defenses will affect different functions. Excessive use of projection interferes with reality testing and thought processes. Aggression turned against the self may temporarily interfere with motility and result in a child becoming accident-prone. Regressive processes, particularly on the side of the ego, can imply a serious disturbance of very many ego functions.

If in a given case there is no particular conflict or type of defense that would explain the existing state of affairs, it is of great value when the Profile discloses a marked inhibition or lack of proper functioning of the ego as a whole. This suggests some sort of arrest in development; by looking to the other headings in the Profile, it becomes possible to find pointers to the real causes of disturbance.

We may ask: how will the faulty functioning of one function affect the development of the others? How does the ego attempt to compensate for this, and what is the result in terms of the final structure? This developmental approach which traces the lines of development of specific ego functions is bound to provide answers to these questions. The same approach is also valid in relation to the secondary interference of defenses with ego functions at different ages and stages of development, and to the manner in which this interference affects further development.

CASE ILLUSTRATION

Ego Apparatuses: Arthur's ego apparatuses seem to be intact. There are no symptoms or signs of primary defects there.

Ego Functions: There are also no signs of primary deficiencies in his ego functions. Arthur is a highly intelligent boy, who cannot at present make full use of his very good potentialities. He has an IQ of 137. Nevertheless his schoolwork is poor and his learning capacity seems to be impoverished. There is no doubt that there is an important secondary interference of his defensive system with many of his ego functions.

Defenses: Arthur's defense organization consists mainly of repression, regression (to anal and oral levels), reaction formations, very marked passivity, clinging and dependence, turning aggression against the self, and withdrawal into illness. This group of defenses is mainly directed against his phallic oedipal wishes for both parents as well as against his aggressive drives. This defense organization is in any case far from effective at present, resulting in anxiety and symptom formation.

Secondary Interference of Defenses with Ego Functions: It is not difficult to see how such a vast and excessive use of these types of defenses has led to an interference with his schooling and learning processes. His marked passivity plays a specially important role here.

Arthur's tendency to control his aggression, partly by means of turning it against himself, seems to interfere with his motility leading frequently to falls and accidents, where he hurts himself. The function of speech is interfered with by his oral aggression and the defenses against it, particularly in a given set of circumstances, i.e., when he has to read in a loud voice at school.

C. Development of the Total Personality or Age-Adequate Responses

GENERAL COMMENTS

For didactic and methodological purposes we artificially isolated the drive development from the ego development and assessed each independently.[3] Now, under the heading of Development of the Total Personality, we aim to see the whole personality, reacting to what Anna Freud has called *life task.* This reaction is partly dependent on the stage of development reached at any given

---

3. At present, one of the aspects of our research program on the Developmental Profile consists of the application of a number of *developmental lines* to our cases. This has been suggested by Anna Freud (1963) who points out: "Far from being theoretical abstractions, developmental lines, in the sense here used, are historical realities which, when assembled, convey a convincing picture of an individual's personal achievements, respectively of his failures in personality development."

moment. Life tasks are situations with which the child is confronted at different stages of his development. Many of these are common to everyone, but some may not be so usual or apply so generally.

Examples of life tasks that will confront children at different times are: going to nursery school at three and a half years; the birth of a sibling; the death of a close relative; hospitalizations (of the child himself, the mother, etc.); separations from the parents; moving house, etc.

We expect that the child's reaction differs at different ages, according to the means the child has acquired through the course of development to deal with such situations. (An excellent example is given by Gauthier (1960).) In these situations the personality as a whole reacts to the particular life task under consideration. The child as a whole adapts himself to the new situation and during this process makes use of all the resources at his disposal.

We can learn a great deal about each individual child. We can obtain information about his ego development and his capabilities, the sorts of defense he can mobilize, his capacity to tolerate frustration, his possibilities of sublimation, of toleration for anxiety and his ways of dealing with it, his ability to accept substitute or neutralized gratification with enjoyment, the progressive forces present in him as contrasted with the regressive ones and so on.

CASE ILLUSTRATION

In Arthur, the age-adequate achievements are lacking in the main. He has remained closely attached to the family (one positive element here is his ability to go biking with a friend). He prefers the family (both father and mother) to look after him and his body as if he were a small child.

The relationship to the parents, particularly to the mother, has remained highly sexualized. His interests in literature are sexualized.

VI. REGRESSION AND FIXATION POINTS

GENERAL COMMENTS

As previously described, we look here for signs that reveal

fixation points in pieces of significant behavior, fantasies, and in certain symptoms.

In some cases the fixation points will show themselves as precipitates in the character structure. Observation of the different imprints which the various libidinal phases left on the character structure can be very relevant. They may manifest themselves either directly as the characteristic traits of any given phase or through corresponding reaction formations, for example, excessive cleanliness instead of dirtiness.

The relevant material is classified under the subheadings: Oral, Anal, and Phallic.

As has been mentioned, there is a link between this heading and drive development. It is obvious that the various aspects of the Profile are intimately connected. Therefore there is a constant need to correlate the material recorded under each heading and to consider how each completes and qualifies the other. This process of correlation helps us to think in an organized fashion. In addition and even more importantly, each section provides checks of the material in the other sections, and the sections pose questions to one another that are relevant to the consideration of the case. This brings out apparent or real contradictions in the material. It constantly forces our minds to translate clinical observations into our conceptual frame of reference and vice versa.

In working with the Profile, the following questions and thoughts occurred to me in relation to the heading Regression and Fixation Points: what, if any, will be the difference between fixation points coming about as a result of deprivation and frustration (extreme cases being institutionalized children) and those which are a consequence of excessive gratification (those overwhelmed by stimulation or intense seduction)? Is there any difference in diagnostic or prognostic significance between these two possibilities?

Deprivation or frustration experienced early in life will under certain circumstances severely damage the child's possibilities for development, and these damages may not be reversible. What will be the counterpart of intense deprivation if we are dealing instead with excessive gratification or stimulation? Will the outcome be similar or even comparable?

Deprivation (intense frustration) or excessive gratification, when it occurs later in life and development, does not seem to have the same significance once a certain stage of development has been reached. After this point it looks as if, in some cases, intense stimulation (excessive gratification) is a more dangerous element than frustration as far as further development is concerned.

A further observation of interest in regard to fixation points is that these points may be almost all that remains of later levels and stages of development, once massive regressive processes have taken place (both on the ego and libidinal sides). Generally, the existence of strong fixation points is a potentially dangerous situation, because when faced with obstacles during later stages of development the libido that has remained behind pulls back the forward-moving libido.

In one of our cases we could observe that this whole process had been reversed. In view of this experience it might be justified to assume that fixation points also exert a forward pull (in this case, toward development) on the libido which, due to regression, has gone back to the very earliest stages. If further observations and clinical material were to confirm these speculative thoughts, we would be forced to add a new dimension to the function of fixation points. Side by side with their potentially pathogenic role in cases of neurosis, in other cases of more severe regressions and disorganization of the whole personality we would have to view fixation points as anchorage points in stages of higher development that had to be abandoned. They would not only be indicators of the stages reached, but would favor (by their "pulling" attraction in the descriptive sense) the forces of recovery. If this is the case, the presence of the fixation points in severe cases of regression would have prognostic value.

CASE ILLUSTRATION

As already pointed out, Arthur has very important fixation points at the oral and anal levels to which part of his libido has regressed.

Oral Level: According to the mother, Arthur slings his food down, eats at an abnormal rate, and is always hungry. He still sucks his thumb when he is at home. He is supposed to have bitten the side of his wooden cot so that the wood was chewed away. At three he used to bite other children at the nursery. Now he screams and yells and has an inhibition to read in a loud voice at the school.

Anal Level: The mother described the toilet training as difficult. Arthur retained, and still does, his bowel movements. He has bowel movements only at home, and he constantly comes home with his pants soiled. He is said to be obstinate and to have a violent temper that may well be the imprint of this phase of development on his character. The relationship with the mother has a sadomasochistic character.

Phallic Level: The relationship with the mother is still highly sexualized. He giggles and says, "ooh," when he sees his mother not fully dressed. He is always making jokes about girls and laughs about nude pictures with his mother. Arthur's battle at the oedipal stage is still going on; as a result of this, part of his libido has regressed to the previous phases. It is also noticable in the intensity of his positive attachment to the father, which has defensive aspects but which is undoubtedly linked with the intensity of his bisexual conflicts and therefore primary in character. The father himself plays an important role in this connection: he bathes Arthur on weekends.

VII. DYNAMIC AND STRUCTURAL ASSESSMENT (CONFLICTS)

GENERAL COMMENTS

This heading is subdivided into (a) External, (b) Internalized, and (c) Internal Conflicts.

(a) Much of the material that one feels tempted to include under External Conflicts belongs in fact in Section III, Family Background and Personal History, and in Section IV, Possibly Significant Environmental Influences. Entries under this subheading are prominent in the profiles of those cases in which a final structure of the personality has not been achieved (superego). The conflicts are between id-ego agencies and external authority figures. This may be due to the age of a child who is still too young to have completed his structural development, but it applies equally to those cases in which an arrested ego development makes final structure impossible, figures in the outside being used as both ego and superego auxiliaries. A similar situation is present in certain cases of defective superego development, in which the conflict takes place with external figures or with society (certain types of delinquent, etc.).

(b) The subheading, Internalized Conflicts (between id, ego, and superego), is of great significance. In itself it indicates that a final development in the structural sense has been reached. Fear of external authority has been internalized and has become fear of superego.

Guilt feelings appear and become the measure and expression of tension between the ego and superego. The presence of guilt in the material is a pointer to the existence of the superego as a functioning mental agency.

The internalized conflicts must be described in metapsychological terms, and a dynamic, economic, and structural analysis must be made of the conflict or conflicts involved (either of a libidinal or aggressive character). For this purpose it is necessary to refer back to the information examined and collected under the other headings, mainly those under defenses and fixation points, describing which drives are defended against and so on.

(c) The subheading Internal Conflicts is meant to cover conflicts between opposite drives—masculinity and femininity, activity and passivity, etc.

The assessment of this is not always an easy task. The older the child the more difficult it can be to sort out how much belongs to the initial bisexual conflict, how much to environmental influence, and how much to a defensive attitude developed at the time of the oedipal relationship and as a consequence of castration anxiety. Nevertheless, in many cases it has been possible to complete the sorting out successfully.

One is reminded here of Freud who said: "In both sexes the

relative strength of the masculine and feminine sexual disposi-
tions is what determines whether the outcome of the Oedipus
situation shall be an identification with the father or with the
mother. This is one of the ways in which bisexuality takes a hand
in the subsequent vicissitudes of the Oedipus complex" (1923, p.
33).

In view of Freud's statement, it is clear that the outcome of the
oedipus situation will itself be a pointer to what the original
bisexual constitution was like. This can be shown with clinical
material and observation. Moreover, in the area of the drives the
child is not as open to environmental and external influence as he
may be in other areas (ego development).

The process of sorting out thus becomes more feasible. When we
are confronted with an apparently passive-feminine identification
in a boy we can always ask whether what we observe is the result of
the original bisexual constitution or rather the outcome of external influences, or perhaps the result of defensive measures brought
about by castration anxiety, or of an early feminine identification.
Freud gives us an answer in the passage I have quoted. The
passive-feminine identification was possible and is the outcome of
the oedipal situation in a particular child, precisely on account of
the strong feminine element in his constitution. If this had been
otherwise, in spite of everything this possibility would not have
been open for him. Similarly, an early feminine identification
(implying a true modification of the ego on the basis of the
identification) is only open to those children who have an original
bisexual constitution which facilitates such an outcome.

On the other hand, one must realize that in relation to this
problem, as anywhere else in the Profile, the interaction between
endowment and environment cannot be overlooked or underrated.
The concept of "complemental series" is as valid in regard to
bisexual constitution as anywhere else. The influence of the
environment is more prominent precisely in those cases which
have a weaker endowment (e.g., a boy not strongly endowed with
masculinity, and consequently with a relatively strong feminine
element in his bisexual constitution).

In working with the Profile we found that, in order to evaluate the problems belonging to this particular subheading, a good developmental history is a great asset. In it we will look for pointers to the nature of the bisexual constitution, particularly (if it is possible) to its character before defensive measures against castration anxiety had the chance to exploit the basic bisexuality conflict and to form a final picture in which it may be more difficult to discern how much is the outcome of defense and how much is primary.

The possibility of an early identification of a passive-feminine character (with the mother, for example, before the phallic phase), as a consequence of, let us say, compliance with the wishes of the mother for a girl, will not be open if a strong masculine element is present. If it does occur and is an identification (with subsequent ego modification), this fact again constitutes a pointer to the marked bisexual conflict of the particular case. One has to distinguish certain types of "as if" identification, which are the result of compliance, from true identification. In the former, the child's drive, strivings, and fantasies remain masculine.

In the developmental history, data about all aspects of the child's behavior since early life, his physique, his voice and speech mannerisms, the way he walks, his body language in movements, facial expressions, the way he runs, climbs, the way he asks for things, the way he reacts in different situations, his games, and so on, may be possible pointers to his original bisexual constitution.

CASE ILLUSTRATION

External Conflicts: While Arthur's conflicts are mostly internalized, there are some conflicts with the external world that play an active role in his actual pathology and stage of development. This is due to the amount of seduction and external interference with his development (factors already referred to at different points).

Internalized Conflicts: These are libidinal and aggressive in character and mainly centered around the oedipal situation (both mother and father aspects playing an important role), as a result of which part of his libido is now back at oral and anal levels. As mentioned previously, not only the positive oedipal attachment to the mother but the strong oedipal attachment to the father must be noted here. Part of it is defensive, but part is no doubt linked with the intensity of his bisexual conflicts and primary in character. Arthur's conflicts at the oedipal level are frequently expressed in anal and oral terms.

Internal Conflicts: There are numerous hints of conflicts between opposite drives (male, female; passive, active). In both cases these conflicts seem to be partly of a primary character and partly a defense against anxiety provoked by one of the elements of the pair of opposites.

VIII. ASSESSMENT OF SOME GENERAL CHARACTERISTICS

GENERAL COMMENTS

This heading has four subsections: (a) Frustration Tolerance, (b) Sublimation Potential (capacity to accept and enjoy substitute or neutralized gratification), (c) overall attitude to anxiety, (d) Progressive Forces versus Regressive Tendencies. It will be noted that these are mainly, though not exclusively, of great prognostic value. For this reason, they have been singled out from other areas and headings where they might belong. The prognostic value of these subsections relates to the possibilities of further normal development, to treatability by the psychoanalytic method, and to long-term prognosis.

(a) Frustration Tolerance is not always easy to assess. (This heading overlaps to some extent with the two following ones, which are in some ways related.) The lower the capacity of any child to tolerate frustration, the worse he is equipped for life. Frustration tolerance refers to the immediate reaction that follows the postponement or total lack of fulfillment of an instinctual wish. When trying to assess a child's frustration tolerance we cover three points: tolerance in regard to the frustration (i) of libidinal drives, (ii) of aggressive drives, and (iii) of failure when engaged in neutralized activities. It should be kept in mind that frustration tolerance varies at various times in life, from practically none at birth and in the child's early life, to different levels at some later stage. When, for example, regression to the oral phase occurs, the level of frustration tolerance will be very diminished. It must be taken into account that the tolerance of frustration may be different in relation to different component instincts.

(b) Sublimation Potential—the capacity to accept and enjoy substitute or neutralized gratification—is a measure of an important safety valve for mental health. Those who have a good capacity in this area are safer in life.

In most cases the material available for diagnostic purposes gives one some impression of what the child looks like in this area. Accounts of the child's behavior, usually given by the mother, generally suffice for this purpose. In addition, descriptions of work and behavior at school may be useful. The presence of sublimation is another pointer.

(c) Under the heading Overall Attitude to Anxiety, as far as possible a metapsychological description of the facts should be given. In one sense this heading is the other side of the picture described under Internalized Conflicts. There a metapsychological account of the conflict situation was asked for. Here, we want to know about the rearrangements that have taken place, precisely as a result of that conflict, in the structure of personality and in character formation, viewed in dynamic, economic, and structural terms. In short, what is required here is the rearrangement brought about as a result of the conflicts and defenses used in the structure of personality and in character formation, as well as an estimate of the child's basic attitude toward anxiety.

There are great variations in the amount of anxiety which different children can tolerate without resorting to symptoms and defenses. If the child can meet anxiety in an active way, this is a positive factor; this is in contrast to those who will either regress or develop phobic symptoms.

(d) Looking at the Progressive Forces versus Regressive Tendencies, we make an attempt to obtain a feeling of the underlying general tendencies in the child. There may be a tendency to progress and develop in spite of external difficulties and stresses, or the contrary may be the case. Many pathological manifestations can be absorbed by a strong impulse to development.

Frustration Tolerance: Arthur has a relatively low capacity for the toleration of frustration.

Sublimation Potential: So far there is no evidence of his having a high sublimation potential, though the real picture here may be somewhat blurred and interfered with by the undue stimulation and seduction on the side of the parents.

Overall Attitude to Anxiety: Arthur tends to withdraw from situations where toleration and mastery of anxiety are required. This can be observed in the reading inhibition he developed when having to read in a loud voice at school (at home his oral aggression breaks through in shouting and yelling) or in his regression to earlier levels of drive discharge and gratification, resulting from castration anxiety and intolerable oedipal strivings.

His ego overall attitude to this type and amount of anxiety is inefficient; the result has been symptom formation and a tendency to restrict the ego, in spite of very high potentialities.

Progressive Forces versus Regressive Tendencies: There is a pullback, a tendency to regress to more primitive levels of libidinal development and more primitive sources of libidinal gratification. This has involved, on occasions, the temporary regression of certain controls and ego functions already achieved when the frustration period sets in (i.e., speech).

IX. DIAGNOSIS

In this section we are only concerned with a broad formulation of the type of disturbance. Broadly speaking, we can distinguish among normal development and its variations; neurotic (i.e., regressive) processes in development; atypical (i.e., arrested) processes in development; and psychotic and borderline (i.e., malignant) processes.

CASE ILLUSTRATION

Arthur belongs in group (3) of the provisional classification proposed by A. Freud in 1962, showing neurotic conflicts with regression to the anal and oral levels, symptom formation and marked ego restrictions.

DISCUSSION

After using the Developmental Profile for a period of about a year, the diagnostic discussions of a number of cases revealed that it meets the requirements for these procedures. Diagnostic discussions are of necessity limited in time, as far as any one case is concerned, after which a diagnostic decision is attempted. However, this time limitation, so necessary for obvious reasons, has certain dangers.

The Profile meets some of the shortcomings of ordinary diagnostic evaluations in a more appropriate way. It forces us, from the very beginning, to pay attention to and cover each and every area of the personality. A case must be seen as a whole, due attention being paid to every aspect. In this way we avoid some of the dangers implicit in the ordinary procedure, particularly the tendency to focus on a particular symptom or striking piece of behavior. Important as this symptom or piece of behavior may be for the assessment of a child, they should not be considered in isolation, in which case they might acquire quite a different diagnostic meaning and significance. They must be viewed in the context of the whole personality, as part of a total structure, because they can be properly assessed and qualified only in this context.

As far as the time invested in elaborating the Profile is concerned, it can be said to be negligible. Since the Profile is truly a way of thinking and of organizing clinical observations and material, metapsychologically and within the conceptual frame of psychoanalysis, it can be built up as soon as one has finished reading the material available (i.e., social history, psychiatric interview, etc.). I have already commented on the fact that the classification of material under different headings is done for didactic and methodological reasons. The analysis of specific areas, for the time being artificially isolated from other areas with which they are closely interconnected, is only the initial step. This must be followed by the synthesis that the Profile represents.

The Profile is meant to be an extremely dynamic and alive picture of a given person. This requires the selection of relevant clinical material, which will convey meaning and imbue the Profile with liveliness. For those who want to achieve this, an important warning must be given: this is not to work from the headings to the material, a procedure which will never make a Profile, but rather the other way round, from the clinical material to the headings. Working in this way the clinical material will tend to classify itself whenever it is a relevant piece of information under a given section. Frequently, the same piece of material will "place itself" under several headings, making a different and valuable contribution to each and throwing light on the particular personality being examined. This makes the Profile meaningful, dynamic, and alive.

If, on the other hand, one "feeds" the headings simply because they exist, if one goes from the heading to the clinical material, one may be able to collect much information under each heading. But this is static and at times meaningless information. The Profile will lack that integrating thought process that is necessary for the construction of a meaningful picture of a person. It will also lack that which enriches the Profile and ourselves by teaching us to correlate our theoretical model with clinical observations and vice versa. In short, the metapsychological approach is missing, and the process of trying out every possible angle in our own mind is lost. The finished Profile constitutes, after all, nothing more than a summary of our mental activities while reading the material, a sort of summary of our mental exercises in correlation, in assessment, in the translation of clinical observations into theoretical concepts, and vice versa.

It may have been noticed that the headings belong to different levels of concept formation. They are hierarchically different and collect and organize the material at different levels of conceptualization. I have mentioned several times that a close relation exists among the different headings, and consequently among the clinical data that are classified under these various headings. Furthermore, some headings are built up mainly on the information which has already been analyzed in several of the others. For this reason the information which is given in and analyzed by the different headings is not all at the same level or in the same conceptual category. Some headings collect the material in a rather simple way, others organize it at a more complex level of concept formation. Finally when we arrive at the summit of the Profile, we have the metapsychological formulations.

The Profile highlights the various areas of conflict, at times giving a very clear picture of the intensity and magnitudes of the forces involved. It permits us to make some quantitative assessment (in relative terms) of the magnitude of the drives, which are present as the result of a person's endowment, and to make comparisons with other cases. In this way a clearer understanding of the economic aspects is possible.

A good developmental history not only helps us to achieve all the purposes mentioned, it also allows us to understand the vicissitudes of the drives at various developmental stages; vicissitudes which are the result of the interplay with forces and figures of the environment, and later the interplay with the inner representatives and heirs of these external figures and conflicts.

With the information available at any time during the course of treatment, or after completion of treatment, a Profile can be constructed which may be compared with that obtained at the diagnostic stage on the basis of the information then available. This enables us to check on how far our diagnostic assumptions, our understanding of the case, and our predictions were correct, and how much of what later emerged in treatment was visible at the diagnostic stage, and so on. It allows us to check whether our metapsychological assessment of the material at the diagnostic stage was correct and whether it coincides with the assessment we could make after several years of analytic treatment.

The results obtained by the application of the Profile in this way have been satisfactory and instructive. The comparisons of Profiles obtained at the diagnostic stage and after the completion of treatment have shown us that the Profile pinpoints at the very beginning the child's basic personality structure and main conflicts.

We then examined a number of cases in which we knew our initial diagnostic assessment to be incorrect or incomplete. The Profile was applied by a worker familiar with its use but who had no knowledge of the particular case. Again, we were impressed by the results and regretted that no Profile had been available at the diagnostic stage of these cases. The analysis of causes of failure in the diagnostic procedures, in the light of knowledge gained after the analytic treatment of these cases, will lead to improvements.

The Profile constantly feeds back information that can, in its turn, improve our diagnostic techniques and our evaluations of the material. The very nature of the Developmental Profile provides checks on the reliability of our different sources of information (mother, father, etc.). We do not rely as much as we did in the past on a particular account given about a patient and on the accuracy of that account. Rather we rely on the internal picture we construct with all the information about the conflicts and the structure of a given personality. This picture must fit with the one familiar to us from our experience with neurotic, atypical, borderline, or psychotic pictures. Our ideal is to achieve a positive diagnosis. As in general medicine, we attempt to construct a syndrome in which all the symptoms and signs must correspond to and fit with what we know about neurotic conflict or atypical cases. For this purpose we follow the role played by the drives, the different structures of the mind, the mechanism of symptom formation, defenses, the degree of maturity of the systems involved, etc. (the medical equivalent being anatomical, anatomopathological, physiological, and physiopathological considerations, etc.). The whole clinical picture thus arrived at must be properly delimited from others and must be internally consistent. If it is not, the Profile highlights contradictions and inaccuracies and permits us to trace them back to their sources.

Furthermore, the Profile poses questions which must be answered in order to resolve such inaccuracies and contradictions; it asks for more information on specific points, before a correct judgment can be arrived at. In this way the Profile checks itself, or rather, leads us to do the checking. If we obtain an incomplete picture of the structure of a neurotic conflict we will be warned to look more closely and to be prepared for a diagnostic surprise of one sort of another. For example, we may have a child with neurotic conflicts similar to those which any other child might have. But in addition, this child has, within certain limits, a faulty or defective ego. We will see the usual picture of neurotic conflict, but also that the child is not able to deal with the anxiety and the conflict situation in quite the same way as other children with normal egos do. This child will be in greater distress, more overwhelmed by his anxiety, and more helpless. The problem here may be a quantitative one, the ego not being able to cope beyond a certain point.

I have mentioned before that the Profile can be applied at any given point during the course of treatment, yielding a cross section of the personality at that particular moment. It follows that the Profile is thus a useful tool for the assessment of the progress of analytic treatment. Applied at the end of treatment it provides an assessment of changes brought about by treatment (A. Freud 1961). The Profile evaluates the results of treatment by scrutinizing the inner changes and the structural rearrangements brought about by the analytic treatment rather than by assessing certain particular external manifestations. This method examines closely the changes in the defensive systems, the disappearance or diminution of the original conflicts in terms of the relative magnitude of the forces involved, the processes of sublimation that have been favored by the treatment situation, and the like. It also takes into account the ego's new capacities and techniques for dealing with anxiety. In short, it tries to highlight the structural, dynamic, economic, and adaptive rearrangements that may have taken place as the result of analysis.

In a number of cases we have repeated the Profile at the end of treatment (psychoanalytic treatment five times a week for a period of two, three, four, or more years).[4] It cannot be overemphasized that the inner picture may be very different from the one based on an assessment of external manifestations, which can be very misleading. This is well brought out by the case of Arthur whose Profile has been presented here.

Arthur was eleven and a half years old at the beginning of his treatment. A Profile was made with the material recorded after three years of analytic treatment and subsequent follow-up. A superficial assessment might give the impression of a very much improved child, with no apparent trace of the conflicts and anxieties that had brought him into treatment. However, a closer examination, making use of the Profile, showed that most of the main conflicts and anxieties remained even though they were no longer as apparent as at the diagnostic stage.

He is now nineteen years old. His passivity and his tendency to revert to it as a consequence of castration anxiety or disappointment were seen at the diagnostic stage and are still present though they are less transparent. The diagnostic Profile also revealed a disturbed mother-child relationship. At present his relationship to his mother is still a highly sexualized one. His school problems and his learning inhibitions (in spite of his high capacities) are no longer present in their original form, but he has renounced his ambition of becoming an engineer and is at present undertaking a training well below his capacities. His difficulties centering around his aggression are still present.

Arthur's neurotic conflicts and symptoms are no longer as apparent as they were at the diagnostic stage. It seems that he has achieved a more stable equilibrium. However, he has paid the price of having to maintain a number of ego restrictions and limitations. He has also developed a number of rather undesirable character traits. He has not solved his conflicts by inner change but

---

4. The material utilized here consists of the reports made by the therapists on the treatment. At Hampstead we make written reports on every child in analysis at weekly and bimonthly intervals; in addition, each case is presented at least once a year to the general staff meeting. After completion of the analysis a summary of the treatment is prepared by the child's therapist. This material is available for research purposes.

rather avoids them. Thus his interest in girls tends to lead to failure, to fear of competing, and to retreat into passivity. When another boy appears he simply withdraws. Similarly the decision that Arthur has made to enter his father's business is apparently not based on a healthy identification with the father but rather seems to be the outcome of a passive submission to the father's wishes.

We believe that time will confirm the expectations we have concerning the use of the Profile as a research tool. It has already proved its usefulness in many ways. The collection and comparison of large amounts of material obtained from specific cases and many different ones may prove valuable as a means of validating many theoretical assumptions and propositions.

In the experience of those who have worked with it, the Profile has stimulated, improved, and trained our thought processes in the field of psychoanalysis. We consider it to be of value in the training of candidates. It helps the student to learn the metapsychological approach. It sharpens the capacity for translating clinical observations and material into concepts, and helps us to use our theoretical formulations in the scrutiny and evaluation of clinical observations.

It may prove to be the basis on which an analytic classification of childhood (and adult) disturbances can later be built. It brings to such a classification not only a balanced view of the interaction of heredity, endowment, and environment; it also includes the developmental aspects, and the point of view of normality. All of these are basic considerations in any attempt at classifying or evaluating childhood manifestations, either normal or pathological.

Moreover, the genetic point of view has been given its proper place within the Profile. We can thus avoid the frequent mistakes that can occur when the genetic approach is taken further than it can really go, particularly at the diagnostic stage. When treatment has given us a much deeper understanding of the case and the forces and influences operative, it becomes possible to fill the gaps that may exist in this area.

References

Freud, A. (1960). Four contributions to the psychoanalytic study of the child. Lectures presented at New York.
——— (1961). The curative factors of psycho-analysis. In panel, International Psycho-Analytical Congress, Edinburgh.
——— (1962). Assessment of childhood disturbances. *Psychoanalytic Study of the Child* 17:149-158.
——— (1963). The concept of developmental lines. *Psychoanalytic Study of the Child* 18:245-268
Freud, S. (1923). The ego and the id. *Standard Edition* 19:3-68.
Gauthier, Y. (1960). Observations on ego development: the birth of a sibling. *Bulletin of the Philadelphia Association of Psychoanaly* 10.
Spitz, R. A. (1954). Hospitalism. *Psychoanalytic Study of the Child* 1:53-74.

Chapter Two

THE NORMAL CHILD

Normality in children is, to say the least, an elusive concept. There is a considerable problem involved in providing a simple and encompassing definition for a situation of such complexity. It is not in fact possible to deal with the problem at a definitional level. What can be undertaken, however, is an examination of the many variables influencing such an abstract concept as health or normality.

The task is not much easier when adults are considered than when children are the object of study. Freud (1909) considered the line between normality and pathology to be very indistinct; he asserted that any given individual might well traverse it back and forth on several occasions during his lifetime. As a matter of fact, this might well happen on several occasions during each and every day of his life.

Nevertheless, professionals have set forth various criteria to measure the degree of normality or pathology present. For example, among the widely accepted criteria for normality in adulthood are the ability to work well, a good sexual adjustment, and the capacity to enjoy leisure. As useful as such criteria may be, they are not suitable for an evaluation of the emotional or psychological health of a group who range in age from birth to the onset of adulthood.

There are a number of significant differences between children and adults which merit particular attention in this regard.

First, the adult is a "finished product." Obviously all emotional and psychological development does not come to a halt with the attainment of adulthood. However, in one way or another the maturational and developmental processes that define adulthood have for the most part been completed. Whatever its quality, whatever its strengths and weaknesses, the sum total of all these processes is a final "adult product."

With children the situation is totally different. They are in a constant process of very active development. This implies rapid changes taking place simultaneously in all areas of personality along numerous lines of development. The different areas of the personality need to interact with one another constantly in the process of living and growing up. There are balances and im-balances in all these lines of development. At each different age and stage of development this creates a constantly changing disequilibrium in terms of the nature, quantity and quality of the conflicts, stresses, etc. As a result, the emerging phenomena are extermely complex. What is normal during the first year of life may be considered quite inappropriate during the second. Thus, the picture for any given age is much more variable and dynamic than is the case with adults. The developmental point of view is an essential consideration when trying to assess the child.

These considerations apply generally throughout the child's development. In addition, there is the complicating presence of the child's capacity to imagine, to fantasize, and to use defenses that distort the reality of any given situation. These are coupled with the child's ego immaturity, limited capacity for abstract thinking (in the earlier years), and limited fund of information. Together, these factors set the stage for the multiple variations of what is normal at any given age as well as for possible psycho-pathological developments. Furthermore, they highlight the in-numerable weaknesses and dangers involved in the developmental processes and the more than ample opportunities for both normal and abnormal variations.

Second, organic maturation of the brain reaches completion

somewhere before two years of age. Up to that point there exists a special relationship between the genetic potential of any given brain and the amount of stimulation that it receives. Early in life such stimulation comes largely from the mother's ministrations. This input is essential if the brain is to unfold ideally and reach its ideal genetic potential.

Formerly it was believed that only internal, genetically determined embryological maturational forces defined the degree of quality and maturation the brain would gain. Increasing evidence from animal experimentation and "fate experiments" in human infants tend to show in quite a compelling manner that such an assumption is incorrect. These maturational forces alone cannot bring a brain to achieve whatever its ideal potential might be. To reach that ideal potential, external stimulation of the immature brain is required. These patterns of stimulation seem to influence brain development and its quality by at least three different mechanisms (see Chapter 17).

1. Appropriate forms of external stimulation at the right time seem to increase the degree of vascularization in various areas in the brain. Generally speaking, for any organ, better vascularization means better functional abilities.

2. Appropriate forms of external stimulation at the right time seem to increase the amount of dendritization that takes place. This means more potentially available functional pathways and, as such, possibly a "better," more capable brain.

3. Appropriate forms of external stimulation at the right time seem to increase the rate at which myelinization takes place. The relationship between myelinization and function seems reasonably well established though here too there are many unanswered questions.

Conceivably the effect of all the above processes is cumulative and may contribute to what determines the "quality" of the brain for any given human being. These basic organic structures sustain psychological function. They are the biological determinants of later human behavior. It follows that the assessment of the developmental normalcy of a young infant must include considerations of this type.

Naturally, we need to be aware of the limitations in our knowledge of such areas. Our ability to assess "normality" as well as "pathology" is necessarily limited by the state of the art. Indeed, it may frequently prove more difficult to assess "normality" than "pathology" and to conclude that a child is "normal" rather than "abnormal."

Nor is the assessment of the developmental normalcy of a very young infant an easy matter. For example, by six or eight months a child may have unmistakable signs of developmental retardation. We cannot simply conclude that the child's brain is abnormal per se, especially in the common situation when there is an absence of clear neurological signs. We have to discriminate between functional retardation due to a lack of stimulation and a host of other possibilities. The latter will range from malnutrition (either during the pregnancy or early life), to diseases in the mother during the pregnancy that might affect brain development, birth traumas or damage, genetic defects or abnormalities, etc. The diagnostic and prognostic significance of such differential diagnoses is self-evident. In those cases that fall within the so-called critical periods, the brain may be potentially normal. The situation may then still be reversible by the provision of nutrients either in the physical or psychological sense. Where the damage to the organic structure is already established or the damage to the functional capabilities of the brain has become irreversible, a totally different assessment of current and future normalcy will ensue.

Third, although neither adults nor children are islands unto themselves, this is particularly true of children. Every child, especially every infant, is an integral part of a complex system. At the outset, the system consists essentially of baby and mother. Mother, in turn, is dependent on other support systems such as her husband, her family, her own mother, etc. As development progresses such systems modify and enlarge themselves. A more influential role is played in the child's normal (or abnormal) developmental progression by such people as the father, siblings, grandparents, etc. In short, the child develops with a special social system, the family unit. As growth continues, such systems and the elements that constitute them continue to change; in latency, they include teachers and the community of peers. The latter acquire enormous importance by the time the child reaches adolescence.

Inevitably all the elements in such systems serve in some measure to determine the shape of the child's developmental progression (or the lack of it and its multiple variations). Once "behavior" or "pathology" is determined to be outside the normal range for a child of a given age, it is essential to ascertain what is at fault with that youngster's particular system.

Let us consider a case of developmental retardation in a baby nine to ten months old. He was late smiling and holding his head up. His hand-eye coordination was poor, he could not sit appropriately, etc. Such a clinical picture could be explained in various ways including the possibility of some organicity. On the other hand, it might be determined that this is an unwanted child, left very much to himself, his interaction with mother reduced to the most basic functions to sustain life, and in short, neglected, understimulated, and sensory deprived. This would also explain the nature of his developmental retardation.

This situation bears on other aspects of the nature of normality. Strictly speaking this child is "abnormal," not in a "healthy state," since he is developmentally retarded. At the same time there is nothing intrinsic to the child that determined such developmental retardation. The child was "potentially" capable of developing normally, and might still be able to do so. He was normal and in a way is normal now; developmental retardation is a "normal" (though not healthy) response to the conditions of understimulation and sensory deprivation to which he was subjected. If this child were provided with the necessary stimulation, the situation would reverse itself and the child "catch up" developmentally, as Spitz and others demonstrated long ago and Selma Fraiberg most recently. I am ignoring for the moment the possibility that there may be critical periods beyond which some permanent damage to certain aspects of the personality may accrue, even if the child seems to catch up in terms of milestones.

Fourth, conceptually and empirically "normality" implies a very wide frame of reference within which much variation can take place. All these variations are perfectly compatible with "normality." Thus, some children will start walking as early as eight or children to go through what has been described elsewhere (Nagera to the second year of life. The same is of course true of speech. Some children are capable of sentence formation and fluency in the first half of the second year of life; others do not achieve that degree of proficiency until they are three or older. In addition, there seem to be significant but "normal" differences between girls and boys in this area. It is not uncommon for children to move into the phallic-oedipal stage as early as two and a half years of age. Such youngsters show clear concerns, interests, and anxieties in terms of triangular relationships although other similarly normal children who are less precocious may not do so until three and a half or four years of age.

Fifth, to complicate matters further, it is typical for normal children to go through what has been described elsewhere (Nagera 1966) as developmental conflicts. These conflicts are both numerous as well as characteristic for every age and stage of development.

Like any other conflicts of children and adolescents, developmental conflicts create stresses, anxiety and guilt. Typically, they lead to symptom formation and behaviors of various kinds that in and of themselves, or when observed in any other context could be considered "abnormal." Hence, a paradoxical situation emerges where it is "normal" for "normal children" to go through developmental conflicts and produce symptoms and behaviors that the inexperienced clinician or the lay person would consider as clear indications of pathology. It is somewhat surprising that every child psychiatrist and pediatrician will occasionally label such symptoms or behaviors as abnormality or psychopathology in essentially normal children. The best example of this, but not the only one by any means, is what psychoanalysts have referred to as the infantile neuroses. Somewhere between two and a half and five, children of both sexes start to show abnormal manifestations of different degrees of intensity. These behaviors and symptoms are the expression of the typical (and quite normal) developmental conflict for that age group. Thus, these children may start displaying various forms of sleep disturbance (see chapter 13). These characteristically take the form of nightmares or night terrors. They wake up in a panic and attempt to sleep in the parental bed, or have one or another of the parents come to their room or sleep in in their beds, etc. Fears of a large variety of types are common, most typically fears of the dark, monsters, "ghosts," and burglars. This is frequently accompanied by anxious requests that they be allowed to sleep with their lights on, or to sleep in the parental bedroom or to have their bedroom doors open, etc. Related requests are posed for yet another story to be read at bedtime, or another glass of water, or another kiss, or still another trip to the bathroom. A different variation is the fear either of somebody hiding in the room with evil intentions or coming through the window to attack the child and harm or kidnap him, etc. Many other phobic symptoms populate the minds of these children such as fears of animals, especially those that can bite such as dogs, cats, lions, tigers, etc. Much (castration) anxiety is observed, usually expressed as concerns about hurts, injuries, accidents, and possible damage to their bodies. Often there are marked reactions on seeing a crippled person, a blind person, etc. Associated behaviors include an increase in masturbatory activities, brief or more extended recurrences of bedwetting, etc. Many bedtime ceremonials and rituals as well as other forms of obsessive-compulsive behavior are not infrequent.

Depending on the intensity of all this the child is handicapped to some degree while the developmental conflict endures. Similarly, parental concern and reactions to the child will vary with the severity, pervasiveness, and intensity of the symptoms. Often enough there is a disturbing effect on the marital couple's activities.

Thus, for children of such an age and at such a stage of development, a very visible disturbance is considered the "normal condition" provided that it is kept within reasonable limits. Again, we have the paradoxical situation of a child showing plenty of "symptoms" and "abnormal behaviors" that by their very existence actually stamp him or her as a perfectly normal little boy or little girl!

One most significant difference between the manifestations of a developmental conflict such as this and those related to other forms of pathological conflicts is that the former is transitory and the latter permanent. In other words, in the case of the developmental conflicts the developmental imbalances that led to the stresses, tensions, and conflicts responsible for the symptoms are corrected spontaneously as development progresses. However, this is not a likely outcome in any other conflictual situation with the exception of the type of phenomenon to be described next.

Sixth, the children's development is constantly being interfered with in a various ways. Developmental interference (Nagera 1966) has been defined as that action arising in the child's environment which disturbs the typical unfolding of development. Usually, this refers to a gross external or environmental interference with the needs and/or rights of the child. It applies as well to situations in which excessive or unjustified demands are made of the child. Interference also occurs when the necessary demands (according to age and stage of development) are not made of the child. This is especially true with those parents or, more especially with those mothers, who tend to prolong the babyhood of their children. The parents who make, or who fail to make the type of demands we are discussing here tend generally not to take into account the fact that the child may well lack the necessary ego development at that point to comply with such demands or to cope.

Such inappropriate interventions can create stress situations that the child cannot handle. This may result in symptom formation or behavior which is superficially similar to what occurs in the case of neurotic conflicts. Yet there are significant differences between them.

In any case, the type of disturbance created by a developmental interference can sometimes affect development in a positive manner. For example, it might speed it up. (Of course, in any given case, that type of outcome may or may not be desirable.) In general, however, such developmental interferences usually affect development in undesirable ways.

The degree of impact on the child is dependent on various factors. Among these are age, the stage of development, the nature of the interference, and the amount of time it has been in operation. Naturally, the interferences can occur at any point in the child's development. Let us consider a few examples. A severe prolonged postpartum maternal depression may interfere with the mother's ability to care for and stimulate her child appropriately. Such a situation will have a number of repercussions. Another example is recurrent exposure to hunger, either through primary neglect or because of the rigid feeding timetables that were so popular with pediatricians not long ago. Other examples include painful illnesses, prolonged hospitalizations that can act as an interference because of the separation itself or because of the trauma of painful medical manipulations. In particular, surgical interventions such as a simple tonsillectomy or appendectomy (performed between the ages of two and a half to five) may trigger traumatic floods of castration anxiety and act as the nucleus for the pathological growth of an infantile neurosis. Interferences can take the form of rigid toilet training with much conflict between parents and child, or training that is either started too early or unnecessarily postponed. Death of parents, siblings, or other important members of the family can affect the child's development in a variety of ways. A sexually provocative or seductive mother can have such an impact during the phallic-oedipal phase or even during adolescence. In fact there is an inexhaustible list of possible developmental interferences all of which will influence how the child appears in terms of "normality" or "abnormality." There are some interferences that are accidents of fate and others that are actively introduced in the life of the young by the world about them.

To further complicate the assessment of what is "normal," the same type of interference may well produce a wide variety of results and reactions in different children. Clearly, there are some distinct general tendencies related to the nature of the interference and the stage of development. Yet, each case needs an individual evaluation since different genetic endowments, different backgrounds, different previous experiences, different internal circumstances (i.e. a better capacity to handle anxiety, more sublimatory potential and capacity, etc.) will either tend to determine where the damage, if any, will be done, or to reinforce or soften the effects of any particular interference.

The effects of such interferences are various and multiple. Children do react to the stresses created by developmental interferences with "abnormal" manifestations. These frequently resemble the symptoms observed in the cases of neurotic conflicts or neurosis proper (as was also true for the developmental conflicts). Thus, for example, much anxiety can be present on the surface, or multiple forms of regression can be observed affecting either the child's instinctual development (i.e. regression to bedwetting) or his ego. In the latter case the result may be the giving up of certain ego achievements such as speech, regression to baby talk, etc. Further, many other "abnormal" behavioral manifestations or symptoms may be present.

But in spite of this superficial identity there are important differences as well. Many of the "symptoms" resulting from interferences, especially early on in life, are not the compromise formations with symbolic unconscious meanings and contents that are found in the neuroses. They are instead reactions to the stress and anxiety produced by the interference. As such, they lack the advantages that a conflict solution achieves even if it takes the form of symptom formation. In other words, many such symptoms are not responsive to interpretations of content, and are not helped by "treatment" in the form of the various psychotherapies. On the other hand, interventions aimed at the removal of the interference (like advising a parent to stop pressing for premature toilet training) will restore the dynamic equilibrium within the child and improve the mother-child relationship. As soon as that happens, the symptoms tend to disappear. This is a most important distinction from the symptoms of neurotic disorders where no amount of manipulation of the environment, or easing the pressures on the child will remove the symptom.

Thus a child may present clinically as highly "symptomatic and abnormal" but a closer look will demonstrate an essentially normal child, on whom unmanageable stresses have been forced from the outside. The child cannot regulate this excessive tension and reacts by producing symptoms. Such symptoms are not the expression of "abnormality" *but of the abnormal expectations and demands that the child's environment is placing on him.*

Many factors contribute to increase the difficulties of this type of assessment. If the interference has been present long enough or has been severe enough, it may further affect personality development, well beyond the production of transient symptoms and abnormal behavior. This may mean that removal of the interference may resolve those symptoms or behaviors that are due to that stress. Nonetheless, these may be a more permanent impact on certain aspects of development. Indeed, the final form of the child's personality structure may well be decisively shaped by the long-acting interference. Certain forms of interference may affect specific ego functions. If these events occur early in life, those affected functions and the ego itself may take after their form. Such changes may or may not be compatible with eventual "normality." In any case, such interferences may in fact be among the significant factors which shape development. They could account for many individual variations in functioning and for the even wider range of variations of normality. They may also contribute to the outcome of subsequent developmental conflicts, neurotic conflicts, the infantile neuroses, etc. They may play a role as well in the establishment of fixation points at different levels. These in turn create weaknesses in the personality that only become visible at later stages. They appear when the child is confronted by some of the later typical developmental conflicts that impose a heavy burden on personality resources.

Seventh, in considering the criteria of normality an added complication emerges. This concerns some special situations that are bound to influence how the child develops. They are in a way a caricature, or a paradigm of something that to some degree is true of all cases. Consider for example the special conditions surrounding a child raised in the ghetto.

It is inevitable that for any society, "normal" behavioral and ethical standards are substantially determined by the values of the dominant social or cultural group. Since there are many subgroups and subcultures that persist within the larger dominant group, it follows that conflicts between subcultural and dominant cultural values are quite common, particularly for certain groups of children.

This is a pattern of so-called asocial, unethical, amoral, promiscuous, and delinquent behavior present in some ghetto children. This definition is applied by those who assess behavior with the standards of middle class America. Yet, within the ghetto subculture that same behavior may have to be considered "normal" since it has adaptive and survival value both in the psychological and physical senses of the word. Thus, the question of normal or abnormal has to be followed frequently by the question for which cultures, groups, subcultures and according to whose criteria.

Children raised in the ghetto may well have internalized the ethical values and standards or behavior offered them by parents, relatives, and peers in the community, or, in short, by the subculture. According to middle-class standards, behavior that is perfectly "normal" in the ghetto is totally unacceptable and is considered "abnormal."

Cases of this type point to some of the added difficulties in considering normality. The problem here is that normality can be defined simultaneously from various points of view and with different conceptual tools. Thus, a given child may be regarded as psychologically "normal," but from the sociological point of view is considered "abnormal." It is unfortunate that psychiatrists are frequently expected to treat or to correct ills at the root of which we find negative sociological, economic, and/or political factors. Naturally, such influences affect the final form of the human beings subjected to their impact. This bears directly on any given child's final "psychological makeup." Under the circumstances, this personality structure is not only expectable but "normal." Yet, from the sociological point of view the behavior may be highly undesirable or downright inappropriate.

The same thinking applies to the variety of possible physical handicaps that children can suffer. The development of a child born blind can differ significantly from that of a normally sighted infant. The difference will be even more marked if no special efforts are made to provide stimulation to compensate for the lack of sight, or to deal with the ensuing distortions in the parent-child relationship such as parental guilt and the associated reactions.

Thus, when sight is lacking development will deviate in ways that are typical and "normal" for children blind from birth, but are "not normal" for the sighted ones. For example, there are the so-called blindisms in children lacking sight from birth. Similar behaviors would have rather ominous diagnostic connotations, if observed in the sighted child.

As we can see the determination of what is "normal" or "abnormal" for any given age is an extraordinary complex exercise for which there are no reliable shortcuts. The very experienced child psychiatric clinician may find it somewhat easier to make such determinations since he will have automatized the identification of gestalts that are basic to differential diagnosis. Such gestalts are not established magically. They are always the distillate of a laborious, and, at the beginning, very slow process of systematic examination of the child itself, and the child as a function of the multiple variables described briefly above.

On occasion a very gifted and experienced clinician may conclude that a child is or is not normal after a very "limited" examination. In such instances he is employing many unconscious engrams and gestalts that allow him to come to a rapid definition of the problem in a very impressive and accurate way. Asked to explain how he formed his opinion, he would find himself hard put to do so. But if he were to spell it out, he would presently be traversing the many difficult paths of differential diagnosis in the several areas outlined here.

Finally, it is appropriate to underline the value of Anna Freud's contributions in this regard (1945). She rightly questions the reliability of symptoms and behaviors as adequate indicators of normalcy and/or pathology in the case of children and adolescents. She approaches this issue from the developmental point of view and concludes that an assessment of "normality" in children should be closely correlated with the child's capacity to continue his development progression unimpeded. If his developmental path is clear of "unusual" obstacles that may distort it, hinder it, interfere with it, or halt it, the child's potential normality is there. Development itself frequently takes care of much "pathology." Thus, in a sensitive manner, she balances the excessive weight given by some to the actual presence of symptoms and abnormal behaviors at any given time during the child's development.

References

Freud, A. (1945). Indications for child analysis. *The Psychoanalytic Study of the Child* 1:127-149.

Freud, S. (1906). Analysis of a phobia in a five-year-old boy. *Standard Edition* 10:3-152.

Nagera, H. (1966). *Early Childhood Disturbances, the Infantile Neuroses, and the Adult Disturbances. New York: International Universities Press.*

Chapter Three

FIXATION AND REGRESSION

While fixation and regression are essential concepts of psychoanalytic theory, especially the theory of the neuroses,[1] they have not always been clearly separated in practice when one is confronted with actual clinical pictures. In this chapter I shall try to demonstrate that it is frequently possible, at the diagnostic stage, to ascertain how much, in certain neurotic developments or disorders of children, is the result of regression and how much can be ascribed to fixation. I shall discuss some aspects of the clinical and prognostic value of this distinction; describe the different types of fixation and regression that can be observed (but only insofar as this is required by the central theme of this paper—for a fuller account, see A. Freud (1963); and, finally, refer briefly to some of the clinical problems inherent in the effort to distinguish what, in the disorders of children, is due to fixation and what to regression.

A similar evaluation of the psychopathology in the adult is somewhat more complicated, though not impossible. However,

1. For a historical review of the concepts of fixation and regression as postulated by Freud throughout his life, I have consulted the drafts on "Fixation," by Miss Elsa First, and on "Regression," by Mrs. A. Gavshon, prepared at the Hampstead Clinic by the Concept Research Group. The Concept Research Group is presently engaged in scholastic research work on basic psychoanalytic concepts.

an understanding of the problems posed by what one observes in the adult presupposes some clarification and at least a limited discussion of the forms in which fixations manifest themselves in children and of the possible vicissitudes they undergo in the development from childhood through to adulthood.

We know that the term fixation may have several referents. We speak of fixation to a given component instinct, to a phase of libidinal and aggressive development, to a type of object choice, to a type of object relationship, and to a traumatic experience. We further know that all these different forms of fixations are expressions of similar and somewhat equivalent phenomena. For example, the controlling, domineering, obstinate, stubborn, sadistic type of object relationship of the anal phase is only the form in which certain drives express themselves in behavioral terms. This behavior is, of course, largely determined by the activity and predominance of the group of component instincts characteristic of this phase.

Nevertheless, our clinical experience shows that there are differences in emphasis among our cases of fixation. We may feel obliged to speak of a fixation to a component instinct as in some perversions. In other cases we have to talk rather in terms of fixation to a given phase, because there seems to be a more extended type of disturbance related to the phase as a whole and not to a single component instinct. Similarly, in certain cases we may observe that the fixation at the anal level manifests itself in a peculiar type of relationship, which is the only one possible for such children, while in other cases the marked activity of the well-known anal component instincts may be in the foreground. The fact that anality expresses itself in a type of object relationship which is the only one the patient is capable of nevertheless implies that a step has been taken away from the direct gratification of the anal component instincts. Such differences make it incumbent upon us to study what precisely determines the different types of emphasis, modes or levels of expression, and outcomes.

In children we establish the existence of fixation points at any given level by several means. We observe their behavior, games, play, attitudes, interests, fantasies whenever available, or symptoms where present. These will indicate at what level or levels of development the child is functioning. One takes into account the age of the child and the wide range of variations in normal development. A child's environmental circumstances, state of health, tiredness, etc., may indicate, as Anna Freud (1963) has pointed out, the existence of temporary regressions due partly to the such circumstances and states rather than to permanent ones. One similarly tries to evaluate whatever is observed in relative quantitative terms. In the end, and after the necessary corrections have been made, one is in a good position to estimate whether or not a fixation exists and its importance.

To illustrate briefly, we may observe an unusual and extensive activity of a given component instinct at a time when it is no longer age-adequate; that is, when it is no longer normal for such an activity to be an important and permanent area of discharge and gratification.

FIXATION VERSUS REGRESSION

In chapter 1 I advanced the hypothesis, already referred to, that it is possible to determine how much of the drive (libido and aggression) manifestations seen at a particular pregenital stage is present owing to the existence of a fixation point at that level and how much to regressive processes. Fixation points indicate a certain degree of arrest in drive development. In regressive phenomena, on the other hand, the drives have at one point or another reached a higher level of development but were, as a result of conflicts at these higher levels, forced back to earlier developmental positions. The majority of cases lie between these two extremes, showing arrested development (fixation points) which receives regressive reinforcement resulting from later conflicts. I claimed that even in these cases it is possible for the clinician to determine how much can be attributed to regression and how much to fixation. It is clear that since we have no direct and concrete method of assessing either fixations or regressions, this evaluation can be made only in relative quantitative terms, on the basis of a number of clinical facts and observations.

I shall discuss here primarily the cases where a combination of fixation and regressive processes is or has been in operation at some point. The two possible theoretical extremes in this series are represented by cases of massive arrest in drive development and by cases where extremely unusual, severe, or traumatic circumstances have created such intense conflicts that regression ensued even when no obvious or important fixation points existed. (I will discuss the latter type of case below.)

To start with, these assessments are in most instances easier in children than in adults. In the child the forms of expression of drive gratification, on which we base our judgment, remain quite direct or at least close enough to the original drive to permit a relatively ready identification. In the adult a series of displacements and transformations of the original drive expression has taken place complicating their elucidation, as will be seen later in the section on the "Vissitudes of the Form of Expression of Fixations." I believe that when a fixation point exists in a child, it betrays itself by the excessive activity of the component instinct or instincts involved in the fixation. In normal development, when a given phase is reached, the characteristic activity of the phase-specific component instincts is clearly in the foreground, while the activity of those component instincts belonging to the pre-

---

2. In "Analysis Terminable and Interminable" (1937) Freud states that his first account of libidinal development assumed an original oral phase succeeded by a sadistic-anal and in turn by a phallic-genital one. He goes on: "Later investigation has not contradicted this view, but we must now qualify our statement by saying that the one phase does not succeed the other suddenly but gradually, so that part of the earlier organization always persists side by side with the later, and that even in normal development the transformation is never complete, the final structure often containing vestiges of earlier libidinal fixations. . . . All that has once lived clings tenaciously to life" (p. 330f.).

Earlier (1913) he had said: "Another and far more surprising discovery has been that, in spite of all the later development that occurs in the adult, none of the infantile mental formations perish. All the wishes, instinctual impulses, modes of reaction and attitudes of childhood are still demonstrably present in maturity and in appropriate circumstances can emerge once more. They are not destroyed but merely overlaid . . . " (p. 184).

I am grateful to Dr. Hartmann for calling my attention to a statement by Freud which highlights how the problems I am concerned with here relate in a broader sense to the question of the immutability of the id contents. In this passage Freud refers to his previous assumptions, according to which the repressed instinctual impulses themselves remain unchanged indefinitely; however, because of the differentiation of the ego and the id, the whole question receives a fresh impetus and is in need of re-examination. Freud says (1926):

vious phases tends to recede somewhat into the background, more and more so as development progresses and the normally expected overlapping between phases is slowly left behind. When a fixation has taken place, this recession into the background does not occur to the same degree.[2] On the contrary, we then observe an "unusual degree" of activity belonging to the earlier phase side by side with that of the later ones. Moreover, in some cases this persisting activity shapes and modifies the form of expression and activity of the component instincts belonging to the later developmental phases.

Clinically such a situation shows itself openly in the child through symptoms, inhibitions, behavior, interests, play, games, fantasies, etc. Thus, though certain portions of the drives (more or less according to the importance of the fixations) may have reached the phallic-oedipal phase and quite clearly express themselves in phallic-oedipal activity, the manifest signs of fixation to the earlier levels will at no point have disappeared from the developmental picture. Unusual oral activity remains present in one form or another, side by side with the anal component instincts, when the nonarrested libido has been moved into the anal stage of drive development. If no further major arrest occurs during the anal phase, and the move to the phallic-oedipal stage takes place, side by side with the signs of the phallic components

---

"But now our interest is turned to the vicissitudes of the repressed and we begin to suspect that is not self-evident, perhaps not even usual, that those impulses should remain unaltered and unalterable in this way. There is no doubt that the original impulses have been inhibited and deflected from their aim through repression. But has the portion of them in the unconscious maintained itself and been proof against the influences of life that tend to alter and depreciate them? In other words, do the old wishes, about whose former existence analysis tells us, still exist? The answer seems ready to hand and certain. It is that the old, repressed wishes must still be present in the unconscious since we still find their derivatives, the symptoms, in operation. But this answer is not sufficient. It does not enable us to decide between two possibilities: either that the old wish is now operating only through its derivatives, having transferred the whole of its cathectic energy to them, or that it is itself still in existence too. If its fate has been to exhaust itself in cathecting its derivatives, there is yet a third possibility. In the course of the neurosis, it may have become re-animated by regression, anachronistic though it may now be. These are no idle speculations. There are many things about mental life, both normal and pathological, which seem to call for the raising of such questions. In my paper, "The Dissolution of the Oedipus Complex" (1924d), I had occasion to notice the difference between the mere repression and the real removal of an old wishful impulse" (p. 142, n.).

will be those of the oral fixation. However, if a fixation point has been established at the anal phase, then by the time the phallic stage is reached a combination of oral, anal, and phallic components will be present in the clinical picture. The new intensity and relative importance of the oral, anal, and phallic-oedipal manifestations are in some way proportionate to the amount of libido and aggression that has remained arrested at the anal and oral levels, and to whatever amount was left free to reach the phallic phase. It is clear that there is an infinite number of possible variations in terms of the relative strength and importance of each one of these elements, in its own right and in combination with others. Freud (1913) stated: "The strength in which the residues of infancy are still present in the mind shows us the amount of disposition to illness; that disposition may accordingly be regarded as an expression of an inhibition in development" (p. 184). This statement highlights the importance of quantitative considerations in the analysis and study of this type of phenomena. Between normal and abnormal phenomena there are mainly quantitative differences. Certainly quantitative considerations are one of the factors on the basis of which one will establish the presence or absence of fixation points.

As Freud's formulations indicate, the stronger the pregenital fixations, the stronger is the pull exerted from such points on whatever has reached a higher development. Even slight difficulties at the higher levels will quickly lead to regressions when important fixation points are present and exert their strong pull.

Once the phallic-oedipal stage is reached, conflicts at that level (with marked castration anxiety) may or may not induce regression. If regression from the phallic phase takes place, we can observe two results, their relative importance and manifestation being dependent on how much of the libido that has advanced to the phallic-oedipal stage takes the regressive path. If all or most of it does so, the previous behavior and fantasies of an obviously phallic-oedipal nature will tend to disappear from the foreground. In some cases of massive regression from the phallic to earlier levels, one is forced to ask oneself whether a particular child has ever reached the phallic-oedipal stage, since no signs of it are any longer observable by the time the child comes for assessment. This is by no means a rare diagnostic situation. Yet the problem may be solved by a good developmental history of the child. This will make it possible to show that a few weeks, months, or even years ago—that is, just before the massive regression took place— there were in the child's behavior, play, interests, fantasies, etc., signs of his having reached the oedipal stage. In this way the differential diagnosis is made, and regressive processes are distinguished from an arrest in drive development.

The second result of a massive regression from the phallic-oedipal stage to the fixation points consists in an intensification, a sudden reinforcement, of the libido that has remained arrested all the time. The outcome of the further regression is thus an intensification of whatever earlier manifestations of symptoms, fantasies, behavior, etc., were representative of the fixation point or points.

It is understandable that if the regression is not a massive but only a partial one, it will still be possible to observe a child's phallic-oedipal activities, though they will be present to a lesser degree; similarly, the reinforcement of the activities betraying a fixation will be less dramatic. In any case, any previous manifestation of fixations such as thumbsucking, overeating, biting, clinging, demandingness, dirtiness, stubbornness, etc., becomes much more apparent and obvious.

To summarize, the existence of fixation points is indicated by the ever-present manifestations of the earlier phases at the later stages, far beyond the age at which such behavior corresponds to specific stages in development and is accepted as normal. Their intensity and activity will be *proportionate to the amounts of libido and aggression arrested.* The reinforcements and intensifications described above correspond and are *proportionate to the regression* that has taken place. Hence the extreme importance of taking a very careful developmental history of the child, in which one tries to follow as closely as possible the vicissitudes of his drive development and even of the specific component instincts operative in the various phases, especially when there are indications of any kind of interference with normal development.

It is not infrequent that the diagnostician sees the patient long after the regression has taken place and when the whole situation of conflict has settled down. In some of these cases, the attempt to determine when the regressive move took place (betraying itself by the increase in the symptoms, etc.) enables us to recover the accidental factors, the environmental triggering circumstances that started or contributed to the situation of conflict, the very nature of which may thus become clearer.

In some analytic circles the view is held that no such distinction between fixation and regression is possible at the diagnostic stage. As a result no effort is made in this direction, leaving to the analysis the task of sorting out what belongs where.

Still, this distinction is of great prognostic importance, because it is unquestionably easier to help the forward movement of libido which has at some point in development reached the higher stages and then regressed than that of libido which has always been arrested at the earlier stages. Furthermore, I believe, this approach might throw some light on such clinical questions as the choice of neurosis, problems relating to symptom formation, and especially the whole field of the relationship of infantile disturbances to adulthood psychopathology. At the same time the problems involved in the theory of fixation and regression might well be further elucidated.

I shall now illustrate, with a very simple example, how regression and fixation manifest themselves in the clinical material of the diagnostic interview of one of our cases, where no special effort was made to sort out what belongs to fixation or regression. I shall single out, from the clinical picture presented by this four-and-a-half-year-old boy, the elements pointing to his oral fixation, and how they show all through his development up to the present day. In this case it is further possible to point out the regressive reinforcement of the oral manifestations that seem to be due to the unhappy confluence of a number of events in his life, at least one of them of a traumatic character.

J was described by his mother as a hungry baby who had to be given supplementary bottle feedings. He was breast-fed for about six weeks, at which point the mother developed a breast abscess. When the mother tried to reintroduce breast feeding later on, J seemed to prefer the bottle. He was weaned from it with no apparent difficulty at about nine months. At sixteen or seventeen months he showed a marked dislike of chewing and would spit out his food. His mother claims that he always tended to dislike new foods and that he has had different food fads. She recalled a week's visit to Holland when J was twenty-two months; during that time he could eat nothing but cornflakes and toast. At present (four and a half) he still sucks his thumb when he is tired.

It is of interest to observe how the child spontaneously introduced the subject of food in his diagnostic interview with the psychiatrist by referring to his brother Simon: "My brother Simon was really a rascal because he said that you mustn't eat more than three Easter eggs, but Simon ate thirteen of them." At another point during the same interview he started to make a square cage for hens and sang: "Will you lay me an egg for my tea. . . ." (All the above clearly shows the ever-present fixation.)

When he was about three, a number of events succeeded each other: his entry into nursery school, a hospitalization for tonsilectomy, and the birth of a sibling. *Since that time his feeding difficulties increased.* The social history says: "The mother made it quite clear that since his operation the feeding difficulties have seemed worse. He is finicky, but the mother sees to it that he gets a balanced die by preparing meals which she knows he likes." (Here the mother's account clearly points to the regressive reinforcement.)

Finally, psychoanalytic theory assumes that massive conflicts at higher levels of development may force a regressive movement of the libido even in cases where it is not possible to demonstrate the existence of relevant fixation points in the previous developmental phases. Clearly when such fixation points exist they favor regression by the constant pull they impose on the libido that has moved forward. Furthermore, the existence of such clear fixations is an obvious indication to the diagnostician of where the regressing libido will finally stop and settle.

For these very reasons the diagnostician finds himself in a more helpless position when he attempts a similar assessment in cases where development has proceeded close to the ideal of normality and no clear-cut or outstanding fixation points can be noted, and a later traumatic episode has forced a regressive movement. Nevertheless, I believe that in such cases the backward movement of the libido will lead to those component instincts which have proved to be particularly strong in any given personality. That this is so is due not to the existence of fixation points proper but to the normal tendency to revert, when it is impossible to obtain gratification at the higher levels, to these primitive and intense forms of gratification that had previously been experienced. What seems to happen during the backward movement of the libido is a recathexis of those old channels of discharge which in the past have rendered intense satisfaction, while the simultaneous constant attraction of the libido, assumed to exist in cases of well-established fixation points, is here absent.

Clinically, one will observe a clean sheet as far as evidence of fixation is concerned. A careful developmental history will show only slight signs, if any, of fixations at the earlier levels. Nevertheless, at a certain point in the development of the child, for example, at four or five years of age, and perhaps as the result of massive traumatic castration anxiety, regression may start; we can then observe manifestations appropriate to the oral and anal phases, either as symptoms or pieces of behavior that were previously absent, or that were only present at the age-appropriate stage and disappeared as soon as the next step in development was taken or the next phase reached.

VICISSITUDES OF THE FORM OF EXPRESSION OF FIXATIONS

I have been able to study a few children whose development from babyhood or early infancy till adulthood was well known to the Hampstead Clinic. It was partly this study which highlighted and made clear how many of the indicators of fixation points at the earlier stages of development disappear from the surface, that is, from the overt behavior of the child. Having gone underground, they then hide behind what are considered to be normally acceptable forms of gratification and discharge. In this way valuable pointers and indicators of diagnostic and prognostic significance are either hidden from or lost to the unaware diagnostician.

What I am calling the vicissitudes of fixations is in many ways comparable and similar to the vicissitudes of the component instincts in general. The "fixation point" is, after all, the result of the same activities on the instinctual side, only to an abnormal degree and with incorrect timing.

For the sake of simplicity I shall confine myself to the oral phase and to oral fixations, taking as a hypothetical example excessive or constant thumbsucking in children well past the age and stage at which thumbsucking can be considered to be within normal limits.

In such children thumbsucking may sometimes tend to persist until somewhere around what ought to be the latency period. This happens especially in cases where this tendency is a very marked one. Yet even those children who have so excessively and for so long engaged in this type of gratification seem to give it up at some point in their development. At least, thumbsucking seems to disappear from the foreground and is no longer observable in the overt behavior of the child.

A closer scrutiny may show that this abandonment, this giving up of the "habit," conceals a substitution for another socially acceptable form of oral gratification.[3] Such a change releases the ego from a situation of growing conflict between the instinctual demand in the form of thumbsucking and the environment that has turned more and more intransigent to the habit as the child has aged.

It is a confluence of several factors that makes it possible for the child to exchange thumbsucking for another form of gratification

---

3. In the *Introductory Lectures*(1916-1917). Freud says that "we must bear in mind that the sexual instinctual impulses in particular are extraordinarily *plastic*, if I may so express it. One of them can take the place of another, one of them can take over another's intensity; if the satisfaction of one of them is frustrated by reality, the satisfaction of another can afford complete compensation. They are related to one another like a network of inter-communicating channels filled with liquid . . ." (p. 345).

at a certain point in his development, perhaps long before latency or at the beginning of it. His ego growth implies not only that the child disposes over a stronger and more capable structure, which can put forward more acceptable alternative solutions, and perhaps even enforce them; there is also a growing awareness of the environmental demands, particularly of the persons looking after him, and of the need to preserve their love. This is coupled with an increasing concern for these persons' feelings as well as a greater readiness to comply, partly because more and more superego precursors (in the form of environmental demands) have become internalized.

Thumbsucking, which has thus become involved in a major conflict, may now be exchanged for a craving for sweets or for any other form of gratification of oral needs more acceptable to the environment of a child of four or five years of age. Later on some of these intermediate forms of oral gratification will be exchanged for more age-adequate and socially acceptable ones, like smoking, certain types of overeating, somewhat excessive drinking, etc.

In still other cases the exchange takes place within the sphere of the subject's sexual life, where it anchors itself especially at the forepleasure stage of the sexual activity. Kissing, licking, sucking, biting the sexual partner, or specific parts of his body, etc., are highly cathected and by far the most exciting elements of the person's sexual life. Behind some preferences, peculiarities, and pieces of sexual behavior of this type and other similar ones may lie hidden some fixation points which are now secret and become active only in certain sets of circumstances. Though fellatio, for example, is a highly overdetermined sexual practice, the importance of the role it plays in the sexual life of some patients is probably closely connected with significant oral fixations and perhaps especially with the sucking component instinct of the oral stage.

What I have described here for the oral phase and sucking as a specific component of that phase applies to the other phases and the other component instincts. There are socially acceptable and age-adequate equivalents for each, though on the whole there is greater tolerance for the oral and phallic strivings than for the anal ones.

In normal development some component instincts regularly make a contribution to normal sexual life and a person's character structure. This circumstance introduces an added complication into diagnostic problems. Nevertheless it is the assessment of the economic and quantitative aspects which must decide whether we are dealing with normal or pathological manifestations.

The fact that many forms of gratification of the oral component instincts can be quite normal and socially acceptable complicates diagnostic assessments, because marked oral fixations may be hidden under this cover of normal oral activity and discharge. In this way valuable pointers and indicators for the study of characters, personality structure, and the nature of the conflicts are concealed, and elements of great prognostic significance are obscured. The diagnostician will do well, during the assessment of adults, to examine in minute detail all those areas where, behind manifestations which are usually normal, potential pathology may be hidden. He will no doubt do so in the extreme cases of eating leading to obesity, or chain smoking, or habitual drunkenness, but he should not neglect those cases that are far from these extremes. Whenever the existence of oral fixations is suspected or needs to be taken into account, it is desirable to inquire closely into the patient's smoking, eating, and drinking patterns in order to avoid overlooking pointers in these areas.

The diagnostic and prognostic value of such findings can prove especially important when the more or less original and direct forms of expression of childhood orality are no longer observable. It is well known, for example, that many cases diagnosed as hysteria are offered to candidates in psychoanalytic training as relatively easy first cases for analysis; not infrequently, however, as treatment progresses, such cases turn out to be severe depressions; the oral fixations then become manifest and more evident and alarming as the depressive episode develops.[4]

4. In his discussion of the Schreber case (1911). Freud pointed out: "For it is possible for several fixations to be left behind in the course of development, and each of these in succession may allow an irruption of the libido that has been pushed off—beginning, perhaps, with the later acquired fixations, and going on, as the illness develops, to the original ones that lie nearer the starting-point" (p. 78).

A careful diagnostic examination of such patients, and especially the recognition of the existence of earlier fixation points now under cover, would have acted as a warning that behind the observable hysteric-type conflicts at the phallic-oedipal level lie deeper and stronger roots at the oral level. As the result of these fixations, more serious disturbances may develop as soon as the precariously maintained conflict equilibrium (of a hysterical type) at the phallic-oedipal phase is upset by internal or external circumstances.

FIXATION POINTS: SOME CLINICAL PROBLEMS

Some children reach the phallic-oedipal stage after rather troublesome oral or anal conflicts. One can then frequently observe a marked contamination of the later phase by the fixation at the previous ones. A contamination of the phallic-oedipal stage and its fantasies by the oral one and its fantasies will betray itself, for example, in the circumstance that the child's phallic fantasies are expressed in oral terms; intercourse, pregnancy, making babies, etc., are conceived as being the result of activities involving both the phallus and the mouth. Babies are thus made by eating or drinking certain substances; they may come out of the genitals or because the genitals themselves are eaten. In these cases the child's castration anxiety is frequently expressed through fears of having his penis bitten off or eaten up, as can be observed in his fantasies and games, e.g., when animals are constantly biting off or eating up other animals' tails, legs, heads, etc.

Similarly, an important fixation at the anal level will tend to contaminate the child's phallic-oedipal wishes, leading him to conceive of sexuality as an aggressive sadistic fight and attack on the sexual partner.

Sexual fantasies of an oral or anal nature may to some extent be present in normal development since the oral and anal phases even in ideal conditions leave behind some remnant or other. Here again the diagnostic problem will be solved by the quantitative factor which perhaps points to a predominance or even exclusiveness of one or another form of expression.

That phallic-oedipal fantasies are expressed, e.g., in oral terms is not accidental. Such an apparent preference for one or another form of expression of the conflict or conflicts is not a matter of chance. On the contrary, I believe it is determined by the relatively greater strength of the oral component instincts and by the particular fixation points which in comparison with those of other phases are of far greater importance. Consequently they ought to be taken as indicators of the special strength of the oral component instincts and of important fixations that have led to a contamination of the later phases. Similar considerations apply if anal fantasies are predominant.

Regressive processes, especially in their first stages, will intensify this form of expression of the conflict. To my mind, this circumstance affords an indication of where the important fixations have been established and of the points to which the libido will retreat if a more or less complete withdrawal from the phallic phase is going to take place. When such a development occurs, the phallic elements of the previous fantasies tend to disappear and are no longer easily observable. The fantasy then becomes less a combination of oral and phallic elements and turns more into a purely oral type.

Clinically, one must distinguish between true regression to earlier levels and those cases where the conflict, though on the whole at the phallic-oedipal level, is expressed in oral and anal terms on account of previous fixations. These forms of expression can be observed the moment the libido moves into the phallic-oedipal phase. If, on the contrary, the oral or anal expression of the phallic-oedipal conflict is due to a partial regression or to a beginning regressive move, there would be a previous period at which the oral contamination of the phallic-oedipal phase was not so evident or not observable at all in the clinical material.

Perhaps the more frequent case is a mixed one, consisting of a reinforcement and accentuation of the oral or anal contamination of phallic fantasies that were present all the way through. The sudden accentuation or reinforcement indicates the sudden regressive movement, while the previous, not so intense, but clearly present contaminated fantasies indicate the fixation point.

So far analysts have concentrated their attention mainly on the role played by the fixation points in the choice of neurosis and in the mechanism of symptom formation. I believe that no less useful results will be achieved by studying the role played by the presence of fixation points of a very diverse nature in the development of the ego. It is important to know, as I have pointed out in chapter 1, that at some time (ideally at the proper time) the right amount of libido[5] has moved forward and thus made its contributions to the development of the ego and to the personality as a whole; in contrast, where excessive fixations exist, large amounts of libido have remained arrested and were unable to contribute to normal development at the time when that contribution was required.

It is not farfetched to assume that arrests in the drive development of the child will in turn influence in some ways his ego development. Psychoanalysis assumes a very close developmental interaction between the drives and the ego. How, when, where, and why the drives make their contribution to ego development is still a rather obscure area; but we work with the assumption that any development move on the drive side acts as a trigger for a number of chain reactions of developmental processes on the ego side. These in turn will feed back to the drives, which again will further stimulate ego development in certain specific directions. A similar situation of interaction and influence on the drives can be assumed to have its origin in certain developmental processes (maturational and otherwise) that take place in the ego.

In this context it may be useful to refer to the clear influence which any fixation points have on children's sexual theories and on their understanding of the world. It is well known that a child at the oral phase of development understands the world around him largely in oral terms and through oral imagery, just as the child in the anal or phallic stages does so mainly in anal and phallic terms, more markedly so as more of his libido has moved freely forward to cathect the corresponding body zones. It is due to this latter factor that the world is interpreted in oral, anal, and phallic terms, since through the massive cathexis of the zone all

---

5. Whenever I refer to libido, similar arguments of course apply to the aggressive drives.

other mental activities, interests, etc., become to a certain extent subordinated to it, especially so in early childhood.

The child who has reached the phallic-oedipal phase, though preferring to relate to and understand the world and its objects in the terms dictated by that phase of development, has nevertheless complete freedom to use oral and anal imagery when necessary. He has reached a very high and complex level of integration and function on the drive and ego sides. On the other hand, a child whose fixations impose upon him an oral imagery, for example, is dealing with similar phenomena with very different means when he reaches the phallic stage. I do not want to imply that the one form of development leads to a better ability on the side of the ego, since observation of oral or anal characters and their ego performance makes it clear that this is not necessarily the case. Nevertheless, in these unexplored areas of differences in human development, and in the differences in basic personality structures resulting from it, lie the answers to many intriguing and obscure problems of psychopathology in general, and especially to those of symptom formation, choice of neurosis, intrinsic differences among basically hysteric or obsessional patients,[6] as well as answers to problems relating to so-called health and normality, character structure, etc.

In certain types of character organization, for example, in obsessional characters and especially in adults, one frequently observes an extraordinary increase in the defensive system or defensive attitude of the ego against certain component instincts that have received a reinforcement through the regressive process. During the first stages of the regressive process one generally cannot demonstrate any direct manifestations of the regresively reinforced component instincts. In this case the regressive move betrays itself by the increase in the defense activity. Thus, in some anal characters the desirable tendencies to orderliness, thoroughness, and meticulousness (which are well-known precipitates of the reaction formations against some of the anal component instincts in the character structure) can increase to such an extent

6. It is well known that there are in addition very marked differences between two hysterics or two obsessionals.

that the performance of daily tasks becomes impossible. The tendency to orderliness and meticulousness transforms itself, for example, into a compulsion to check and recheck every step so many times that productive work is completely paralyzed.

We have occasionally observed children who relate to a given object, e.g., the mother, at a level that seems to point to a fixation to the anal stage, when chronologically and otherwise one would expect such a child to have left behind that phase. Further observation of the same child discloses that he relates to other objects at a higher, normal level. Clearly, if this difference in his relationships is to be attributed to a fixation at the anal-sadistic level, the fixation is restricted to the relationship with the mother and is not as severe as it would be if this were the child's only possible way of relating to all persons.

Furthermore, I believe that an important and by no means easy differential diagnosis is required here. The study of the role played by the object in this type of relationship is most important. In some of these cases, one gains the impression that the child's ego is adapting to the environment, that he complies with the demands made by such an important object as the mother by forming the only type of relationship that is possible in view of the mother's own psychopathology. This situation can be very different from one in which the ego is forced to an anal-sadistic type of relationship and is itself incapable of forming any other types of relationships. In the one case the ego chooses a type of relationship that it knows to be the only form of communication possible with a given object, or perhaps the only way to get a reponse from that object, while in the other the ego is helpless, having to endure its limitations and having no choice or possible alternative.

Finally, in studying the problems involved in fixation and regression, it is necessary to provide a precise and accurate description of the specific points to which the regression has taken place. Thus it really is not sufficient to say that regression has taken place to the anal phase; a specification of the proper subphase within the anal phase is of clinical relevance. Even within the subphase one needs to know which are the really relevant component instincts or their equivalents in any given case. Certain qualitative differences—in some cases of prognostic value—between neuroses of the same type in different individuals lie hidden behind such details.[7]

References

Freud, A. (1963). Regression as a principle in mental development. *Bulletin of the Menninger Clinic* 27.

Freud, S. (1911). Psycho-analytic notes on an autobiographical account of a case of paranoia (dementia paranoides). *Standard Edition* 12:3-84.

——— (1913). The claims of psycho-analysis to scientific interest. *Standard Edition* 13:165-1920.

——— (1916-1917). Introductory lectures on psycho-analysis. *Standard Edition* 15/16:3-496.

——— (1926). Inhibitions, symptoms and anxiety. *Standard Edition* 20:77-178.

——— (1937). Analysis terminable and interminable. In *Collected Papers*, Vol. 5, pp. 316-357. London: 1950.

7. These and similar problems are at present being studied at the Hampstead Clinic in the "Clinical Research Group" under a project known as "Studies on the Psychoanalytic Theory of the Neuroses."

Chapter Four

VULNERABILITY
AND STIMULATION
IN EARLY LIFE

I begin with the statement that all children are vulnerable. There are, of course, many unfavorable situations that bring vulnerability to the fore, such as child neglect, under- or over-stimulation, child abuse, adoption, disruption of the family organization, and parental death. Hence, I review here some of the developmental needs of young infants, hoping to highlight some of the reasons for their vulnerability. Further, I do so against the background of the present move toward day-care centers so that I can point out what I consider their considerable dangers given the vulnerability of children, especially during the first two years of life (see chapter 17).

If we consider first the dangers involved in this practice to children in the age group of up to 1½ years of age, we have to examine at least three distinct sets of variables. Each one of them plays a fundamental role in the healthy development of the infant ("healthy" implying here not only physical health but including a good intellectual, emotional, and psychological development). The first set of variables comes from the child himself. The second is from the type of environment in which the child lives, including those human objects responsible for his care. The third is the resultant of the interaction between the endowment, the genetic makeup of all humans as a species (and that peculiar to each individual), and the environment (including the human objects).

Those variables that concern the infant itself are in part genetically determined and are essential to certain characteristics specific for the development of the human brain. Thus, comparatively speaking, the infant of the human species is born with an extremely immature, unfinished brain, to the point that it takes 1½ to 2 years after birth to reach the level of maturity that is typical at the time of birth in other mammalian species. It is embryological maturational forces that push brain development in the anatomophysiological sense to its completion. To complete their tasks such forces, though genetically determined, need the collaboration of specific forms of environmental stimulation. In other words, the genetic developmental embryological forces cannot unfold the anatomophysiological blueprint of the brain to its ideal potential without the essential contribution of environmental factors. This environmental contribution is in the nature of a diversity of stimuli that must reach the brain. The function of that stimuli is to trigger and stimulate those genetic embryological mechanisms to complete its task.

Admittedly, this is still an obscure area, but the current evidence is at least quite suggestive, if not conclusive. Different forms of external stimulation (usually contained in the multiplicity of interactions of the mother with her baby) seem to influence the internal, anatomical-maturational processes by at least three different types mechanisms.

The first type of mechanism seems to favor significant increases in a progressive and more complex arborization of dendrites during the first few months of life. The importance of this phenomenon should be clearly understood. More dendrites mean increased and more complex pathways in the brain, and more pathways mean more functional capabilities and better possibilities of performance for that brain. Conel's studies of the cerebral cortex of babies (1939) demonstrated that although the number of cells (neurons) in the cortex is fixed at birth, complex morphological changes continue for long periods of time. Thus he found progressive arborization of dendritic processes during the few months following birth without quantitative cellular increase. The situation here would be similar to a sophisticated piece of electronic equipment that has been poorly wired, where the connections between the systems are not as numerous as they could have been. Such a situation will naturally restrict unnecessarily the functional capabilities of the total equipment. Richmond and Lipton (1959) stated that "since it is now accepted generally that neurons are connected in a network and not merely in a linear series, and that nerve impulses pass about the connections in a circular, more or less continuing fashion, the potential significance of this growing arborization of dendrites for the development of the infant may be appreciated" (p. 80). Thus understimulation of the brain during the first few months of life, for example, may well lead to an inferior quality of brain structure (less dendritization, connections, and functional pathways). Furthermore, such developmental maturational processes as those leading to appropriate dendritization can only occur during a limited period of time after birth. Hence if they do not take place during that critical period, they cannot be brought about at a later date. The damage, in the sense of loss of capabilities and function, is permanent.

The second type of mechanism increases the degree of vascularization in certain anatomical structures of the brain. The relationship between function, functional capacity, and the degree of vascularization of an organ (implying here the amount of oxygen available to the organ) is a well-established medical fact.

The third type favors the process of myelinization. Myelinization and function are very closely related. Here again there is hard evidence from animal experimentation suggesting clearly that environmental stimulation has significant effects upon ultimate structure and function. Richmond and Lipton (1959) concluded that these "types of studies seem to give support to the contention that even after the fetal stage, environmental stimulation (or lack thereof) can modify developing structure in the central nervous system" (p. 82).

Since the first two years of life seem to be the critical period for all these developments, it follows that if the right kind of stimulation is not provided during this phase, the result may be a structure that, though not necessarily "damaged" (in the sense of brain damage), has certainly not developed to its full potential.

If we take into account the possibility of cumulative effects of this type, leading to inferior development in multiple areas of the brain, it is conceivable that the finished brain is one of "inferior quality" for those unfortunate children whose fate it will be to grow, during their first two years of life, under conditions of deprivation and understimulation. Such conditions are typical of a variety of environments including, in my view, most of the existent day-care centers and no doubt those numbered in the thousands, that are to be created.

Provence and Lipton (1962) have clearly demonstrated by means of direct observations of infants, the appalling damage to the personality and more especially to ego and intellectual development resulting from growing under conditions of deprivation and understimulation, that is, by lack of sufficient human contact and interaction during the early stage of the child's development.

Some of such developmental lags can be "undone" by placing such children in a more suitable environment (a good foster home, for example) at the appropriate time. As I have written elsewhere (Nagera 1972),

> It seems to me that in another sense many such children are irreversible and permanently condemned to perform, in terms of his intelligence, at the lower end of normality. To be graphic, it is the difference between somebody digging holes in a road and somebody with the intelligence necessary for a university education. Thus, though "normal," deprivational child-rearing practices may have blunted his original genetic potential to such a point that his best is an IQ of 80, while genetically, and given more favorable circumstances in babyhood, he might have reached an IQ of 120.

Clearly, then, the first step that we must ensure developmentally is that the internal maturational embryological forces unfold as ideally as possible. That, as we have shown, requires external stimulation of the kind and quality contained "usually" in the mother-child relationship. This will ensure the best basic equipment in the form of the best brain that the child's endowment has provided him with. But that condition, essential as it obviously is, is not enough or sufficient in the human species. Most human

behavior and controls are learned—this constitutes a most significant difference from all other species. In the latter most behavior is
controlled instinctually. In other words, it is controlled automatically by innate, inbuilt mechanisms in the brain that trigger
off adaptive responses after the reception of the significant signals
and stimuli from the environment. Self-preservation, mating behavior, preservation of the species, food gathering, and so on are
frequently regulated in this manner. Not so with the human
infant.

To start with, his brain is enormously superior in functional
capabilities to any other species. Evolution has not provided him
with the type of instinctual patterns of behavior described in the
preceding paragraphs and observed in other species. When the
time comes he must—since he is helpless and dependent on
parental care and teaching for an inordinately large amount of
time—use his intelligence to deal with his environment, with
dangers, and with others. His specially developed brain has provided him with the capacity to learn to solve problems in a variety
of ways. In other words, he can choose "intelligently" among
several alternatives, the most adaptive response in a given set of
circumstances. He is not restricted, like other species, to one single
stereotyped solution. He has the capacity for language development as a tool of communication. He can and indeed has established innumerable forms of social organization and culture. He
can store and teach his descendants that culture. He can modify his
environment to suit his needs and thus he has to a large measure
the greatest capacity for survival, in terms of evolution, of any
species known. By the same token he possesses the greatest capacity for destruction intraspecies, interspecies, and of his environment.

All these differences clearly demonstrate that he must start
learning from day one, and at incredible paces if he is going to join
his social group and its organization in an adaptive healthy
manner. This learning is predicated on an active and constant
interaction from birth onward with human objects. The intensity
of the contact needed to achieve this aim is generally lacking under
the institutional conditions of foundling homes, orphanages, and

most likely in ill-devised day-care centers. To use a comparison, it is not enough to have acquired the best computer possible (the best brain possible for a given child), it is also necessary to program it wisely and efficiently. The best computer, if mishandled and badly programmed, will be an inefficient piece of equipment.

We have enough evidence in the field of human development to state that the best programmer of the human brain and of much of human behavior is a good mother-child interaction in the first few years of life. Once that basic and early programming has been achieved many others (in the forms of teachers, etc.) can participate successfully in the further programming and teaching of the human brain. (None of this should be taken literally. *Programming* is a graphic word of some explanatory value, but as a term it possesses connotations that are inappropriate and insufficient to describe human development; still, it expresses graphically some of the problems at hand.)

One essential factor in this regard is the constancy of the object—the constancy of care of the object ministering to the child. The child's brain, at the same time that is developing and acquiring more complex capabilities, must be exercised. It must be exposed to innumerable experiences, not only so that it receives essential stimuli and continues to grow, but so that it organizes itself, learning slowly to distinguish (given its capacity to think) inside from outside, self from object, and the body parts under its control and command, as control is progressively acquired. Similarly, he must go successfully (if normality is to be achieved) through the process of separation-individuation as described by Mahler and must learn to use his ego apparatuses as these become structured as well as to understand the innumerable complexities of its environment. Most important, he must learn to establish very early controls over its own primitive reactions and feelings. To further complicate the problem, all these developments must take place in a situation where the infant is not excessively subjected to undesirable forms of stimuli either. Thus in the earliest stages it is imperative that the child (the child's brain) not be subjected to overwhelming, traumatic forms of experiences that it cannot handle and that are enormously disruptive in terms of personality organization. Such stimuli, capable of overwhelming the necessary homeostatic equilibrium in the child, can come from outside, for example, from excessive handling or mishandling, excessive cold or heat, multiple sources of unorganized sounds and other undesirable stimuli impinging on the baby for prolonged periods of time and enforced separations. It can come from the inside when the baby is left to suffer from hunger or from pain unduly.

Granted the kind of background that is ideal for human and brain development, that is, neither excessive nor insufficient stimuli, but the right happy medium, the child still needs some constancy of objects to organize its experiences, to understand its world. An example may clarify this. When a newborn baby is sufficiently hungry his pleasure-pain equilibrium is disrupted. A disturbing feeling interferes with his well-being. This automatically leads to clear signs of distress on the part of the baby that are picked up by the baby's mother. This, in turn, activates the behavior of the healthy mother, who immediately relates to the baby and his need. Usually, the mother has a very ritualized, stereotyped procedure while going about getting ready to satisfy the baby's hunger and thus alleviate or remove his distress. She might go and see her baby, talk to him, manipulate him to ascertain the cause of the cry or other signals released by the infant (he might be wet or uncomfortable for a variety of reasons). Then she may go to the kitchen to fetch bottles and prepare the baby's milk. All this time the child is receiving a variety of sensory stimulation, the steps of the mother while she moves about, her voice if she talks to him (this tends to be stereotyped, too), sounds produced by opening the refrigerator, closing it, the handling of bottles, glasses, spoons, pans, and so on. The baby, who must have been quite disturbed by his first few and new experiences of hunger, learns that after all this stimuli that reaches him, satisfaction arrives and his hunger and distress disappear.

Naturally, once he has established these links in his mind (after a few good experiences of satisfaction) one can observe how his crying stops automatically as soon as he can hear the noises resulting from the mother's activity in the preparation of his food.

Thus at this point the internal distress is not a frightening, disturbing experience of discomfort, but one associated with relief and satisfaction. In short, despair becomes hope. Further, he has made in some primitive form the first connections between cause and effect and has learned that control pays, that waiting and being attentive can bring rewards, and so on. Obviously, these first steps in the organization of the mind and of the inner world of feelings and affects, of learning and knowing something for the first time, is possible, or more feasible and easier, if the object who ministrates to the child is constant. Her stereotyped and routinized behavior, the sameness of the behavior allows the baby to find his bearings, to know the situation or rather to identify it as similar to previous experiences, and consequently to predict the outcome. A constant change of caretakers with different ways, different manners of ministering to the baby, in short, the lack of sameness at the appropriate times will, I think, make it much more difficult for him to find his bearings, learn about the situation, predict the outcome, acquire early control structures, and be confident and relaxed in the face of the internal distress. Clearly, sameness, familiarity, and repeated similar experiences lead to learning and to primitive understanding and organization in the mind. Without these early and primitive processes of organization and integration later learning becomes difficult. Constantly changing the system by means of which we attempt to teach something to any child is disruptive and makes the mastery of the tasks more difficult, confusing, and hopeless.

This simplified example, relating to feeding and its significance for mental organization and structuring, can be multiplied ad infinitum in terms of what is happening constantly in the context of the mother-child interaction. Therefore, I believe that in the early stages of the process of the organization of the mind the existence of essentially one caretaker for the child, the existence of sameness in certain experiences, though not in all, is of enormous significance. After some time, that is, after the ego structure has achieved a certain level of organization, the child is able to deal with more complex tasks, even if some of the variables involved are changed frequently. The need for constancy of the caretaker still exists at somewhat later stages, but that need is then based on factors other than the need for organization in the mind and for the organization of our first mental processes.

The examples I have selected show clearly the close interaction between biological factors and psychological factors. In this dependence lies the superiority of the human infant as well as its vulnerability.

References

Conel, J. L., (1939). *The Postnatal Development of the Human Cerebral Cortex.* Vols. 1 et seq. Cambridge: Harvard University Press.

Nagera, H. (1972). Social deprivation in infancy: implications for personality development. In *Handbook of Child Psychoanalysis,* ed. E. Wolman. New York: Van Nostrand Reinhold.

Provence, S.A., and Lipton, R.C. (1962). *Infants in Institutions.* New York : International Universities Press.

Richmond, J.B., and Lipton, E.L. (1959). Some aspects of the neurophysiology of the newborn and their implications for child development. In *Dynamic Psychopathology in Childhood,* ed. L. Jessner and E. Pavenstedt. New York: Grune and Stratton.

Chapter Five

SELF AND OBJECT

Various authors describing the earliest stages in self- and object-representation formation do so in terms of self-object matrix, out of which self and object will finally become differentiated (Jacobson 1964, Kernberg 1975, 1976).

Naturally enough, later pathology (narcissistic, borderline, and psychotic) is explained on the basis of such a model. Invariably, these theories place the accent on failures in the mother-child relationships, or on failures (more or less dramatic depending on the author), of the world of objects, as Kohut (1977), for example, has recently postulated. In my judgment, this is at times an incorrect formulation because it ignores many intermediary steps, such as the cognitive development of infants. It is thus a sort of descriptive shorthand, but it is pregnant with dangers of inter-pretative errors. I believe this can be so even on those occasions where in fact the psychopathology can be explained on the basis of unsatisfactory mothering, or poor early object relationships (as is indeed frequently the case). On the other hand, such causative interpretations (in terms of failure in object relations) are applied as etiological explanations for *all* cases that descriptively fit one of the above-mentioned clinical pictures, when in fact many of them are the result of a variety of ego failures. Thus, we can correctly understand the mechanisms involved in such pathology only if we consider a multiplicity of other factors.

Coming back to the self-object matrix, we find that such formulation substantially ignores well-established facts about the cognitive and ego development of children. Yet, the way the ego cognitive organization acquires structure, contents, and significant meanings does have considerable psychological impact on the later emotional structure of the personality and its conflicts, on its assets and deficits.

How does it happen then that the infant separates self from objects and how is that process significant to later psychological life?

We are thus faced with the problem of trying to map out and understand in as much detail as possible, how the self-representations are acquired, and built up from birth onward (and perhaps earlier). Out of that very gradual building up, a concept of "self" will evolve as a psychologically viable and operative entity.

The same line of argument applies to the development in the infant's mind of the concept of objects. But for such mappings of the development of the concept of the self and of the object, we must keep as close as we can to what we know about the level of cognition possible in the newly born. In other words, what is his true cognitive capacity at this point and how much of what is theoretically postulated by authors dealing with the development of the self-representation and the self is actually possible? The same question might also be asked regarding the concept of "objects" and "object-representations." Otherwise we may fall into the error of assuming that the newly born infant's level of mentation, his capacity to process stimuli, and his actual functional abilities are far beyond what is in fact the case. This reification of his functional abilities, can lead only to incorrect formulations, to a sort of mythology that has no bearing on what is really happening in the infant's mind.

Beyond this, we must look closely at how the infant's cognitive capacities slowly and gradually unfold during the first months of life. It follows that our models of how self- and object-representations are built, and the concept of self and object finally acquired, must be closely correlated with this unfolding of the child's cognitive capacities.

With this in mind, I will present now a highly condensed summary of some of Piaget's view about the cognitive capacities of infants and how they develop during the first two years of life.

According to Piaget (1967) the reflex behaviors that are described as the typical type of mental functioning during the first month of life begin to be modified immediately; and during the next three months rapid and important changes take place. Significantly, according to him, the earlier reflex activity now becomes integrated into somewhat more organized perceptions and habits, leading to new observable behaviors partly acquired through "learning" by experience. By nine to twelve weeks, for example, thumbsucking becomes a habit and reflects the increased hand-mouth coordination. Clearly, habituation to thumbsucking cannot be explained by the reflexes described above but it can be understood by the child's discovery of sensorimotor relationships while acting on an environment, the existence of which is unknown to him. Of course, the fact that the newly found activity yields pleasure is of importance in forming the habit. He can also follow moving objects with his eyes (eye coordination) and his head in the direction of sounds (eye-ear coordination).

Piaget points out that from the fifth week onward, an observer has the distinct impression that the child seems to "recognize" some persons in some ill-defined way, and yet there is no evidence that the child has any notion whatsoever of a "person or of an object." Piaget believes that what the infant "recognizes" is a sort of animated perceptual presence, but that this does not imply an awareness of the substance and permanence of that perceptual presence in the outside world. It also does not imply even a beginning dissociation between self and external world (p. 21). Yet, as I see it, the fact remains that he can now make certain distinctions that he could not make before. He can "recognize" the nipple from which milk flows as different from other suckable things. In some sense, we can speak here of some process of adaptation to external reality (Piaget calls it accommodation), as long as we are aware that he has no knowledge of external reality except through the presentations made by it through perception. In other words, it is not differences in external things themselves that he recognizes but differences in the marks that perception leaves in the infant's "perceptual reality." These types of behavioral changes are among the first observable signs that an internal organization is taking place. They imply some adaptation to the world outside (the existence of which is unknown to the infant). In any case, what is important is that the child is now making primitive sensorimotor differentiations and acquiring limited sensorimotor coordinations.

Another maturational development that helps the infant's processes of differentiation of self and objects is that he can now move his head toward the source of sound, and look at the "objects" he hears. This indicates a new coordination between vision and hearing. Around this time the infant starts to follow the path of an "object" (a thing) with his eyes until it disappears from his view. As the background to all that I have described so far, I should add that Piaget has demonstrated that up to this point, (stage 2, 1-4 months), the infant's behavior essentially lacks intentionality, in the sense of willfully initiating behaviors directed at certain goals. Behaviors are in fact still primarily reflexive (though modified) and goals are set off only after behavior sequences are begun.

During the next stage (Piaget's stage 3, 4-8 months), one can observe the appearance of intentional behavior in the infant. His behavior can now follow a sequence clearly aimed at the goals he means to obtain. Indeed, he specifically selects the means that will obtain his goals.

During this stage the infant's behavior becomes more and more oriented toward "objects" (things and persons) and toward events beyond his body. Thus, he now grasps and manipulates anything he can reach. Another observable new characteristic is the infant's tendency to actively repeat any new interesting or unusual experience.

Effectively, before this stage, he had been unable to distinguish himself from other "objects" on a sensorimotor level. Similarly, he was unable to coordinate his hands, with his eyes and mouth, at least in part because of lack of maturation of his central nervous system (for an exploration of this problem from the psychoanalytic point of view see Hoffer 1949).

Piaget believes that the fact that at this time the child begins to anticipate the positions that objects will follow while moving through his field of vision indicates that the child is developing a beginning awareness of the permanence of the objects. Yet, in spite of this, the infant still continues to see himself as the cause of all activity, indeed he sees himself as the cause of all events.

Toward the end of the next phase, (stage 4, 8-12 months), certain behavior patterns emerge that demonstrate the first clear acts of intelligence. The infant begins to use means to obtain ends. One can see an intentional selection of such means to obtain his ends, i.e., a pillow may be moved out of the way to reach for a toy. He shows an "initial" ability to anticipate events. Objects (things outside himself including people) start to acquire a new measure of permanence. While previously he ignored "objects" the moment they were out of his field of vision, by the twelfth month he starts to search for objects that he sees disappear. This seems to imply that they have acquired some kind of existence or permanence outside the actual perceptual moment. Perhaps, because of the above, he begins to realize that other "objects" in the environment can themselves initiate activity and be responsible for the causality of things.

It is during this phase that the infant acquires the sense of the constancy of the shape and size of the objects. This is in contrast with the earlier stage in which any change in distance from a given object was "understood" as a change in the object and not in the point of view of the subject (relative to the object). It is not until this time (the eighth or ninth month) that he starts to explore the perspective effects occasioned by the actual displacement of objects.

During this period (stage 4) and even toward the end of the previous one, the child begins to distinguish between his own movements and those of the objects, while before he could not distinguish between movements of the object and those of his body.

But even more important is the fact that in the mind of the child objects start to acquire a substance and permanence they did not previously have. Thus, if before this stage we hide a rattle in which he is interested under a blanket while he looks, the infant does not search for it. In other words out of sight, out of existence. But somewhere between the eighth and the tenth month of age, the infant will begin to search for the object when hidden under the blanket, finally retrieving it. This seems to suggest that in the infant's mind objects now exist after they disappear from his sight. Yet, there is still much to be acquired in this area since the infant will look for the object where it "usually" disappears and not necessarily where he saw it disappear. It is not until the infant reaches twelve months that he becomes capable of looking for the object where it actually disappears and not where he was used to see it disappear.

Concomitantly, a child develops some awareness of its dependence on human objects for satisfaction, since he begins to understand that he cannot accomplish certain things without some help. Thus objects for the first time start to be seen as the actual causes of certain activities (pp. 25-26).

This particular stage is of special significance for all later development. Piaget describes it as the "practical intelligence" or "sensorimotor intelligence". For him, intelligence is observable long before language development—before words are used as the tools and symbols of thought processes. This practical intelligence applies instead to the manipulation of objects and utilizes only perceptions and organized movements in action schemes. On this basis, the infant is not contented anymore with reproducing and repeating familiar movements or activities that he finds interesting but he now uses many variations of such movements and activities with an exploratory aim. Piaget gives the example of the child who throws objects to the floor from his high chair, now in one direction, now in another, in order to study direction and trajectories. When the child combines and coordinates various such schemes (reciprocal assimilation), he begins the period of practical intelligence properly speaking.

As the result of all these advances in intellectual development, there is an enormous transformation in the way things are represented in the mind, finally leading to a differentiation between self and external world. Thus, the infant now arrives at the conception

that objects (things and persons outside the self) do have a permanence and are substantial. In other words, there is now in the
child's mind an actual belief or knowledge according to which the
thing perceived corresponds to something that continues to exist
even though he can no longer perceive it. As mentioned earlier, by
the third month of life, he can already "recognize" certain familiar
sensorial (perceptual) pictures, but the fact that he can recognize
them when they are present does not mean that he can place them
somewhere when they are outside his perceptual field. Thus, he
"recognized" persons and was aware that screaming made them
reappear, but this is not proof that he attributed to them either
permanence or substantial body in space when he could not see
them.

To make this point Piaget (1967) reminds us that at the beginning, when the infant starts to grasp all he sees, he shows no
searching behavior if the desired objects are covered by a han-
kerchief, even if he saw us cover the object. Later on, he would
search for the hidden object, but only where he saw it disappear the
first time. If we hide it under some other corner of the handkerchief
he cannot find it, in spite of the fact that he saw us hiding it under a
different corner of the handkerchief. As Piaget says (p. 26) it is as if
the object was part of a global gestalt and not a mobile element by
itself. But, according to him, this search for the object is the criteria
that allows us to recognize the beginning of the exteriorization of
the material world. In my own words, that there is something out
there and not inside me. This move from inside to outside is a good
example of a first step in the final elaboration of the external
universe.

In Piaget's conception, the concepts of space and spaces are
constructed in much the same way as the concept of "objects." At
the very beginning, there are as many spaces—without any coordination among them—as there are sensory-perceptual fields or
areas. Thus, there is a bucal space, a visual space, a tactile space,
etc. But each such space is centered on, or strictly linked with the
infant activities and movements of which it forms an integral part,
with no existence of its own. Furthermore, the visual space, for
example, does not know (or recognize) to start with the same

depths that the infant will perceive later on. By the end of the second year, there has developed a concept of a general space that contains all other spaces, the relations between objects, and the child's own body. The elaboration of the space concept is essentially the product of the coordination of movements. According to Piaget, one can see here the close relation that exists between this development (coordination of movements) and the so-called sensorimotor intelligence or practical intelligence (p.27).

In terms of the concept of causality, Piaget says that at the beginning, causality is strictly related to the infant actions or activities. In other words, he makes "everything" happen. This he describes as "magical causality." It is not until the second year that the child fully recognizes other causal relations (p. 27).

Piaget concludes that when certain objects (things and persons) are clearly differentiated as belonging outside the self, the awareness of the self becomes more affirmative. In other words, there is a sense of an interior pole of reality, opposed to that other objective and external pole of it. On the other hand, by analogy with the me (ego) the objects (things and persons) are conceived of as active, alive, wilfull, and conscious (the analyst's animistic stage). The choice of the object is thus correlated to the intellectual construction of the object (p. 30).

From eighteen months onward, and thanks to the development of language, profound changes take place. The child can now reconstruct past events in verbal form and anticipate his future actions by means of verbal representations. Three important consequences derive from this:

1. An exchange of meaningful communications between individuals, that is, the beginning of the socialization of action.
2. An internalization (Piaget uses the term interiorization) of speech, that is, the beginning of thinking proper with the support systems of the internal language and its symbols
3. An interiorization of action.

Piaget rightly remarks that while language is not definitely developed, interindividual interactions are limited to imitation of body gestures and postures, and to global affective relationships without well-differentiated communications. With speech, the infant shares his internal life, and at the same time, it is built up consciously, to the same extent that it can be communicated (p. 34).

STAGES IN THE DEVELOPMENT OF THE SELF

1. *The Autoerotic Non-self Non-object Stage*

At the very beginning there is no conception of the self; but many processes that will determine its appearance begin by the time the child is, on average, three months of age. These are very slow and gradual processes, with no sudden or clear demarcations from one day, or one week to the next. Further, there is considerable overlapping between stages, until finally one of them supersedes the other and becomes dominant. Some remnants of the earlier stages are frequently carried along to the later ones.

The "autoerotic non-self non-object stage" corresponds in Freud's timetable of libidinal positions to what he described as the "phase of autoerotism," a phase that precedes the "phase of primary narcissism" (see chapter 6).

Let us now try to characterize the conditions that exist at the autoerotic non-self non-object stage.

The ego as an organized system is not yet in evidence, though we can observe in operation some of the functions that will later be taken over by the ego and be under its control. At this point, they occur as isolated manifestations with little or no correlation and integration between them. Among these are perception and perceptive processes both of external and internal stimuli. Though perception is functional and effective, actual aperception is minimal or perhaps nonexistent to start with. Memory impressions are constantly being formed and laid down, feelings in the pleasure-unpleasure series are perceived, etc. These memory impressions are at first sensorimotor in character; at times specific affects are associated with them.

The picture observable on the side of the drives during this stage of the non-self closely resembles the state of affairs described for the ego. Each component instinct that has already appeared on the scene with each erotogenic zone is on its own, as isolated nuclei of libidinal activity, as disconnected points of excitation and discharge; in brief, as zones independent of one another. This is partly related to the total lack of organization and integration of the ego we have just described (and that most of us assume to be the state of affairs at birth).

It will follow from the above that the newly born infant not only has no conception of himself and so of the "self," but that a similar situation applies to of what constitutes the not me, or the non-self, and the world of objects. All this is nonexistent for him, there is no such conception in his mind.

It seems that all we can postulate at this point in development is the existence of a "primitive mental apparatus." This apparatus is capable of registering certain impressions, that presumably create a certain "mental state" or "feeling state" that can be recognized. This apparatus is also capable of triggering certain responses, most of which are, at the very beginning, automatic or reflexive.

One of the basic endeavors of such a primitive mental organization or apparatus is to recover a basic feeling of homeostasis. That is, recover the homeostatic equilibrium (and its accompanying feeling) that has constituted up to this point the basic line for that living organism. We assume he is accustomed to it and can recognize it and deviations from it.

At this point increases in tension are felt as unpleasure and decreases as pleasure. But at the same time this mental apparatus is, as yet, unable to differentiate among the source or sources of unpleasurable or pleasurable stimuli. He also cannot dissect the different elements or component parts of any particular stimulus.

It must be taken into account that a newborn child comes from a very protected environment, the mother's uterus. Though some stimuli may reach him here, these are minimized and not many in comparison with what is to come later on, a genuine bombardment of it. Consider too that in the uterus things are automatically regulated by means of very efficient servomechanisms that coordinates the mother's body and the child's. We can assume that under normal conditions he will have experienced few, if any, needs, and would have had little or no opportunity, to learn or exercise whatever skills he already possesses.

Thus, in a manner of speaking, he is born like a blank screen. He has no concept of his body and its parts. He does not know that he has a head, arms, legs, a mouth, and genitals. In terms of the latter and under more normal conditions, none of these organs has had an opportunity of being exercised (and experienced). This will come about as he experiences needs, is fed, and as a result defecates, urinates, etc.[1] In terms of the head, arms, legs, etc., he presumably has registered some sensations; for example proprioceptive or tactile sensations, since he moves some *in utero* (the traditional kicking). But this of necessity must be very limited in nature, given on the one hand the inmaturity of the areas of the brain that control these different body parts, and on the other the limited opportunities for exercising whatever skills he has. He can certainly "feel" body parts but has no willful control over them. It seems reasonable to assume that the registrations he has made of his body are part of the global gestalt that we described earlier as his basic feeling of homeostasis. Within the limits of that feeling (we assume a certain flexibility to it) he feels eupathic (Sandler, 1960) and safe, that is, biologically safe and in a state of psychological quietness. When such limits are transgressed he is biologically unsafe, loses the eupathic feeling, and responds accordingly.

Think now of his first experience of hunger and the activation of his body organs (including his mouth) that accompanies this process. This new set of sensations will fall on that blank screen and produce a new idiosyncratic feeling state, a new mental state, previously unknown to him. At this point his basic homeostatic feeling, the one he is normally familiar with, the one that allows him to know not only that he is but what he is, is replaced by a totally new feeling state. A new "awareness" has come to be and new memory traces are laid down. Now, suddenly there is a new

1. There are occasional exceptions. It is said that some infants have sucked fingers in utero. It is certain too that children may have passed meconium *in utero* (especially under distress delivery conditions). But for all practical purposes, all this can be ignored.

and different feeling state; at such a moment that is all he knows about himself.

He will react with his limited repertoire to this new biological stress; to this reaction an average expectable environment (and mother) will produce a suitable response. Thus, he will be fed, a situation for which he is endowed with the necessary biological prerequisites (sucking ability, rooting reflexes, etc). This again produces a new series of feeling states at the conscious level until finally his homeostatic equilibrium, his basic feeling is restored. He is back to the status quo previously familiar to him, but something has been added to this known state. He has received new and strange stimuli both from inside (hunger and all the phenomena associated with it) and from outside (food, mother's ministrations); he has had a new awareness, new feelings, a new mental state; and some memory traces of the experience taken as a whole may have been laid down. I say taken as a whole because he is not quite yet capable of discriminating what aspects of the experience are contributed by his own body and what by the outside agencies. This will come later as the experience repeats itself many times; until the infant starts to show that he has made certain associations which have predictive value for him. For example, after his intial whimpering and as a response to the mother's voice and the noises that she produces as she goes about preparing his food, he calms down. He knows, as it were, that the right sequence is taking place, that relief is on the way, though he does not know much more (realistically) about the actual meaning and component parts of the total experience. At this early stage, it is as if he gains the impression that by doing certain things (whimpering, random movements, sucking movements, etc.), he can bring about the relief of his tension, and/or distress, thus reinforcing the "belief" in his magic and omnipotence that the limited capacity of his ego and its peculiar form of functioning promotes. Remember that he knows nothing of the world, or of the existence of objects, outside of his feeling experiences.

It is important to recognize that once the child's hunger has reached a certain pitch his basic feeling and basic mental state are successively replaced by the "feeling of hunger" (and associated phenomena), the experience of being fed, and that of regaining homeostasis with a pleasurable bonus added to it. Clearly, with sufficient repetition of these various stimuli he recognizes that he is not only the basic feeling known to him from his intrauterine life but that basic feeling plus this new one. Though at first the one may replace and abolish the other, the child soon behaves as if he recognizes that they occur in a sequence and that he is both feelings. Similarly, as his ego abilities develop, he may include in this mental schema of himself those parts of his body that participate in the experience (e.g. his mouth) toward which his brain sends certain automatic activating messages. But his "concept" of the mouth is very different from what the adult observer will tend to conceptualize. It is no more, early on, than a number of sensorimotor coordinations. The child, in his limited awareness, is or has become this increased gestalt of sensations plus the feeling states that accompany it. The external observer could translate this by saying that at the times described the infant is building and getting to know some aspects of himself that concern his mouth. In this way he is laying down the bricks for the development of the knowledge of what he is, of himself. In other words, laying down the first bricks of what later will become the "self." At this stage it could be described as a mouth self. What I have discussed so far in relation to hunger and feeding must be considered as a prototype that repeats itself constantly in relation to many other areas of the body. They similarly contribute to his gradually but constantly increasing knowledge about himself, and toward the building of a body image of sorts, one based originally in sensorimotor coordinations and schemas. These intial images are no doubt highly distorted at the beginning, given his brain's immaturity, the mechanisms and principles that seem to regulate mentation at this point, and the limited functional capacity of his ego. But as the latter develops, the necessary corrections are gradually made and the necessary interrelations of the different parts are established.

If we consider other important bodily functions related to biological needs, we might proceed as follows. After feeding, a new part of the infant's body gets activated, produces new sensations, and leads to another new feeling state. His regained home-ostasis is interfered by this new set of sensations, as he finally has a bowel movement with all the concomitant sensations. Young infants do not generally get very disturbed by this unless they have some degree of pain (colics), constipation, etc. But be that as it may, the "external agencies" clean the child, thus introducing a large variety of new stimuli.

At the very beginning of life when this occurs, this novel set of sensations comes to the foreground (in his consciousness), and for the moment that is what the infant is aware of about himself. At that point he is the new sensation. Later on, and very gradually as the experience repeats itself, it will become part of a continuum of sensations. In other words, it is as if the child at some point recognizes this continuum, and furthermore, that he can be at any point on it. But of course, by then there is an increasing awareness that he is all of this experiental continuum. Each of these new sensations has a different body reference, a different body projection, something that makes it quite distinct from the others. Given time and the repetition of these different experiences (with the sensorimotor schemas associated with them), the developing ego will start to build up associations, body references, projections, and locale for all of them.

Links will be established among these experiences, a primitive mapping of the body will occur, and thus gradually a primitive body self begins to develop. At the same time, some primitive rudiments of some of the psychological aspects of the self start their own fabric both in relation to the beginning body scheme and independently from it.

A similar case can be construed in terms of the infant's wetting. We have concentrated on the role bodily needs play in the development of the self because they seem to us to be central to it. It is clear, however, that in such development many other sources of stimulation, from inside and outside, play significant roles. For example, there is the mother's need to relate to and stimulate her infant. She can do this in mulitple ways; talking, cleaning, bathing, singing, touching, kissing, playing, carrying, etc.

Up to this point, we have described a variety of feeling states that appear for the first time after birth in relation to various forms of stimuli, from the body itself, from outside, or from both. We have also described how, at the very beginning, they succeed one another as isolated phenomenon that the infant has no means to correlate. Each one of them is independently the potential beginning of an element of the body self and gradually will become a significant brick in the fabrication of the self.

It is our view that somewhere around the third month these various elements have come to form a recognizable whole that constitutes the first, very distorted, and very primitive representation of the self. At this point the cathexis and attention that was going to each one of these experiences as they took place, begins to go to this primitive self in which these experiences seem to take place. It is at this point that the stage of primary narcissism has been reached, and the phase of autoerotism left behind.

Before moving to the next stage, I want to highlight the following points:

1. It is not far fetched to postulate that during this autoerotic non-self non-object stage every feeling of unpleasure that disturbs the mind—whose only aim at this point is homeostasis—must be felt like a disturbance coming from outside.[2] This is very understandable since the child has no sense of a self, not even of a body self; there is no body schema or body image at all. Similarly, there is no awareness of any external objects in the psychological sense. Given the principles of mental functioning that rule his mentation, i.e. the principle of constancy and the pleasure principle, and given the lack of knowledge of the self, it is more than easy to disown for a time, as coming from outside, whatever disturbs his basic original homeostatic eupathic feeling. There only exists in fact the capacity to register pleasure and unpleasure and some memory traces of these experiences as they accumulate. But note that these memory traces have to be acquired; they are not there from the beginning.

2. "Outside" means here outside the mental apparatus (or rather its recognizable and familiar basic original feeling state of homeostatis, the eupathic feeling which at this point is all the infant knows about himself), including the infant's body that may well be the actual source of the unpleasurable feeling.

2. At some point the organism—or rather this mental apparatus—will learn to differentiate between external and internal stimuli by various means. For example, as Freud pointed out, one can escape from certain stimuli by taking flight but not from others, finally identifying the former with external stimuli and the latter with internal ones.

3. At some point during this stage it becomes possible for the mental apparatus of the child to identify certain patterns with which it has been confronted, patterns that have led to sensorimotor representations associated with pleasure or unpleasure in the mnemic systems. These patterns are identified not only through the perceptual activities of the ordinary senses, but also through proprioceptive perceptions, like the position of the body when held at the breast or for feeding as well as the recognition of tactile experiences—sounds, postural tone of the mother, warmth of her body, etc. The recognition of such patterns can now be associated with an oncoming experience of pleasure.

I wish to underline that the above is quite distinct from such phenomena as the smiling response to the human face which seems like an atavic instinctual form of response.[3] It becomes possible when a certain anlage gets activated as the ego reaches a certain stage of maturity (10 to 12 weeks). Yet, we know that that response is triggered off specifically by the three obscure dots representing the two eyes and the mouth. Spitz and Wolf (1946) clearly demonstrated that the infant will respond with a smile to a mask with three dark dots on it. This indicates that some of the child's reactions, functions, and mode of response are during this stage, closer to being conditioned reflexes. But in spite of this one can see the beginnings of what will later be a highly complex psychological response. For the time being they are still primitive and not based on his ability to recognize objects (in the psychological sense) either outside his body or in his own body. It is a relatively moot question what happens with all these experiences (good or bad) that register during the "objectless" stage. I fully

3. I say *atavic* and *instinctual* because of the parallel (for example) with the regurgitation of food in the case of birds when parents see the appropriate pattern in the open beak of the infant bird.

agree with Anne-Marie Sandler (1975) when she objects to those psychoanalysts who assume that very young infants are capable of the most complex mental functions and thought processes. As she remarks: "This is not to say that the first year is unimportant in later development. On the contrary, it is of crucial importance: for the significant patterns of sensory-motor behavior and the extremely important and infinitely varied feeling states developing, in even the first weeks of life, can persist through the mental life of the individual. In other words, a sensory-motor schema is formed which persists but is reorganized and observed in later phases" (pp. 367-368).

There is much in these various modes of response that is closer to reflex phenomena, to biological responses. The pause introduced by the activity of the mind (in higher forms of symbolic thinking) is not yet developed, with the exception, presumably after some experiences of satisfaction, of the possiblity of dealing with certain types of needs and tension by means of hallucinatory wish fulfillment. Even Freud's formulation of the hallucinatory wish fulfillment need not be understood of necessity in any complex terms. It suffices to assume that what is hallucinated by the young infant is the sensorimotor patterns and coordinations related to the activity, for example in sucking, as well as the feeling state associated with them (Freud 1911b).

2. *The Primitive-Primary-Narcissistic-Self Stage*

We described at the end of the previous section how a primitive self, mostly a body self got organized. This was possible thanks to the gradual development of the ego, partly related to to the physical maturation of the brain, and partly by being subjected to stimuli that act as a growth nutriment, as well as giving an opportunity to acquire, practice, and exercise skills, to accumulate knowledge, and to organize structures.

I believe this primitive-primary-narcissistic-self stage is generally reached around the third month of life. But this is just the very beginning of the stage, which itself continues at least up to the end of the first year of life or a little later (12-15 months of age).

This phase that I describe here as the "primitive-primary-narcissistic-self stage" coincides roughly with Freud's stage of primary narcissism, and precedes the stage of object relations.

During this stage, the activity of the component instincts and erotogenic zones as manifested through autoerotic activities no longer occur as isolated manifestations of tension and discharge phenomena, taking place in a random fashion anywhere in the body, and totally independent of each other. The limited awareness and lack of organization typical of the previous phase (autoerotism) has now been modified. Some degree of differentiation and structuralization has occurred and this has led in the direction of the first steps in organizing and forming a self image, particularly its body image component. This constitutes the beginnings of what we acknowledge to be one of the functions of the ego, the establishment and maintenance of the self; indeed, the development of the body image marks at the same time the very beginning of the ego as an organized system.[4] It should be noted that with this beginning of structuralization the autoerotic activities (manifestations of excitation of the component instincts and erotogenic zones) occur in a new referential frame—that of the body image as now known and recognized. It is for this reason that the impingement of tension, caused by the drives or component instincts looking for gratification in an auto erotic manner, or other painful stimuli can no longer be easily viewed or felt as an attack from outside the basic original feeling state.

During that first stage, the child can cathect only the experiences of pleasure and unpleasure and the memory traces that are formed out of these experiences. The degree of organization of the mind and the lack of a body image, of a concept of the self, make it impossible during the first stage (autoerotic non-self non-object stage) to cathect the body, at least that part of the body that brings about the pleasurable sensations, the cathexis goes to the experience itself.[5] Yet, a little later, by the second stage (primitive-

---

4. "The ego is first and foremost a bodily ego" (Freud 1923, p. 26).

5. This brings to mind some "borderline" children who do not recognize objects but the functions that they perform for them or the experience these objects provide them with. They refer to the therapist as the therapy, and to the lady that provides orange juice as the orange juice lady.

primary-narcissistic-self), when the beginning of the self is already present, the body, particularly that part of it involved in the experience of pleasure, can be cathected, since it can now be identified by the mental apparatus as a pleasurable part of itself. I said "pleasurable" because it seems possible that at least early during this second stage of the primitive-narcissistic-self, there is still the tendency to disown unpleasurable feelings. At some point later on, even the unpleasurable or painful sensations will have to be acknowledged and contained as belonging to the self. Otherwise, the establishment and development of reality testing will be permanently interfered with. This will also be true of the necessary shift from functioning according to the pleasure principle to functioning according to the reality principle.

I believe Freud (1914) had this type of phenomena in mind when he noted "that a unity comparable to the ego, cannot exist in the individual from the very start; the ego has to be developed. The auto-erotic instincts, however, are there from the very first; so there must be something added to auto-erotism—a new psychical action—in order to bring about narcissism" (p. 77).

Furthermore, now that these tensions and consequently the pleasurable sensations that accompany their relief (through a given autoerotic activity, for example) are identified with one's own body, the body is recognized as the "me" and as that which yields the pleasure, thus making it possible for the infant to cathect it. It is thus that Freud's stage of primary narcissism is reached (the position of the libido is now in the self), a stage that coincides with my stage of "the primitive-primary-narcissistic-self."

The concept of the self and the body image take a long time to evolve. They are at first quite distorted and far from accurate representations of one's actual physical and psychical reality. One's actual physical and psychical reality can only be known better (but never completely) at a much latter developmental stage. Indeed, we should add that the self is never static. On the contrary, it is modified all through life though certain aspects of it may have some degree of permanence from very early on.

It is clear that the nature of stimuli that now impinges on the mental apparatus and the processes that handle this information, sensations, stimuli, etc. have become much more "psychologically" significant and meaningful than they were before (at the earlier autoerotic non-self non-object stage).

For the infant to maintain this stage of primary narcissism, and its accompanying homeostasis, as well as for the self to continue to evolve, the infant is nearly totally dependent on the external environment. Thus, during the first (auto erotic non-self non-object stage) and second (primitive-primary-narcissistic-self) stages the mother as the child's biological object fulfills a large number of essential functions. She acts as a barrier against undesirable or excessive stimuli for the infant, and is the provider of all of his essential physical needs. She is the most important regulating factor in the constant struggle for the recovery of the basic original homeostatic eupathic feeling, which is forever being disturbed by external and internal stimulation.

She provides too, innumerable forms of stimulation and forms of body contact which are essential as an important contribution for the normal development of the infant. These are required ingredients for the development of the body image and as such of a healthy self as time goes on. Her role as the triggering and releasing agency of many other processes furthering drive and ego development must never be underestimated. With the increasing delineation of the body image and the self that takes place during this stage,the outside (not self or not me) becomes quite distinct from the self. This is a distinction of great significance but it does not imply that the child can clearly distinguish where in the not self (not me or external world) different things belong. This type of process starts early and proceeds very slowly during this second stage. From this point onward and due to his further ego development, experiencing and learning during the nine months or more of this stage, he embarks on the long and arduous task of coming to understand not only some of the constituent elements of his external world, but also of the interaction between it and the primitive self. Of course, the non-self (external world) is only vaguely hinted at at the beginning of this process. Yet, ill defined as it is in the child's mind, these vague hints of an outside help considerably in the further and more precise delineation of the primitive-primary-narcissistic-self by gradually excluding certain things and including others.

Given the dominant role that his mother plays in his life—as the most significant element of that essentially unknown external world—it is natural that from a given time onward he would develop (at first in an obscure manner and later more precisely) an increasing psychological interactional awareness of her existence and her essential functions. In this way she begins to draw larger and larger amounts of cathexis and interest. When this shift has acquired sufficient momentum, we arrive at that stage that Freud described as the stage of object relations signifying that the libidinal position has shifted once again. In other words, from cathecting only the self, libidinal cathexis now moves outside the self, to the external world and its still ill defined objects.

In terms of the development of the self, we arrive at what I would describe as "the interactional—self and other—quasi-object stage" the final outcome of which will be the development of object relations.

3. *The Interactional—Self and Other—Quasi-object Stage*

The beginnings of the type of phenomena that characterizes this stage have to be looked for early in the previous phase we have described. But at that time it occurs only as occasional single isolated manifestations that do not get linked to one another. In other words, they are like questions with different, closely interrelated contents posed to the mentational abilities of the child at different moments in time. They tend to contradict the achieved status quo, posing conceptual problems that puzzle the infant, problems that he must answer satisfactorily at some later date, as he matures, learns, and develops.

As many of these originally isolated events acquire a more specific meaning in the child's mind, one that is closer to its "real" meaning, many of them gel together. In this new light they acquire a significance in terms of their correlations and relatedness. Slowly but surely, as that happens, "new understandings" develop. This process further permits the infant to dissect from aspects of the self things that do not in actuality belong to it, but that were assimilated to it by virtue of the global nature of the sensorimotor experience of the young infant, and of his limited capacity for fine discriminations among the constituent elements of any given sensorial experience. Similarly, certain things that were originally exteriorized because of their painful or unpleasurable nature must be accepted as parts of the self, at some point.

In any case, many events, happenings, etc. make it clear to the young infant that certain aspects of it cannot really be placed on the self as they were before (when mentation was more primitive and less discriminatory), so that they belong somewhere else, on that vague outside that is starting to materialize but that remains very imprecise. An example of what I have in mind here is the fact that young infants can "recognize" certain people, and that these so recognized are different from others. Spitz (1957) believes this is possible from the third month onward, Piaget (1967) from the fifth week. But as Piaget points out (p. 21), we cannot for this reason assume that the infant has any notion of a person, or an object. All he is recognizing is certain animated sensory perceptions, but this proves nothing regarding their substantiality or regarding a separation between him and the external world, the object world. Piaget adds a little later (p. 25) that it is easy to demonstrate that early on the infant does not perceive objects (things or human) properly speaking. He does recognize certain familiar sensorial pictures, but the recognition while they are sensorially present is not at all equivalent with placing them in "some place" (that is, with their being substantial and somewhere) when they are outside the perceptual field. Yet, there can be no question that at such points there has been a change of some kind in the child's perception, a new obscure awareness of something. This is a first but incomplete step in the direction of further differentiation.

According to Piaget (1967) there are four fundamental processes that characterize the intellectual revolution of the first two years of life. They are all highly relevant to our subject but for our purposes I will discuss only one of them. I refer to the construction of the category of objects (the concept of objects).[6] Early on in life, the concept of objects is a practical category related to pure action (sensorimotor coordinations), and does not as yet take the form of a thought or a thinking notion. This concept or practical category once fully established, a process that takes up to the first eighteen months of life, it is characterized by the substantial permanence that is attributed by the infant to the sensorial pictures. That is, the infant has developed a concept according to which the aperceived figure corresponds to "something" that will continue to exist even when one is not perceiving it any longer.[7]

This awareness or recognition is a necessary prerequisite to the permanent cathexis of objects, to genuine—in the full psychological-cognitive sense—choice of objects and object relationships.

Indeed, according to Piaget, it is not until nine to twelve months of age that the infant clearly shows a "searching" behavior for objects that move out of his perceptual field. Objects have become permanent and substantial. They are somewhere "out there" (though not seen at the moment). You will remember that Piaget stated that this is precisely the criterion that allows us to recognize the beginning of the exteriorization of the material world, a step in the elaboration of the exterior universe. In other words, a consciousness of the self starts to develop as an internal, subjective pole of reality, in contrast and opposition to that other external and objective pole of reality constituted by the external world and its components.

Given the importance of the concept of the object in psychoanalysis and all the formulations that are derived from it, and given that it is generally agreed that before that stage what gets cathected is a particular sensorimotor experience (the object being part of the mixture and going unrecognized), it may be valuable to examine briefly, once more, Piaget's views about the construction of that concept by the infant from the very beginning of his extrauterine life.

6. Piaget's use of the term *object* may refer to either things or humans. It is usually clear in what follows which he is referring to. Frequently, I'll leave in brackets to avoid possible confusion which he refers to in any specific case.

7. This seems to occur at around 8 or 9 to 10 or 12 months of age.

Piaget believes that the object concept is not innate but must be acquired. In other words, the idea that objects are more or less permanent and substantial and that they are not destroyed when they disappear from the infant's perceptive field is not an inherited characteristic. He thinks that an awareness of objects will develop out of the infant's sensorimotor experiences very gradually during the first year of life. Thus, the infant has to construct for himself the external world and the universe of objects (things and humans) through his own experiences.

During the first month of life then, the infant has no object concept. "Objects" coming in contact with him are, as Wadsworth (1971) says, quoting Piaget, merely something to suck, to grasp, or to look at, and this evokes only an undifferentiated reflexive response (p. 39).

During Piaget's stage two (1-4 months) the child develops an awareness of objects that was not present during the first month. Thus, he can focus on objects and track an object moving through his field of vision. Further, he can now turn to look at the objects he hears, showing the coordination between vision and hearing. The infant does not have the concept of the constancy of the shape and forms of objects so that a new angle or more distance between subject and object are not understood as a change in perspective but as an actual change in the size or form of the object. There are still no signs of any active searching for objects (things) when the desired object is covered with a handkerchief, even when the infant has carefully followed with his eyes every one of the movements made in hiding the object.

During stage three (4-8 months) the infant is capable of anticipating the positions objects will pass through while they are moving in his perceptive field. Since he "knows" where the object will be in the trajectory before it gets there, it would seem that in some as yet obscure and very primitive way he is developing a sense of its permanence.

During this stage, the infant starts to acquire the ability to distinguish between movements of the object and those of his own body, in contrast with the previous phase when such distinction was not made. It is in this distinction that the beginning of the searching for objects when they disappear is to be found, according to Piaget and Inhelder (1956). As they say, "It is in terms of this grouping of movements, and the permanence attributed to the object, that the latter acquires fixed dimensions and its size is estimated more or less correctly, regardless of whether it is near or distant" (p. 11).

By the end of stage three (8 months) infants can anticipate the positions at which falling objects (things) will rest, thus demonstrating a better knowledge of some aspects of their behavior, but there is still no active searching behavior for hidden objects.

By stage four (8-12 months) the infant definitely acquires the concept of the constancy of shape and size of objects. According to Piaget and Inhelder (1956), by eight or nine months he really explores the perspective effects of actual displacements (p. 17).

It is at this stage that a new dimension in the object concept develops. Up to this point, if an object such as a rattle is hidden under a handkerchief while the infant looks, he does not search for it. But now he actively searches for and retrieves the rattle hidden under the blanket. To do this, the infant has to acquire the concept that objects continue to exist after they disappear from perception. Nevertheless, at this point, the infant searches for the object where it generally disappears and not necessarily where he saw it disappear. Thus, he has no ability to understand what Piaget calls sequential displacement.

In Piaget's stage six (18-24 months), the child moves from the sensorimotor level of intelligence (practical intelligence) to representational intelligence. By now the child can represent events internally and this newly acquired ability is reflected in the child's object concept. Thus, he can not only find objects when he sees them being hidden, but he will search for and find (and in a sequence of places) objects that he does not see being hidden, a fact that shows his liberation from immediate perception. The development of this latter skill can in fact be seen as early as the fourteen and fifteen month of life. In my observation this is about the time at which the child develops object constancy in Anna

Freud's sense of the term (1968).[8] Indeed, it seems, quite reasonable to assume that object constancy cannot be developed appropriately before the object can be represented in the child's mind, and before the knowledge of its substantial and permanent nature (out there) is well established. For an excellent discussion of some aspects of the problems involved here, see Fraiberg (1969).

I have thus chosen to select this point in development as the beginning of "genuine" object relations on the following premises:

1. There is a "sufficient" distinction (though not absolutely precise and/or complete in all respects) between the self and the external world.

2. There is a "sufficient" awareness of the existence of objects in the external world, though it is not absolutely precise and/or complete in all respects.

3. There is a "sufficient" awareness of the relative importance in regard to the self of the various objects identified in the external world at this time, though that distinction is not absolutely precise and/or complete in all respects.

4. There is "sufficient" evidence that one object has acquired a particularly significant and relevant position in regard to the self, and vis-a-vis the other objects, namely, the mother or mothering person.

5. That object now draws the most cathexis and interest from the child, and has acquired the characteristics and qualities that I described as "object constancy" and the "primary object."

This formulation is consistent not only with psychoanalytic theory and psychoanalytic observations, but with the tenets of cognitive development, the development of the concept of the object, the external world, causality, and intentionality, as substantiated in Piagetian theory.

---

8. This means that the object has suddenly become important per se, in contrast with the previous need-satisfying stage where the object was valued for its function. From the moment the child reaches object constancy, the child is permanently attached to the object whether the object satisfies or not, whether it is good or bad. I believe it is at this point that the concept of "primary object" crystallizes, after a long line of development in that direction. Once that happens, that object cannot be substituted without traumatic consequences for the child.

Of course, in all the above I have referred to the course of normal development, and we are all aware that there are many children that for one reason or another do not develop object constancy, or only in a limited manner. Similarly, some children do not develop a clear, distinct, and preferred "primary object." I believe that the large number of reasons that may explain the failures in cognitive development, the development of a "clean" concept of the self and of the object, the development of object constancy and the attachment to a primary object are the reasons that underlie certain types of psychotic, borderline, narcissistic, and neurotic disturbances, depending on where the defect lies and its severity.

It should be clear that with the development of the object concept and its location in the not me (the external world), and with the resultant and concomitant establishment of object constancy we have reached a functional and definitional beginning in terms of object relations.

Object constancy implies of necessity a fusion of the good and bad object representations (in the sense of Jacobson, Kernberg and others) since it means that the child continues to be attached to the object irrespective of the object being good or bad, or satisfying the child's needs or not. But this has to be taken as a base line that can be temporarily obscured by the vicissitudes of the multiple interactions between subject and object. In other words, certain aspects of the object behavior may be denied, displaced, or are subjected to the vicissitudes created by the infant's ambivalence, hostile or aggressive feelings, shifts from love to hate, various drive demands, level of frustration tolerance, egocentrism, etc. Thus, the base line described above gets more or less temporarily submerged or distorted under the weight of one or more of all these possible influences in the course of normal development. If there are important unfavorable circumstances of various types, that distortion or submersion may become more permanent, with consequent damage to personality development and possible multiple consequences in terms of later psychopathology. But it is important to realize that the damage thus accrued is on the basis of conflictual situations as they arise in the interactions between the subject (drives, needs, etc) and the object. This is quite different from pathology resulting from damage to the actual apparatuses (and/or cognitive structures) for organic, hereditary, or other reasons, or those that are the result of insufficient opportunity to receive stimuli, to practice and acquire skills, to acquire knowledge etc, in the process of the interaction with an expectable environment.

References

Fraiberg, S. (1969). Libidinal object constancy and mental representation, *Psychoanalytic Study of the Child* 24: 9-48.

Freud, A. (1968). Panel Discussion, 25th Congress of the I.P.A. Copenhaguen, July 1967, International Journal of Psycho-Analysis, Vol. 49, p. 506.

Freud, S. (1911). Formulations regarding the two principles of mental functioning. *Standard Edition* 12: 213-226.

———. (1923). The ego and the id. *Standard Edition,* 19: 3-68.

———. (1914). On narcissism: An introduction. *Standard Edition* 14: 67-104.

Hoffer, W. (1949). Mouth, hand and ego-integration. *Psychoanalytic Study of the Child* 3/4: 49-56.

Hoffer, W. (1950). Development of the body ego. *Psychoanalytic Study of the Child.* 5:18-24.

Jacobson, E. (1964). *The Self and the Object World.* New York: International Universities Press.

Kernberg, O. (1975). *Borderline Conditions and Pathological Narcissism.* Jason Aronson: New York.

———. (1976). *Object Relations Theory and Clinical Psychoanalysis.* Jason Aronson: New York.

Kohut, H. (1977). *The Restoration of the Self.* New York: International Universities Press.

Piaget, J. (1967). *Seis Estudios de Psicologia.* Barcelona: Editorial Seix Barral.

Piaget, J., and Inhelder, B. (1956). *The Child's Conception of Space.* London: Routledge and Kegan Paul.

Sandler, A.M. (1975). Comments on the significance of Piaget's work for psychoanalysis. The Internattional Review of Psychoanalysis 2:367-68.

Sandler, J. (1960). The background of safety. International Journal of Psychoanalysis 41:352-356.

Spitz, R.A. and Wolf, K.M. (1946). *The Smiling Response:* Genetic Psychology Monograph 34.

Wandsworth, J.R. (1971). *Piaget's Theory of Cognitive Development.* New York: David McKay Co.

Chapter Six

AUTOEROTISM, AUTOEROTIC ACTIVITIES, AND EGO DEVELOPMENT

Autoerotism and autoerotic activities lie at the base of the sexual theory, itself. They are important elements in the discharge of tension aroused by the sexual drives (component instincts) all through development, and are the very first manifestations of sexual activity out of which adult sexuality will develop.

This being the case, it is puzzling that not enough attention has been paid to the concept of autoerotism. As a result of this relative neglect, there is a great deal of confusion and misunderstanding and sometimes even a failure to grasp many of its implications. In turn this misunderstanding has led to reformulations, new theoretical propositions, and ever more confusion.

A revision of some aspects of the concept of autoerotism inevitably leads us into other areas of confusion among analysts, but I believe some light is thrown on them once the phenomenon of autoerotism is clearly defined and properly placed among Freud's other theoretical formulations. One such area of enormous confusion relates to the term *object* and the use Freud made of it.

Though many factors are responsible for some of the misunderstandings, two of them are perhaps of particular relevance and deserve to be mentioned here.

First, not enough distinction is made between autoerotic activities viewed within the frame of the "phase of autoerotism" (in

Freud's timetable), and autoerotic activities considered in the broader frame of sexual development, long after autoerotism as a phase in libidinal development has been left behind. Secondly, not enough attention is paid to the fact that some aspects of the sexual theory were developed after the original appearance of *Three Essays on the Theory of Sexuality* in 1905. Freud made many additions to the *essays,* in some cases many years later, that is, when further work in other areas had thrown new light on certain aspects of the original formulations. It should not be forgotten then that different portions of the *Three Essays,* though closely related to each other, are sometimes found on close analysis to belong to very different levels of concept formation and of development in psychoanalytic theory. This makes it necessary when quoting from such material to take into account the context and background against which they first appear, in order not to distort their significance.

The implications of autoerotic phenomena for understanding and developing theoretical formulations in relation to the early stages of ego development are obvious. A clarification of the meaning of autoerotic phenomena will also throw some light on the theory of narcissism. I am inclined to think that it is not possible to deal with the questions inherent in this theory until the ground has been cleared of these misunderstandings of Freud's assumptions in relation to autoerotism and the use of the term "object," both in relation to autoerotic phenomena and in a more general sense. Very many of the alleged contradictions in the area of narcissism either disappear or fall into proper perspective once the difficulties due to misconceptions about autoerotism and autoerotic activities are overcome.

Finally, I want to call attention to, and will try to distinguish, three different types or levels of autoerotism and autoerotic phenomena which can be seen at three different stages in the development of the personality. They are, of course, closely connected with each other. Although the phenomena remain basically the same, there are important differences among these three types or levels of autoerotic manifestations.

I think these differences were implicit in Freud's mind when he established the timetable: autoerotism, primary narcissism, object relationships. I hope to show that he explicitly distinguished the "phase of autoerotism" and the autoerotic activities then present; further, these first autoerotic activities do not have quite the same organization and complexity as those present in the next stage of his timetable, primary narcissism.

THE CONCEPT OF AUTOEROTISM AND AUTOEROTIC ACTIVITIES

"Autoerotism" is a term used by Freud to describe a phase in libidinal development, while "autoerotic" is a term used to describe a specific type of sexual activity and gratification.

"Autoerotic" sexual activity and "autoerotic" forms of gratification can be observed during the phases of "autoerotism" and "primary narcissism" and not infrequently side by side with other forms of sexual gratification characteristic of more advanced phases of development such as that of "object love."

I believe an autoerotic activity can best be described as an objectless instinctual activity seeking for a particular kind of pleasure. This pleasure is normally brought about by a special handling, stroking, or other type of manipulation necessary to produce the gratification. In this way the excitation in the corresponding erotogenic zone or the excitation of a particular component instinct (expressing itself through an appropriate erotogenic zone) is reduced.

Autoerotic activities are observable during early sexual development in all erotogenic zones—mouth, anus, and genitalia.

Freud's first mention of the term appears in a letter to Fliess (December 9, 1899) in which he says: "The lowest of the sexual strata is auto-erotism, which renounces any psychosexual aim and seeks only local gratification. This is superseded by allo-erotism (homo- and hetero-), but undoubtedly survives as an independent tendency" (Freud 1887-1902, p. 303f.).

Though Freud borrowed the term from Havelock Ellis who introduced it in 1898, he used it in a different sense. He insisted frequently that autoerotism is an objectless condition. In the *Three Essays* he says: "It must be insisted that the most striking feature of this sexual activity is that *the instinct is not directed towards other people, but obtains satisfaction from the subject's own body. It is auto-erotic.*" (1905, p. 181; italics mine).

In 1920 Freud added a very significant footnote to this sentence: "Havelock Ellis, it is true, uses the word 'auto-erotic' in a somewhat different sense, to describe an excitation which is not provoked from outside [whether directly or indirectly] but arises internally. *What psycho-analysis regards as the essential point is not the genesis of the excitation, but the question of its relation to an object*" (italics mine).

It is now necessary to determine how far this "objectlessness"— the main characteristic of autoerotic activities—is carried in Freud's formulation. This is by no means an easy task. Careful consideration in this respect seems to indicate that neither the cases in which there is a physical biological dependence of a component instinct on an object in the external world, nor the cases in which there is an object in the external world, nor the cases in which there is an object choice through the agency of the ego (though mainly operative in fantasy) are truly autoerotic manifestations. That seems to be the reason for such statements as: "At a time at which the first beginnings of sexual satisfaction are still linked with the taking of nourishment, the sexual instinct has a sexual object outside the infant's own body in the shape of his mother's breast. It is only later that the instinct loses that object. . . . *As a rule the sexual instinct then becomes auto-erotic.*" (1905, p. 222; italics mine).

It is clear that the object referred to in this statement is the biological object of the oral component instinct. It must be noted that Freud is quite specific in pointing out that the relation here is one between the *sexual instinct* and its *sexual object* and not between the child's ego and its object: "the sexual instinct has a sexual object outside the infant's own body." He further stated that it is only later *when the instinct loses that object* that the sexual instinct becomes autoerotic.

From this and many other similar statements one is forced to conclude the following: Freud thought that the relationship to an object determines whether a given sexual activity is autoerotic or not; this excludes from autoerotic phenomena all cases in which the physical-biological relationship of a component instinct to an object still exists and in which gratification is dependent on this relationship. Sucking at the mother's breast is consequently not an autoerotic activity, in contrast to sucking one's own finger, which is an autoerotic activity.

Similarly, when there already exists a relationship to an object on the ego side (even in fantasy, as, for example, in masturbation during the phallic phase), we cannot speak of pure autoerotic activity but must consider the phenomenon a composite in which a fantasy has inserted itself into the previously pure autoerotic activity.

Freud (1908) linked fantasies with autoerotism when referring to masturbation. He mentioned that during a period of masturbation the fantasy was evoked in conjunction with some active behavior for obtaining self-gratification at the height of the fantasy (p. 161). A very clear example can be taken from Little Hans's own comments when he said: "I put my finger to my widdler just a very little. I saw Mummy quite naked in her chemise, and she let me see her widdler" (1909, p. 32).

In current usage one would refer to this type of masturbation as an autoerotic activity. Strictly speaking, however, one could not call this autoerotic, since by now the activity is a highly complex composite of which the relationship to an object in fantasy is an important part. Thus the cases in which there is a relationship through the agency of the ego with an object are not truly autoerotic manifestations either. Strictly speaking, a true autoerotic activity is taking place only in those cases in which the object of the component instinct is the subject's own body or a part of it.

During this early period in the development of psychoanalytic theory Freud had not yet asked the question whether the child had any psychological awareness of his own body. This question of self-awareness was taken into account a few years later, starting in about 1909 with the introduction of "narcissism" as an intermediary libidinal position on the way from autoerotism (as the first libidinal position) to that of object love. The autoerotic activities are now seen in a new and psychologically more meaningful context: "Recent investigations [e.g., Freud 1910, p. 100] have directed our attention to a stage in the development of the libido which it passes through on the way from auto-erotism to object-love. This stage has been given the name of narcissism. What happens is this. There comes a time in the development of the individual at which he unifies his sexual instincts (which have hitherto been engaged in auto-erotic activities) in order to obtain a love-object; and he begins by taking himself, his own body, as his love-object, and only subsequently proceeds from this to the choice of some person other than himself as an object" (1911, p. 60f.).[1]

During the phase of autoerotism each component instinct that is aroused is seeking gratification quite independently of any other. According to Freud, in the next stage of libidinal development (narcissism), the different component instincts somehow become unified and take the self as a love object. Consequently the type of sexual gratification during the phase of primary narcissism is autoerotic as well, the object being one's own body and not an external one as in the following phase of object love. "One's own body" as an object is now a psychologically meaningful experience, owing to the degree of development we assume to have been reached at the stage of the narcissistic libidinal position.

The difference between the autoerotic activities of the phase of primary narcissism and those of autoerotism, as I see it, is that those corresponding to primary narcissism are less close to the biological realm of phenomena than those belonging to the phase of autoerotism in which there is no awareness of the self as is the case in primary narcissism. As Freud said, "the ego cannot exist in the individual from the start; the ego has to be developed. The autoerotic instincts, however, are there from the very first, so there must be something added to auto-erotism—a new psychical action—in order to bring about narcissism" (1914, p. 77).

Furthermore, it must be noted that Freud considered it important clinically that the regression in dementia praecox extends not

1. This sentence was also added as a footnote to the *Three Essays* in 1910.

merely to narcissism (as in paranoia) but to a complete abandonment of object love and a return to infantile autoerotism. The dispositional fixation point must therefore be situated further back than in paranoia, and must lie somewhere at the beginning of the course of development from autoerotism to object love (1911, p. 77).

It may have become clear by now that the first accounts of the phenomena we are concerned with here were mostly of a descriptive nature and given by Freud against the background of his theory of infantile sexuality as formulated in his *Three Essays* (1905). Considerations pertinent to ego development, its possible relationship to, and mutual influence on, autoerotic phenomena were not so explicitly in the foreground at this stage. Ego psychology as we know it today was not developed until many years later.

In any case, with the introduction of the theory of narcissism the first such links were established, but unfortunately, as with some other aspects of psychoanalytic theory, this formulation was never integrated with the later, more advanced conceptualizations of ego developmental psychology. A modest attempt in that direction is made in the last section of this chapter.

It may be worth while at this point to remark on how some analysts after Freud have added to the confusion by, in my opinion, misinterpreting some aspects of Freud's formulations. The statement that "the sexual instinct has a sexual object outside the infant's own body in the shape of the mother's breast" has not infrequently been taken to imply a psychological relationship of the type that only the developed ego is capable of. It seems obvious that what Freud had in mind here is that *the sexual instinct* and *not the child's ego finds an object.* Furthermore, this is a readymade biological object for the particular instinct, characteristic of the species. This will be the biological prototype of the finding of an object later on in development by the ego.[2]

2. These biological prototypes should not surprise anybody who has noticed similar statements made by Freud in the *Three Essays.* For example, in two footnotes added in 1924, he mentions Abraham's paper of 1924, pointing out how the anus is developed from the embryonic blastopore—a fact which seems like a biological prototype of psychosexual development. Another one refers to the phallic phase having, according to Abraham, its biological prototype in the embryo's undifferentiated genital disposition which is the same for both sexes.

In the same type of statement, Kleinian theory assumes that object relationships are mediated through an agency which would have to be a highly developed ego structure present "from the beginning."

Freud's final point of view in this question can be clearly seen in the following statement from the *Outline*: "A child's *first erotic object* is the mother's breast that feeds him, and love in its beginnings attaches itself to the satisfaction of the need for food. To start with, *the child certainly makes no distinction between the breast and his own body;* when the breast has to be separated from his body and shifted to the 'outside' because he so often finds it absent, it carries with it, *now that it is an 'object,'* part of the original narcisistic cathexis" (1940, p. 89f., italics mine).[3] Kleinian theory can consequently dispose—and in fact does so implicitly—of the whole range of manifestations covered under autoerotism and autoerotic activities.

Lastly, another important source of confusion is due to the fact that at the time of the *Three Essays* Freud postulated that infantile sexual life "exhibits components which from the very first involve other people as sexual objects. Such are the instincts of scopophilia, exhibitionism and cruelty, which appear in a sense independently of erotogenic zones; these instincts do not enter into intimate relations with genital life until later, but are already to be observed in childhood as independent impulses, distinct in the first instance from erotogenic sexual activity" (1905, p. 192). It is not always realized that later on, partly as the result of the introduction of the narcissism theory, Freud modified the formulation given above. He said: "For the beginning of its activity the scopophilic instinct is autoerotic; it has indeed an object, but that object is part of the subject's own body. It is only later that the instinct is led, by a process of comparison, to exchange this object for an analogous part of someone else's body" (1915, p. 130).

AUTOEROTISM AND EGO DEVELOPMENT

The autoerotic activities proper to the phase of autoerotism and those autoerotic activities that supersede this phase must be con-

---

3. This very argument and other similar ones are to be found in several places in Freud's writings. Compare. for example, *The Introductory Lectures* (1916-1917, p. 314).

sidered against the background given by the stage of ego development reached.

In accordance with my introductory premises, I shall describe three different types or levels of autoerotism and autoerotic phenomena which can be observed at three different stages in the development of the personality.

First Type

The phenomena described under this heading correspond in Freud's timetable of libidinal development to the phase of autoerotism. At the very beginning the ego as an organized system is not yet present, though some of the functions that will later be taken over by the ego and form an integral part of its organization are already present. Yet at this point they occur as isolated manifestations, with little or no correlation between them. Among these are perception and perceptive processes both of external and internal stimuli, memory impressions that are constantly being formed, feelings of the pleasure-unpleasure series, etc.

Similarly the picture on the side of the drives during this phase of autoerotism resembles that of the ego side. Each component instinct that has already appeared on the scene with each erotogenic zone is on its own, as isolated nuclei of libidinal activity, as disconnected points of excitation and discharge; in brief, as zones independent of one another. This implies of course the total lack of organization and integration on the side of the ego that we assume to be the state of affairs at birth.

Again at this stage all one can postulate is the existence of the mental apparatus, whose basic endeavor is to recover homeostatic equilibrium whenever it is lost by tension arising in the organism itself or coming from outside. The increase of tension, as is well known, is felt as unpleasure and vice versa. At the same time this mental apparatus is still unable to differentiate the source from which the stimuli of an unpleasurable or pleasurable nature arise.

Later on the organism—or rather, this mental apparatus—will be able to differentiate between external and internal stimuli by different means; for example, it will have learned that one can escape from external stimuli by taking flight, but not from internal ones. It may not be too far reaching to postulate that at this very primitive stage every feeling of unpleasure that comes to disturb the mind— whose only aim at this point is homeostasis— is felt like a disturbance coming from the outside (outside here means outside the mental apparatus, including the body that may well be the source of the unpleasurable feeling).

There is no awareness of any objects in the psychological sense, neither external nor internal (the body or part of it). There exists only the capacity fo feel pleasure and unpleasure and gradually also memory traces of these experiences. Yet even these memories must be acquired through experience: they are not there from the beginning.

At a given point during this phase it will become possible for the mental apparatus of the child to identify certain patterns with which he has been confronted, and which already have created representations associated with pleasure or unpleasure in the mnemic systems.

The identification of these patterns comes about through perception (not only through the ordinary senses, but also through proprioceptive perceptions, like the position of the body when held at the breast, etc., as well as the recognition of tactile experiences, sounds, warmth of the mother's body, etc.). The recognition of this pattern can now be associated with the oncoming experience of pleasure. Recent experiments have made it clear that there is no recognition of individual objects (e.g., the mother); the child will react similarly to any object that repeats the pattern he is familiar with. Similarly, the child will react to a mask that contains the pattern he can recognize (Spitz and Wolf 1946).

At this stage the child's reaction, functions, and mode of response are closer to the animal being, and of the nature of conditioned reflexes. Yet one can see the beginnings of what will later be a response through highly complex psychological ways. At this point they are still primitive and not based on his ability to recognize "objects" (in the psychological sense) either outside his body or in his own body, which later in development will become an object.

This mode of response is closer to the reflex phenomena, to typical biological responses. The pause introduced by the activity of the mind is not yet developed, with the exception—presumably after some experiences of satisfaction—of the possibility of dealing with certain types of tension by means of hallucinatory wish fulfillment.

Second Type

This second type of autoerotic activity belongs no longer to the phase of autoerotism that I have described above but to that of primary narcissism. The changes that now have occurred on the ego side make the autoerotic activities appear in a different light.

The autoerotic activities remain basically the same, since by autoerotic we understand the capacity to satisfy certain component instincts in one's own body. Yet one must distinguish this second phase (primary narcissism) from the phase of autoerotism, just as one must distinguish autoerotism as a phase in libidinal development characterized by the absolute dominance of autoerotic activities of a particular kind (due to the stage of development of the child) from autoerotic activities which occur later on when the development of the child has proceeded further; these autoerotic activities now take place in a different setting, and by virtue of this fact have acquired certain qualitative differences which distinguish them from activities occurring during other phases.

During this phase the autoerotic activities no longer occur as isolated manifestations of tension and discharge phenomena, taking place anywhere in the body and totally independent of each other. The lack of awareness and organization typical of the previous phase (autoerotism) is now modified. A certain degree of differentiation and structuralization has taken place, through the first steps in the formation of the body image. This constitutes the beginnings of what we acknowledge to be one of the functions of the ego, the establishment of the self; in fact, the development of the body image is the very beginning of the ego as an organized system ("The ego is first and foremost a bodily ego"—(Freud 1923, p. 26). With this beginning of structuralization the autoerotic activities now occur in the frame of reference of the body image.

The impingement of the tension caused by the drives or component instincts looking for gratification in an autoerotic manner
can no longer be viewed or felt as the same attack from outside as
they were in the previous phase, against the homeostatic equilibrium of the mental apparatus.

During the first stage the child can cathect only the experiences
of pleasure and unpleasure and the memory traces that go with
them, or rather, that are formed out of these experiences. The
degree of organization of the mind and the lack of a body image, of
a concept of the self, make it impossible at that stage to cathect the
body, at least that part of the body that brings about the pleasurable sensation; the cathexis goes to the experience itself. A little
later, when the beginning of the concept of the self is present, the
part of the body involved in the experience of pleasure can be
cathected, since it can now be identified by the mental apparatus as
part of itself.

I believe Freud had this type of phenomena in mind when he
said: "that a unity comparable to the ego cannot exist in the
individual from the very start; the ego has to be developed. The
auto-erotic instincts, however, are there from the very first; so there
must be something added to auto-erotism—a new psychical action—in order to bring about narcissism" (1914, p. 77). Considerations of that kind may have led him to the original formulation of
the timetable: autoerotism, primary narcissism, object relationship.

Furthermore, now that these tensions and consequently the
pleasurable sensations that accompany their relief through a
given autoerotic activity are identified with one's own body, the
body is recognized as the "me" and as that which yields the
pleasure, thus making it possible for the child to cathect it, and
bringing about primary narcissism.

The development of the self takes a long time and phenomena
related to it must be viewed according to the stage of its development. In fact, it could be said that the self is constantly being
modified all through life, even though its basic structure remains
more or less permanent after a certain point.

It will be clear that the libidinal gratifications at this stage of primary narcissism are autoerotic in character, just as they were in the previous phase of autoerotism. Nevertheless there are certain differences due to the level of organization that the mental apparatus has reached. The nature of their impingement on the mental apparatus differs from that of the previous phase of autoerotism, and so does their whole relationship to it. They have become psychologically significant in a way that they were not before.

Yet, in order to maintain this stage of primary narcissism the child is extremely dependent on the external environment. During these early phases of autoerotism and primary narcissism, the mother as the child's biological object performs for him a number of essential functions. She acts as a barrier against undesirable or excessive stimuli for the child and is the provider for all of his essential physical needs. She is the most important regulating factor in the constant struggle for the recovery, at least to a tolerable degree, of the homeostatic equilibrium which is forever disturbed by external and internal stimulation.

Furthermore, she provides for certain types of stimulation and forms of body contact which are required as an important contribution for the normal development of the child. They are essential elements, for example, in the development of the body image and of a healthy self at the appropriate time. Her role as the triggering and releasing agency of many other processes furthering drive and ego development must never be underestimated. With the increasing delineation and awareness of the child's "self" that has developed during the stage of primary narcissism, the mother becomes distinct from the self. From then onward an ever-growing psychological awareness of the existence of the mother and her essential functions develops, drawing to her larger and larger amounts of cathexis and interest.

Yet even in the best environments and with the very best mothering, the child inevitably must suffer frustrations, It is the frustrations which, according to Freud, force the next step in development and away from the phase of primary narcissism. Though frustrations are inherent in this phase, further development and maturation cannot proceed without the many ministrations of the mother.

Third Type

Gradually we have moved into the next phase in ego development which already allows for true object relationships. A relationship to an object though starting with the beginning of life is
at the very first established on a "need-satisfying basis." Out of this
primarily biological link with the external object will slowly
develop a psychological relationship through the agency of the
"ego." "Need satisfying" thus gives way in due time to "object
constancy," the relationship to the object growing more and more
complex and acquiring new facets and forms of expression as
development proceeds further (Hartmann 1952, Hoffer 1952, Anna
Freud 1952).

In any case at some point in the development of the mental
apparatus the role played by the autoerotic activities is again
modified and made more complex by the addition of a new
dimension provided by the development of the ego. This new
dimension is marked by the appearance of an object-related fantasy life which now attaches itself to the autoerotic activities.

For the special purposes of this chapter I shall choose an
example belonging to a state in development long after "psychological object relatedness" has been firmly established. The example is masturbation as it occurs in the phallic-oedipal phase or
later. When Freud speaks of the "choice of an object" during this
stage, he is of course referring to the choice of an object for the
satisfaction of the child's phallic strivings, coming to the foreground anywhere between two or three and five years of age. But
now the satisfaction takes place in fantasy. This can be considered
the forerunner of later stages in sexual development, where gratification of the sexual impulses in normal conditions requires a
partner to produce the release of tension.

Thus Freud said in the *Three Essays:* "It is in the world of ideas,
however, that the choice of an object is accomplished at first; and
the sexual life of maturing youth is almost entirely restricted to
indulging in phantasies, that is, in ideas that are not destined to be
carried into effect." In a footnote added in 1920, he continues:
"The phantasies of the pubertal period have as their starting-
point the infantile sexual researches that were abandoned in

childhood. No doubt, too, they are also present before the end of the latency period" (p. 225f.).

Freud considered a regression to the stage in development in which the object is still in the world of ideas important for the differential diagnosis between paraphrenic affections and the transference neurosis: "in the former, the libido that is liberated by frustration does not remain attached to objects in phantasy, but withdraws on to the ego" (1914, p. 86).

At the stage in development "in which the object is still in the world of ideas," the activites remain fundamentally autoerotic; they do not require the active participation of the object or its body (physically speaking), the gratification comes from one's own body. Yet in fantasy this autoerotic activity is object-directed. Masturbation at the phallic phase is generally still referred to as an autoerotic form of gratification which, on the one hand, is accompanied by fantasies that are object-directed, and on the other does not require the presence of the body of the object. In "Hysterical Phantasies and Their Relation to Bisexuality" (1908), Freud said: "At that time the masturbatory act (in the widest sense of the term) was compounded of two parts. One was the evocation of a phantasy and the other some active behaviour for obtaining self-gratification at the height of the phantasy. This compound, as we know, was itself merely soldered together. Originally the action was a purely auto-erotic procedure for the purpose of obtaining pleasure from some particular part of the body, which could be described as erotogenic. Later, this action became merged with a wishful idea from the sphere of object-love and served as a partial realization of the situation in which the phantasy culminated" (p. 161).

The transition from the second to the third stage is no doubt a very slow and gradual one and at this point can be referred to only in the vague terms I have so far used.

SUMMARY

Each one of the stages in the development of the ego and the self makes some contribution to the nature of the autoerotic phenomena, and they in turn play an important role in the development of the ego and self.

In the evaluation of autoerotic phenomena careful consideration should be given to the contribution of these different levels of integration and complexity and to the use made of them, first by the organism (biological being) and afterward by the ego (at the stage of the psychological being).

Though an autoerotic type of gratification can be forced onto the ego in certain situations of conflict or frustration at any time in life, it is also possible that in other cases the ego makes use of this type of phenomena for very constructive purposes. One is reminded here of persons who seem to be better able to concentrate, study, or work when at the same time they engage in some kind of autoerotic activity like curling of the hair, sucking their tongues, handling of the penis, etc.[4]

References

Abraham, K. (1924). A short study of the development of the libido. In *Selected Papers*. London: Hogarth Press, 1927.

Freud, A. (1952). The mutual influences in the development of the ego and the id: introduction to the discussion. *Psychoanalytic Study of the Child* 7:42-50.

—— (1962). Assessment of childhood disturbances. *Psychoanalytic Study of the Child* 17:149-158.

Freud, S. (1887-1902). *Origins of Psychoanalysis*. New York: Basic Books (pp. 115-116). From *Standard Edition* 1:173-280.

—— (1905). Three essays on the theory of sexuality. *Standard Edition* 7:125-248.

—— (1908); Hysterical phantasies and their relation to bisexuality. *Standard Edition* 9:157-166.

—— (1909). Analysis of a phobia in a five-year-old boy. *Standard Edition* 10:3-152.

—— (1910). Leonardo da Vinci and a memory of his childhood. *Standard Edition* 11:59-138.

---

4. Spitz and Wolf (1949) described observations of children in whom some specific autoerotic activites served the purpose of object relationship with their abnormal mothers.

——— (1911). Psycho-analytic notes on an autobiographical account of a case of paranoia (dementia paranoides). *Standard Edition* 12:3-84.

——— (1914). On narcissism: an introduction. *Standard Edition* 14:67-104.

——— (1915). Instincts and their vicissitudes. *Standard Edition* 14:111-140.

——— (1916-1917). Introductory lectures on psychoanalysis. *Standard Edition* 15/16:3-463.

——— (1923). The ego and the id. *Standard Edition* 19:3-68.

——— (1940). *An Outline of Psychoanalysis*. New York: Norton, 1949.

Hartmann, H. (1952). The mutual influences in the development of the ego and the id. *Psychoanalytic Study of the Child* 7:9-30.

Hoffer, W. (1952). The mutual influences in the development of the ego and the id. *Psychoanalytic Study of the Child* 7:31-41.

Spitz, R.A., and Wolf, K.M. (1946). The smiling response. *Genetic Psychology Monograph* 34.

——— (1949). Autoerotism; some empirical findings and hypotheses on three of its manifestations in the first year of life. *Psychoanalytic Study of the Child* 3/4:85-120.

Chapter Seven

INSIGHT IN CHILDREN AND ADULTS

The definition of insight in *Webster's New World Dictionary,* Second College Edition, is as follows: "1) the ability to see and understand clearly the inner nature of things, esp. by intuition. 2) a clear understanding of the inner nature of some specific thing. 3a) *Psychol.* awareness of one's own mental attitudes and behavior, b) Psychiatry. recognition of one's own mental disorders" (p. 729). The first three definitions with slight modifications are representative of the use of the term in psychoanalysis.

The term insight is frequently used as synonymous with understanding or knowledge; it is also used as a synonym of comprehension, of introspection, of a sudden realization or understanding, etc.

The value of insight in psychoanalysis is well established and has been discussed frequently. Richfield (1954) for example, says: "The criterion of whether a given form of psychotherapy is analytic has been made to rest upon the undoing of neurotic defenses through the achievement of insight, especially through the insight gained by the interpretation of resistances and derivative impulses expressed by the patient in his transference" (p. 390). More recently, at the Anna Freud Symposium in Detroit, November 1978, Blum, Neubauer, Anna Freud, and Hansi Kennedy have discussed extensively the question of insight and its implications for child and adult analysis.

129

Nevertheless, insight remains an obscure subject. The origin of the term itself is not easy to trace. Further, over the years it has acquired a variety of meanings. Sandler et al. (1973) believe that the term was borrowed from psychiatry. It is not without interest to point out that the term does not appear in the general index of the Standard Edition. Blum (1978) found the term in a passage of the *Interpretation of Dreams*. Personally I know only of a handful of occasions in which the term appears in Freud's work.

There are not only different degrees of insight, but many varieties of it. Thus, for example, we hear of deep, emotional, experiential, or psychological insight as a contrast to superficial, verbal, or intellectual insights. Richfield (1954) says about them: "If, for example, a person is aware that various psychological factors interfere with his social adjustments and the fulfillment of his capabilities, his recognition that he needs help in overcoming his adaptive limitations is considered to be a manifestation of insight. Such insight is helpful in diagnosis, classification, and prognosis, but it is considered to be of comparatively insignificant therapeutic importance. These insights are generally considered to be 'verbal' or 'intellectual' and to differ significantly from what has been termed genuine 'psychological' insights.

"'Psychological'" insights are said to consist of some understanding or appreciation of the motives and genesis of symptoms, but among this group of insights important differences are to be noted" (p. 392).

Of course there is as well the question of patient's insights vis-a-vis the therapist's insights. In both cases, but particularly in the latter, the meaning is frequently that of understanding. But the word itself has some kind of mystical connotation.

Reid and Finewsiger (1952) concluded that "any instance of insight necessarily entails some cognitive act by which the significance of a pattern of relations is grasped. Insight is said to be cognitive as distinguished from the conative or affective states which do not, as such, express inferences, make claims as to truths, or yield knowledge" (p. 396).

The same authors distinguish among three groups of insight, the intellectual, the emotional (with a subvariety), and the dynamic insight—they are defined as follows:

Intellectual insight. "By 'intellectual' insight is meant a cognition in which neither of the terms in the relation whose significance is grasped by the act of insight is an emotion. Since it is granted that any insight is by definition intellectual, this variety is called 'neutral.' The insight is neutral with respect to emotion" (p. 397).

The emotional insight. "This is said to be one in which some relevant emotion is a part of the subject matter grasped by the patient."

This type is to be distinguished from the type of insight that makes the patient conscious of some fact which then "cognitively mediates" an emotion. In other words, "an emotional response is released or set off by an insight which, unlike the first variety of emotional insights, need not itself be about an emotion" (p. 397).

The dynamic insight. In their opinion this is the "summum bonum of analysis." "Such insight is 'dynamic' in the systematic freudian sense of penetrating the repressive barrier and making the ego aware of certain hypercathected wishes that were previously unconscious" (p. 398).

It is said of it that it leads to therapeutic changes "through the 'economic' shifts brought about with their consequent alterations in the unconscious cathexes on 'thought-contents' at various levels of organization in the symbolic behavior of the patient" (p. 399).

Richfield (1952) proposes instead of the above the terms "descriptive insights" and "ostensive insights" with meanings similar to Russell's knowledge by description and knowledge by acquaintance.

Myerson (1960, 1963, 1065) introduced the concept of modes of insight implying not only the type of insight but the process that leads to it. Thus, in 1965 he referred to analytic insights and the reality oriented insights.

One other important problem that is not well understood is the very significant differences in the therapeutic results of the various forms of insight. Indeed, insights do not always lead to an improvement in the patient's condition; they may lead to a significant deterioration of it. The best example of this is that of the negative therapeutic reactions.

Kris (1956) described the "function of insight" as the end product of a multiplicity of combined ego functions. He addressed the following as essential:

1. An ego capacity for self-observation particulary reflective or critical self-observation
2. An ego capacity to control the discharge of affects
3. An ego capacity to tolerate unpleasant affects
4. An ego capacity for controlled ego regression
5. An ego capacity to utilize the synthetic and integrative capacity for the purposes of insight

In the same paper Kris (1956) added that in terms of insight there are enormous differences among individuals. "It is as if in every case the function of insight was differently determined, and its impact differently embedded in the balance of the personality" (p. 450).

THE REASONS FOR THE DIFFICULTIES OF ACQUIRING INSIGHT IN CHILDREN

At the Detroit Symposium Mrs. Kennedy (1978) described some of the reasons that in her opinion interfere or make it impossible for the child to acquire insight, particularly in children under four or five years of age. To those she discussed I have added others that seem to me relevant. The list that follows is valuable because we can immediately note that many such reasons very significantly influence the adult's capacity for insight, an aspect that will be discussed in detail later on in this chapter.

1. The child's inability to tolerate painful affects as well as his automatic tendency to avoid them. This includes children in the latency period.
2. Related to the above is his tendency to turn painful affects

into their opposites, e.g., sadness to joy, as often happens in the case of a parent's death.

3. Related too to the first two points is the fact that the small child's mental processes are governed by the pleasure principle. The change to the reality principle takes years and even then it remains for some time in an unstable condition when in the presence of significant conflicts or anxiety.

4. The child's limited capacity for reality testing (distinguishing his fantasies from reality) as well as his limitations in assessing and understanding external reality. Naturally, all this is very variable and depends on the age of the child. It is usually not much of a problem as latency advances.

5. The level of cognitive development at the various ages explains, among other things, the restricted capacity of the child to assess, understand, and process external reality. It also makes for a constrained capacity to understand the relations of cause and effect. In the small child that capacity is essentially nonexistent and it only develops very gradually. It is generally well established during the latency period but much more so toward the end than towards the beginning.

6. The specific characteristics of children's thought processes at certain ages. Small children's thinking is characterized by concretism, magic, and animism. The capacity for abstract thinking increases with age and is usually well established by latency though for some time there is some overlap between them. Furthermore, the capacity for abstract thinking can regress to concrete thinking as long as the former is not well established or under the influence of traumas, conflicts, and anxiety.

All this allows us to understand the little patient that Mrs. Kennedy (1978) refers to who says happily to her therapist, " 'Let's throw all the hurts out of the window' and proceeded to enact this with much satisfaction." Or the four-year-old Rose Mary when she suggests to the therapist that they ought to lock the monsters (of her fantasy) in the drawer "so they will starve and be dead."

7. The typical tendency of the young child toward action. For this reason, his impulses and affects are retranslated immediately, without a reflexive pause, into specific behaviors, such as an embrace, a kiss, a kick, spitting, etc.

8. The restricted ability of the child to tolerate frustrations, postpone gratifications, accept substitutes, and to sublimate. Progress in these areas is slow, but by latency all of them should be significantly present. Nevertheless, there is much variability as to the levels reached and in some cases observable deficits persist into adulthood.

9. In children, and more particularly so in the very young, the developmental processes take place simultaneously and multidimentionally. Thus, there is no real distance, no space among them in many cases. If we add their lack of concepts concerning time, such as before, now, after, or yesterday, today, tomorrow or in the past, the present, or the future we can understand that things are felt as compressed by the child. Given that in adult life the passage of time spaces events and experiences, and given that in analysis references to the past (and its roots) play such a significant role, we can see the difficulties that this introduces in the treatment of young children.

10. The limitations of language in the young child and the consequent restrictions in his capacity for verbalization. As the result of this, it is not easy for him to translate his needs, impulses, affects, wishes, and experiences into thoughts, and similarly to verbalize them. Thus, we can understand better not only his difficulties in "manifesting" insight but his difficulties in free associating as well.

11. The limited capacity for experiential, critical, sustained self-observation.

12. The egocentric tendencies of the child, particularly strong during the early stages.

13. The inability to regress in a controlled manner at the service of the ego.

14. The fact that for the child, many of his impulses and wishes are nonconflictual, though adults may consider them inappropriate given the child's age.

15. The child's need to use defense mechanisms such as displacement, negation, and externalization to deal with conflict and anxiety. This is true too of the latency period and can persist in a more moderate form during adolescence. By that time the tenden-

cy to externalize is replaced in good measure, due to the ego advances, by the rationalizations and intellectualizations typical for that stage.

16. The belief of the young child in the omnipotence and omniscience of the adults.

17. The lack or relative lack of motivation in many of them for treatment.

Most of the variables mentioned above result from the degree of ego development reached at various stages with its concomitant functional capacities. As time goes by and as the child grows and develops he progressively approximates the functional skills of the adult.

Mrs. Kennedy (1978) believes that once the latency period is reached the child is functionally capable (at least to a degree) of acquiring insight. I share her opinion. Yet, as she says, the special characteristics of development during this stage are such that the latency child has to vigorously oppose many of the processes that will make insight possible as well as the insight itself.

The adolescent is of course quite capable of insights but given some of the characteristics of the stage, he too—like the latency child—must fight against it.

Perhaps more important is the fact that all the variables mentioned for the child, where they are present for reasons of the stage of development, can also be seen in isolation or in various combinations in adult patients. This is due sometimes to specific ego deficits acquired during development that could not be mastered, and at other times because some functions get caught in conflictive situations that if unresolved satisfactorily will seriously interfere with such functions in the adult ego. It is these two sets of reasons that explain why many adult patients are as resistant to the acquisition of insights as children are, and in many cases for the very same or similar reasons. It is my opinion that the careful study of the variables or factors in development that interfere with the acquisition of insight in children will help clarify many of the difficulties in this regard that we frequently observe in our adult patients. Here then, we can see another important contribution of child analysis to the analysis of adults. As Kris (1956) said: "the complexity of ego functions which participate in the process of gaining and using insight may well account for the wide variations of the impact of insight on individual cases" (p. 453).

CLINICAL COMPARISONS
BETWEEN CHILDREN AND ADULTS

Mrs. Kennedy's paper (1978) and my own experience as an analyst for children and adults have convinced me that the study of the specific difficulties that interfere with the acquisition of insight in children lead us to find the prototypes of similar difficulties observed in our adult patients.

Thus, for example Kennedy (1978) while discussing some children's characteristics that of necessity interfere with their capacity to acquire insight says that, "Under the immediate impact of strong feelings the young child will be quite unable to reflect; and he will often need to be controlled." This is the reason why, as she points out, "The analyst's constant endeavor to put the child's wishes and feelings into words aims at channelling actions into thought and verbal expression." All the above is particularly true of children under five years of age since by latency the child is capable of exercising much better control in this regard.

A little reflection show us some of the parallels with adults. The adult too, under the impact of strong emotions cannot function efficiently in analysis, and it is for this reason that in patients undergoing "emotional crises" of various types analysis may not be indicated for as long as it is present. In those patients already in treatment such crises may and frequently do become a temporary disruption for the analytic process. One reason for this is that the capacity for reflective or critical self-observation may be lost temporarily, absorbed as the patient is by the crisis itself. Obviously, in such circumstances the capacity for insight is highly compromised.

One other parallel that can be established is the one with the tendency of many adult patients for acting out. Naturally, the sources for acting out are many and variable; but in many cases they are related to immaturities or deficits of the adult ego that are for the child perfectly normal and the reason for his behavior. I am referring here to the imperative character of his drives and the limited controls he can exercise over them, his low frustration tolerance, his poor capacity to accept substitutes and to use sublimation.

But it is precisely all these variables that favor the tendency to act out in those adults that retain such characteristics. The tendency to act out is one of the greatest enemies to the capacity for insight both in children and adults.

Let us now consider the child's capacity for self-observation. Unquestionably, it is present in children three, four, and five years of age though it may differ somewhat from that of the adult. The child can certainly tell us his feelings, but in contrast with the adult he cannot do so in the sustained, consistent, and controlled form of the latter. He does it in the form of short-lived sudden flashes and eruptions. But the child up to the age of four or five is much more in contact with his needs, feelings, wishes, and impulses than the latency child, the adolescent, or the adult. He is not only more in touch with them but communicates them readily. He tells us how much in love he is with his mother, or how he hates his father, or how he would like his younger sibling to be sent back, etc. We can understand this ease in communication between his ego and his id, if we consider that his super-ego is still not fully structured and functional and consequently somewhat tolerant of these impulses. It is possible too that such behavior is due to the combination of the imperative nature of his impulses and limited superego structuralization.

What the child of this age certainly lacks is the capacity for self-observation in a reflective, critical, and sustained manner.

But, are children of this age incapable of insight? I do not think so, though it manifests itself in a different way and has imposed on its form of expression the limitations resulting from the degree of ego development and all those functional characteristics (such as fleeing from pain, etc) that are so well described in Mrs. Kennedy's paper.

There is no doubt that the latency child and the adolescent not only possess the capacity for self-observation but that they can do it in a reflective and critical manner. Nevertheless, the developmental characteristics of these two stages are such that not infrequently they are forced to fight this function and the acquisition of insight.

Self-observation, especially reflective self-observation, is one among many ego functions involved in the acquisition of insight, a fact well established by Kris (1956). It is perhaps the only one that has been studied in some depth, for example by Hatcher (1973) in his paper "Insight and Self-observation." More efforts in this direction will help clarify some of the existent confusion.

If we consider briefly the adult situation in this regard we know that the capacity for reflective, critical self-observation is one positive indicator for analyzability. We know as well that when this function is damaged either by primary reasons (ego deficits, marginal intelligence, etc.) or by secondary reasons (type of conflicts and defenses, etc.), treatment progress would be compromised due to the constrictions that such factors impose on the acquisition of insight.

Another variable already mentioned is the normal child's tendency to actively avoid conflictual and painful situations and the universal tendency to externalize and negate such events. All analysts are well aware of many adult patients who retain these characteristics and behave, both in life and in the analytical situation, in a similar fashion. It seems as if such patients have a fixation to these stages, a fixation that favours the utilization of these mechanisms well past the developmental stage where they are legitimate and normal. In such patients, sooner or later we come across the conflicts, traumas, and events that in the genetic sense explain this abnormal tendency. Of course, we all know the difficulties that the excessive use of externalization can create in terms of the acquisition of insight.

Mrs. Kennedy (1978) makes reference to the fact that if the conceptual skills of the child remain tied to magical thinking both the treatment process and the capacity for insight are influenced by it. She mentions for example a little girl, six years old, who says about her therapist: "If he was really clever he would do magic."

We are thus reminded of the type of adult patient who expects the therapist to improve or cure them "magically," angrily rejecting every effort he makes to have the patient observe himself, free associate, or make use of the interpretations. These are patients that will wait indefinitely for the therapist's "magic" and do not wish to work or suffer in order to resolve their emotional difficulties.

The same happens in the case of the child's belief in the omnipotence of adults. Thus, our inability to make things better quickly, to reduce the conflicts and anxieties, as well as our inability to gratify many of his needs, is erroneously interpreted, as Mrs. Kennedy (1978) remarks. To him, we simply do not want to help, with the consequent aggressive and hostile reaction. Of course, this is true too of those adults who have retained such a belief and thus add themselves to the number of patients that expect to be cured by "magic" means.

Other child patients are incapable of talking during the sessions for some time because they feel extremely anxious, guilty, or ashamed. This leads to a conscious withholding of information or a deliberate distortion of the facts for varying periods of time. It is my opinion that no adult analyst can avoid a déjà vu experience in relation to all the above.

Now, let us look for a while at the role that egocentrism plays in children. We know that it is very marked up to the age of four or five. During this time every event is interpreted in reference to the child's ego. Such a tendency diminishes gradually after this age but is still present to a lesser degree up to the age of ten or eleven. A more or less important remnant of this is retained into adulthood where it attaches itself to the narcissistic elements present in any given personality whether normal or pathological. In some cases the persisting egocentric component is significant and as such influences the type of personality, its pathology, the capacity for insight, and even the prognosis of the patient.

This egocentrism is a highly distorting factor that among other things interferes with understanding causality (cause and effect) and with the capacity to evaluate objectively external reality. Naturally, failures in this regard are an important obstacle to the acquisition of "genuine insights." Genuine insights differ from "false insights"—those connections patients make, either spontaneously or after an interpretation by the therapist for defensive purposes. In other words, the patient's intention is to avoid genuine or significant insights. In this way they distort the aims and contexts of the interpretation, and manage to establish a number of false connections which are aimed at reconstructing, in the genetic sense, a concatentation of events by means of which they try to explain and justify their behavior, their symptoms and psychopathology, etc. Typically, these false reconstructions and the subsequent false insights are designed to absolve the patient from all responsibility, mostly through massive externalizations, where the "guilt" is placed on environmental factors or on the human objects of that environment.

The therapist is in fact surprised by the patient's persistence in this behavior as well as by his reaction when the therapist tries to point out his error, what he is actually doing and the reasons for it. This reaction is one of rage and hostility coupled with accusations that the therapist is incompetent, stupid, or incapable of understanding the patient. Such a situation can be observed in various degrees of malignancy in patients with a variety of narcissistic problems where the idea of the self as perfect must be maintained at any prize. This is true of some borderline patients with narcissistic problems, and even of some neurotic patients with a large narcissistic component, but in this latter case the patient's reaction is not as malignant and he responds to the appropriate interpretations.

Let us look now at the limited capacity of children for regression at the service of the ego, something that we require of adults during psychoanalytic treatment. Such regressions seem contrary to the basic purpose of development during childhood, since the trend is to leave behind, bury, and master wishes, needs, gratifications, and behaviors that become inappropriate as the child moves forward in his development. It is frequently said for this reason that at this age and in some ways analysis runs contrary to the developmental tendencies. To this we must add that the child's ego control over his impulses is precarious, particularly where it has been acquired recently. The ego fears any regressive tendency, feeling uncertain of its capacity to remain in control. This state of affairs, typical for children, applies to some adult patients with specific ego deficits, a situation that makes them fearful of losing control over their impulses in general. In another kind of case, the ego fear is more specific and related to certain conflictual areas where ego control is maintained only at great expense. Naturally, when the analysis approaches such areas the ego strongly opposes the regressive tendency out of its fear of losing control.

Frequently, with children (and some adults) we can observe—either spontaneously through the regression or as the result of inappropriate content interpretations—a breakthrough of instinctual impulses, a sudden onrush of frightening phantasies with a total, or near total disruption of the ego.

If this happens frequently, the child may run away from his session in a marked state of excitation, even a panic, or in a more controlled manner by asking the therapist permission to go to the toilet, etc. The adult patient may stop treatment on the basis of various excuses and rationalizations, or more dramatically, in a kind of phobic state about the treatment and/or the therapist. In this group are included borderline patients with ego deficits, in whom certain types of content interpretations produce a paradoxical negative reaction. That is, the interpretations do not reduce the nature of the conflict or the anxiety present, but have the effect of a seductive action and as such increase anxiety at times to traumatic proportions. It is this that explains the phobic reactions produced by some patients. Of course, this is more acutely experienced in the case of children given the limited abilities to control strong affects and impulses and given the demanding imperative quality of their needs. As Mrs. Kennedy (1978) says: "Under the immediate impact of strong feelings the young child will be quite unable to reflect; and he will often need to be controlled."

One important difference between children (especially the small child) and adults is that in the former many of his needs, impulses, and wishes are nonconflictual. The adult world may take objection to them either because of the age of the child or because of educational demands that are considered necessary. Obviously, this makes it more difficult to generate insight. But even in this area we notice some similarities with the adult. I am referring here to those patients where a given instinctual impulse or group of them are ego syntonic. Thus, the ego and superego attitudes toward them do not favor the process of insight in their regard. Certain types of perversions are typical examples of what I have in mind.

One other basic difference between children and adults concerns the area of motivation whose importance can hardly be overestimated. By contrast with adults, many children are poorly motivated. This is partly due to the fact that many children's symptoms are ego syntonic and as such may disturb other people but not the child himself. But more important still is that the child's situation is covered by a protective shield.

Thus for example, if the child's symptoms interfere with his ability to work and adjust at the school, the teachers and parents may become concerned but there are no direct, immediate consequences for him. In sharp contrast, if the symptoms of an adult lead to an interference with his capacity to work, the consequences are enormous and immediate. Given that this is the way he supports himself and his family, we can understand the significant disruption that takes place automatically. We can understand too why there is such a marked difference in motivations.

Here we can consider Mrs. Kennedy's example (1978) where the child remarks to his therapist: "You will think that I did this because of such and such a reason but you are wrong, I did it because of this, that or the other, etc." This type of phenomenon commonly occurs in the treatment of adults. The same is true of those interpretations that are actively refused or simply ignored and where nevertheless the subsequent analytic material shows meaningful changes or where even symptomatic and behavioral changes may be observable; or those children where the need to comply is so prominent that they accept interpretations without any understanding; or those small patients that refuse to speak about specific subjects during the sessions because they would be reminded of painful events that they want to avoid; or those children during the latency period or adolescence that identify with the analysing function of the therapist but only in order to apply it to others; or the children's preference for external solutions that alter the world or the objects in it (making everything pleasant) to the internal and most painful solutions; or finally the special difficulties that the handling of the transference poses in some cases. But none of this fails to bring to the analyst's mind innumerable similar examples from his adult patients. All this leads me to the conclusion that the differences between children and adults in terms of the forces or resistances that oppose the phenomenon of insight are at best minimal and possibly nonexistent. The only difference is that the child is entitled to these reactions as a developmental right, a right to which the adult is no longer entitled. One has the definite impression that some among the multiplicity of reasons that can interfere with the manifestation of insight in children prolong themselves into adulthood in one area or another and in various combinations according to the vicissitudes of each individual's development. And this is so in spite of the fact that many of the ego deficits observable in the child (related to the stage of development) have been superseded in the adult.

We cannot but be surprised at the great complexity of the processes that lead to the acquisition of insight, the large number of variables that are involved in it and in consequence, the ease with which the process can be disrupted or stopped.

Of course, in children many of these factors or variables are active simultaneously and may become cumulative in their effects, thus blocking the possibility of the child's production of insights similar to those of the adult in ideal conditions. In adults it is generally one or another of these various factors that interfere with the process but rarely all of them acting simultaneously.

The situation is further complicated because we take as the definitional model of the insight the phenomenon that becomes manifest in the adult under ideal conditions. This adult form we apply to the child, concluding that the child is not capable of insights. It is my opinion that the child does produce insights, but that they are quite different from the ones observable in the adult. The difference consists in two things: on the one hand, in the child's case the experience cannot be verbalized and certainly not with the adornments and elaborations that some gifted adults produce; on the other hand, all the many factors already mentioned are strongly opposed to the contents of the insight becoming conscious. If that is so why do we expect children to verbalize their insights, and why do we conclude from their inability to do so that the child, especially the latency child, is not capable of producing insights? It seems to me more logic to conclude, given that the processes that lead to insights and the consequences of it are observable in children, that the child produces insights but that they have their own characteristics and references and are naturally different from those of the adult.

As Anna Freud (1978) says: "With children the bulk of their resistance, or at worst their total unwillingness to be analyzed thus stems from their ego's age-adequate preference for clinging to its own methods for safeguarding or re-instating well-being and for their inclination to reject all others. Analytic insight belongs to the latter category, and it taxes the therapist's technical skill and ingenuity to lead his patients towards accepting it."

THE ROLE OF THE PRECONSCIOUS EGO IN THE ACQUISITION OF INSIGHT

The acquisition of insight is an ego function. It results from ego activities that combine in various ways a multiplicity of its functions to achieve this aim.

Our actual knowledge of these functions is poor; this is particularly true of the organizational levels reached at the various ages and in the early stages of development. This applies too, to the synthetic and integrative functions of the ego that play such an important role in the production and acquisition of insight. We can only be certain that the degree of structuralization reached in the young child is limited, a fact which of course influences and determines his functional capacities.

It would be very helpful from the structural point of view if we could determine which contributions are made to the process of insight by the unconscious ego, the preconscious ego, and the conscious ego. It is my opinion that the greatest contribution to the phenomenon under consideration comes from the preconscious ego. I am referring here to the processes that lead to the insight and not to the end product, the insight itself in terms of the contents that finally reach and define themselves in the conscious ego. I believe with Kris (1956, p. 447) that "some and perhaps all significant intellectual achievements are products or at least derivatives of preconscious mentation" (see also Kris 1950). If we accept this proposition and the need to differentiate between the process and the end product, we must accept too that our present knowledge of the functioning of the preconscious ego is in general very limited but even more so in the case of young children. Thus, it would be valid to ask at what point or at what age the preconscious ego acquires the functional characteristics typical of the later stages. Could it not be the lack of certain functional capacities of the preconscious ego (and to some degree of the conscious ego) that determine the child's inability to acquire insights of the adult type during the first three, four, or five years of his life?

Yet, if this is true, how can we explain the enormous successes that frequently follow the treatment of children in this age group? Possibly, the best answer is to be found in the last paragraph of Mrs. Kennedy's paper: "The analyst's interventions organize and articulate what the child is experiencing. Whenever the analyst interprets and expresses 'his insights' in terms that the child is capable of understanding, some new integration will take place. . . . The need to be compliant, the wish to please the therapist and to get approval, will help reinforce a wish for understanding and this will ultimately contribute to treatment outcome." Of course, she applies the above to children in general, while to me it seems particularly relevant for children under three or four years of age. The factors she mentions, along with a few more that I will ignore here, are the ones that may explain the therapeutic success. But on the other hand we must note that her statement applies in its entirety to the adult situation as well. This perhaps helps us understand the significant improvements that we frequently observe in adult patients who cannot be characterized by their capacity to acquire insight.

It is essential to distinguish the actual occurrence of insights from their outward manifestation. It is the latter that analysts seem to have chosen as their paradigm. For this reason the external manifestations of insights (verbalizations for example) have been given undue weight at the expense of the very substance of the phenomenon that takes place internally and silently.

By the time the child is four or five years of age the general tendency seems to be to assume that the activities of the preconscious ego are representative of the later stages, though somewhat limited still by the ego characteristics of the stage.

Once we have accepted that insight may be the product of preconscious mentation, it is appropriate to inquire about the basis of the difficulty latency children have in manifesting insights on the adult model.

I think it possible and perhaps even necessary to postulate that the difficulty, at least in part, consists in raising the end product (the actual contents of the process of insight, the insight itself) to conscious ego levels. In other words it seems that the preconscious ego of the latency child is basically capable of all the functions (though with some limitations) that in the adult lead to insights. Nevertheless, for some reason the actual contents of the insight rarely if ever reach the conscious ego. Could this perhaps be the difference between the latency child's and the adult's capacity to produce insights? If this were so, the reason the latency child cannot verbalize or communicate insight to the therapist is that it does not reach consciousness. We have already seen many of the reasons that could, either by themselves or combined in various ways, explain why the work of the preconscious ego cannot reach a conscious level in the child or even why he actively opposes the presence of such contents in consciousness.

Earlier, I stated that it seemed possible to me and perhaps even necessary to postulate that the difficulty in the latency child consists in his inability to raise the relevant preconscious contents of the insight into consciousness. Two important clinical arguments or reasons support this thesis. The first one is that though the child cannot make insight manifest in the way adults do, the outcome of our interpretations, even when actively rejected by the child, is often a significant change: an improvement, a modification, or even an erradication of symptoms; and a correction or a lifting of ego restrictions; and no less important, a restoration of the normal processes of development.

The second reason comes from our experience with adults. Though it is generally true that adult patients with limited capacity for insight usually carry a more conservative treatment prognosis, all analysts are familiar with exceptions to this rule. There are patients in whom the conscious manifestations or expressions of insights are very transitory, minimal, or nonexistent, that nevertheless improve markedly. (I mean here those patients where the actual changes are legitimate and the result of the interpretative work, but I am excluding those cases where the improvement is a transference phenomenon or due to the patient's excessive utilization of the multiplicity of noninterpretative elements that form part of the analytic procedure whether we like it or not, such as corrective emotional experiences, support, etc.)

Kris (1956), referring to the various degrees of consciousness reached by the insight said: "Interpretations naturally need not lead to insight; much or most of analytic therapy is carried out in darkness, with here and there a flash of insight to lighten the path. A connection has been established, but before insight has reached awareness (or, if it does, only for flickering moments), new areas of anxiety and conflict emerge, new material comes, and the process drives on: thus far-reaching changes may and must be achieved, without the pathway by which they have come about becoming part of the patient's awareness" (p. 452).

All the above may suggest that insight as defined for the adult (reaching consciousness and verbalization) is a process with two stages. The first stage takes place in the preconscious ego (and as such is unconscious). This is applicable not only to the process that of necessity is always unconscious but to the contents of the end product, the insight itself. In a second stage (that may or may not follow the first one automatically) that content is raised into consciousness.[1] The latter is characteristic for many adult in-

1. Here Freud's concept of another type of censorship (with a different function) between the preconscious and the conscious ego suggests itself.

sights, but not so for children. But as we have noted the large majority of adult insights do not reach consciousness, though they contribute in a very positive way to the treatment progress, reduce conflict and anxiety, etc. Suddenly we now face a contradiction in the definition of insight (in the sense of it being conscious), something similar to what happens in the case of the unconscious sense of guilt. Nevertheless, such a contradiction is in itself no argument against the reality of the mechanisms involved; it only means that the term chosen to describe the process is unfortunately quite inadequate.

Another important consideration follows naturally from the above: there are qualitative differences between various types of insight, particularly between insight that reach consciousness and those that remain unconscious in the dynamic sense. This is so much so that at present, rightly or wrongly, the non plus ultra among insights is the one in which consciousness partakes fully. This is the ideal of the psychoanalytic and dynamic therapies, at least at this point.

INSIGHT AS A NEGATIVE FACTOR

Up to this point we have mostly considered the positive value ascribed to the insight in the analytic and dynamic therapies. Yet, there are exceptions to this rule. The prototype here is the negative therapeutic reactions where the response to interpretations producing insight is not, as we would expect, a diminution of anxiety, shame, or guilt, or a step toward symptomatic improvement, but just the contrary. Instead of improving, the condition of the patient worsens and deteriorates markedly, a response that repeats itself with every new acquisition of genuine insights.

Genuine insights, false insights or pseudoinsights can be and frequently are used by patients as a resistance, as a defense mechanism, with very detrimental results for the treatment.

Kris (1956) has described this in detail. Thus for example, he refers to patients who are inclined to accept all the analyst's interpretations and "insights" about the patient. In these patients, the integrative function is in itself operative, but not in an autonomous form. In fact, its aim is to win the analyst's praise, or love, or a "fusion" with him/her. In other words, it is not only that the aim of insight is sexualized, but that the process itself is sexualized. In some cases, primitive phantasies hide behind this fusion. The danger of this type of insight, as Kris (1956) points out, is that it does not last beyond the period of the positive transference.

Other patients produce genuine insights with the sole aim of replacing the analyst and his function. These patients frequently have conflicts around the polarity activity-passivity, or severe passive-homosexual longings where the therapist's interpretations are felt as an intrusion, in fact "a penetration." The latter must either be actively rejected, or the patient must produce his own interpretations and/or insights, thus avoiding the "penetration." Still other patients will behave in a very similar fashion when they are riddled by conflicts around competition or conflicts with their aggresion that are never expressed directly, but only by means of an intellectual contest where they try to beat their adversaries.

We referred earlier to tht type of patient that distorts the interpretations of the analyst, recombining its elements to produce his own "insight" or rather false insight. Externally this false insight may be accompanied by all the qualitative characteristics of the genuine insight including the classical "aha!" Naturally, this patient is endeavoring to avoid the genuine insight that for one reason or another represents a serious danger to him. Many such cases are severe in nature and frequently borderlines. These false insight are sometimes so intense that they acquire many of the characteristics of a delusional idea or an organized delusion. When this is the case, treatment reaches a dead end. Every effort of the analyst to find a solution to the impasse lead to a paradoxical response. One is looked at as dull, with no empathic capacity, unintelligent and as such not able to understand the patient and his problems. In the end, when it is no longer possible to keep control over the situation the patient abandons the treatment in rage and frustration. Frequently, this type of patient will reenter treatment with another therapist. All seems well up to the point where the central conflicts are again approached. At that point, the cycle repeats itself so that this type of patient would have been in treatment with three, four, or more therapists at different times during his life.

There is the case too of the "brilliant" patient capable of producing "magnificent insights" that manages to seduce the analyst, who in turn rewards the patient with his own "magnificent insights." The treatment then becomes what can only be described as an "orgy of insights." Such situations are a massive exercise in intellectualization that in reality do not lead anywhere. Analysts who conduct second analysis may once in a while come across what I have described. What is surprising is that the patient has vivid recollections of many of his insights, that were genuine enough in terms of contents, and yet the symptoms, behaviors, character, and inhibitions present were not modified at all. This shows that though the insights may have been genuine in terms of the contents they were not experiential but intellectual in character. As you will expect, this patient will try to reestablish the "orgy" of his first analysis with the second analyst. If the latter is not seduced and confronts the patient with the defensive character of his behavior, the patient feels humiliated, becomes enfuriated, and complains that we cannot understand, or are stupid and lacking in talents. This type of resistance must be thoroughly dealt with before the analysis can proceed on its normal course.

The experience of patients in their second analysis frequently highlights the tendency to forget or repress the insights that resulted from the first analysis. On occasion this is so marked that the second analyst may well wonder what became of the first four or five years of analysis. Nevertheless, as the reanalysis progresses the patient can and does recover many of the original insights. I wish only to add that children too tend to forget, at times completely, the contents of the treatment as time goes by. But here too we observe a great similarity with many adults.

As Kris (1956) says: "It seems that insight with some individuals remains only a transient experience, one to be obliterated again in the course of life by one of the defenses they are wont to use" (p. 453).

References

Blum, H.P. (1978). Insightful development and creative insight. Unpublished paper presented at the Anna Freud Symposium, Detroit, November.
Freud, A. (1978). The role of insight in psychoanalysis and psychotherapy. Unpublished paper presented at the Anna Freud Symposium, Detroit, November.
Freud, S. (1900). The interpretation of dreams. *Standard Edition* 4/5:1-63.
Hatcher, R.L. (1973). Insight and self-observation. *Journal of the American Psycho-Analytical Association* 21:377-398.
Kennedy, H. (1978). Some thoughts on the role of insight in child analysis. Unpublished paper presented at the Anna Freud Symposium, Detroit, November.
Kris, E. (1950). On preconcions mental processes. *Psychoanalytic Quarterly* 19. 540-560. Reprinted in *Psychoanalytic Explorations in Art.* 303-320 New York: International Universities Press.
Kris, E. (1956). On some vicissitudes of insight in psychoanalysis. *International Journal of Psycho-Analysis* 37:445-455.
Myerson, P. (1960). Awareness and stress: post-psycho-analytic utilization of insight. *International Journal of Psycho-Analysis* 37:445-455.
Neubauer, P. (1978). The role of insight in psychoanalysis. Unpublished paper presented at the Anna Freud Symposium, Detroit, November.
Reid, J.R. and Finensiger, J.E. (1952). The role of insight in psychotherapy. *American Journal of Psychiatry* 108:726-734.
Richfield, J. (1954). An analysis of the concept of insight. *Psychoanalytic Quarterly* 23:390-408.
Russell, B. (1912). *Problems of Philosophy.* New York: Henry Holt and Co.

Part II

DEVELOPMENTAL CONSIDERATIONS: EGO APPARATUS AND STRUCTURE FORMATION

Chapter Eight

THE EGO APPARATUS: CONSIDERATIONS CONCERNING THE SOMATIC ROOTS OF THE EGO

THE TERMS APPARATUS AND EGO APPARATUS

The term *apparatus* is frequently encountered in psychoanalytic literature. It is used in a variety of ways, usually forming compounds such as the mental apparatuses of the mind, ego apparatuses, etc. As is indicated in chapter 9, it was Hartmann who, in 1939, introduced the term "ego apparatus," though Hartmann as well as others, especially Rapaport, have used "apparatus" interchangeably with "structure." In the same publication, Hartmann stated that the further development of "inborn ego apparatuses" takes place, to some extent, in what he called the "conflict-free sphere of the ego." He said:

The newborn infant is not wholly a creature of drives; he has inborn apparatuses (perceptual and protective mechanisms) which appropriately perform a part of those functions which, after the differentiation of ego and id, we attribute to the ego [p.49]. The human individual, at his birth, also has apparatuses, which serve to master the external world. These mature in the course of development [p. 50]. We know that maturation processes are not entirely impervious to environmental influences. Yet they are independent factors which, both before and after birth, bring the inborn apparatuses successively into play, and determine at least grossly the rhythm of developmental processes. [p. 104]

[Later, in 1952, he stated:] Generally speaking, the apparatus serving perception, motility, and others that underlie ego functions, seem, in the infant, to be activated by instinctual needs.... But they are not created by the needs. These apparatus, as well as those that account for the phenomena of memory, are partly inborn; they cannot be traced, in the individual, to the influence of the instincts and of reality, and their maturation follows certain laws which are also part of our inheritance. They will gradually come under the control of the ego; on the other hand, they act on the ego and its subsequent phases of development. [p. 167]

According to Hartmann, the inborn ego apparatuses include perception, laying down of memory traces, motility, thinking, and consciousness.[1]

Hartmann (1939) clarified the relationship between ego apparatuses and adaptation when he stated that "adaptation (speaking now mainly about man) is guaranteed, in both its grosser and finer aspects, on the one hand by man's primary equipment and the maturation of his apparatuses, and on the other hand by those ego-regulated actions which (using this equipment) counteract the disturbances in, and actively improve the person's relationship to, the environment" (p. 25), adding that the "psychoanalytic study of those primary disorders of ego apparatuses which result in failures of adaptation has barely begun" (p. 39f.).

Hartmann further maintained that ego development and drive development are partly based on somatic maturational processes.

Let us consider first the somatic processes of maturation: just as the phases of libido development depend upon somatic maturation

---

1. With regard to the system of consciousness Gill (1963) stated: "In present-day terminology, *Cs.* would be described as a primarily autonomous ego apparatus, as are the apparatuses of perception and motility" (p. 66). On the basis of the observation that *Cs.* can be stimulated in abnormal conditions and during sleep, for example, by contents invested with drive energy and organized according to primary process, Gill adds the interesting comment that "In a sense, then, we may say that these apparatuses belong not to the ego but to the entire psychic apparatus, even though they are usually under the control of the ego" (p. 66).

processes (for instance, the anal-sadistic phase develops "obviously in connection with the cutting of the teeth, the strengthening of the musculature, and the control of the sphincters" [Freud 1932, p. 135]), so ego development too is connected with the somatic maturation of certain apparatuses [p. 46 f.]. [He wondered] whether or not the defense processes are influenced by the maturation and exercise of the apparatuses of the conflict-free ego sphere. . . . It is possible that the developmental rhythm of these apparatuses is one of the determinants of the sequence in which defense methods arise. [p. 106]

Furthermore, Hartmann saw ego development as a complicated process of differentiation in which primitive regulating factors are increasingly replaced by more effective ego regulations: "Differentiation progresses not only *by the creation of new apparatuses to master new demands and new tasks, but also and mainly by new apparatuses taking over*, on a higher level, functions which were originally performed by more primitive means (p. 50; my italics). He also thought that the study of the disorders of automatized actions due to organic brain disease would, for example, "give us important information about the function of the somatic apparatuses involved in action, while we learn about the function of the mental apparatuses involved from developmental psychology and from psychoanalysis (particularly of psychotics)" (p. 88).

The closest Hartmann came to defining his concept of mental apparatus is in the following statement (1939): "'Mental apparatus' is a particularly fitting description of the preconscious automatisms (and not only of those which pertain to action); however, since it implies structure and formedness, as all concepts of apparatuses do, it is hardly applicable to what is occasionally termed the automatic character of the id" (p. 100). He remarked that little attention had been devoted to the study of somatic and mental apparatuses, stating that:

If we take the conflict-free ego sphere into consideration and if we want to develop a general psychology of action, the study of these apparatuses becomes imperative, because otherwise all our statements about action include an unknown.

[He made it quite clear] that the apparatuses, both congenital and

acquired, need a driving force in order to function; and that the
psychology of action is inconceivable without the psychology of
instinctual drives [pp. 100 f.]. [The] psychology of the ego apparatuses seems to me a good example of the interlocking of conflict and
adaptation (and achievement). . . . [p. 107]

He insisted (1939), following Freud (1937), on the crucial role
that hereditary factors play in the ego's constitution and apparatuses. Thus he says: "Let us now return to the inherited ego
characteristics in general" (p. 105). Similarly, in "Psychoanalysis
as a Scientific Theory" (1959), he points out that "It is likely that in
man not only instinctual factors are in part determined by heredity, but also the apparatus of the ego underlying the functions just
mentioned" (p. 329).

At times it is not clear whether Hartmann means to include
"physical apparatuses" as an integral part of the ego organization.
Some of the statements to be found in his monograph (1939) seem
to point in that direction, for example: "The functions of all the
mental and physical ego apparatuses mentioned can become
secondarily sources of pleasure" (p. 46; italics mine). A similarly
ambiguous statement is the following: "The use of a term is after
all a matter of definition; the term 'automatism' here is applied
only to *the somatic and preconscious ego apparatuses . . .* " (p. 90;
italics mine). At other times he clearly specifies that the somatic
apparatuses are used by the ego, thus implying that they are
outside the ego organization. He says, for example: "The ego uses
somatic apparatuses to execute actions. I will discuss first the
motor apparatuses . . . " (p. 87), and on p. 100: "In action the ego
uses both somatic and mental apparatuses." Or: "The individual
does not acquire all the apparatuses which are put in *the service of
the ego* in the course of development: perception, motility, intelligence, etc., rest on constitutional givens" (p. 101; italics mine).
But the question remains: are these somatic and mental apparatuses an integral part of the ego organization or are they outside of
it and only used by the ego organization when appropriate?

Further, Hartmann (1939) has used the term apparatus in referring not only to ego apparatuses in general or to the inborn ego
apparatuses in particular (p. 49f.) but also to physical (p. 100) or

somatic ego apparatuses (pp. 87 and 90), mental ego apparatuses (p. 100f.), congenital ego apparatuses, acquired ego apparatuses (p. 101), and inherited ego apparatuses (p. 105), etc. Further, he quotes (p. 100) Bleuler who coined the term "occasional apparatus" to explain the process of abreaction.

Although questions such as those raised above are occasionally a source of contention and argument in analytic discussions, they seem to me to be more rhetorical than of fundamental significance. There are advantages in considering the ego in purely psychological terms and in viewing it as being in charge of the control and organization of the multiplicity of functions of which humans are capable. There is also no reason not to consider all the somatic apparatuses whose functions finally come under the ego's control and are placed at its service as outside the ego organization properly speaking. The ego remains a psychological agency that uses, organizes, and controls all the functions that these apparatuses can perform according to specific sets of rules and regulations that take into account the demands of the other agencies (id and superego) as well as those of external reality. But the decision to define the ego in these terms must not obscure the fact that the qualities, abilities, and functional capabilities of any particular ego are nevertheless determined to a large extent by the basic nature, quality, and intrinsic characteristics of all those physical organs that lie at its root. Obviously, no ego organization could exist were it not for the functions that can be performed by these underlying somatic organs or structures. It is equally obvious that because of this dependent relationship the damage to any of these somatic apparatuses (i.e., the organs of vision or of other brain structures, etc.) leads to atypical and deviant ego organizations. Hartmann (1952) stated that: "In the ego's relationship with the body, we can now describe three aspects: the postulated physiological processes underlying activities of the ego; those somatic apparatus that gradually come under the control of the ego and which in turn influence the timing, intensity, and direction of ego development; and, third, but not necessarily independent of the two others, those special structures that underlie what we call the body ego" (p. 169).

Although I have singled out a few ambiguous quotations from Hartmann's *Ego Psychology and the Problem of Adaptation,* it is clear to me that the study of Hartmann's work shows beyond doubt that his conception of the ego is in line with Freud's formulations and that the ambiguity referred to results only from the difficulties inherent in the attempt to show the dependent relations between the ego agencies (as a psychological construct) and the somatic structures that underlie them.

Brenner and Arlow in their monograph *Psychoanalytic Concepts and the Structural Theory* (1964) showed a marked predilection for conceptualizations in terms of functions. Thus, they rarely use the term ego apparatus and instead usually refer to ego functions. These authors use the term apparatus primarily in expressions such as psychic apparatus, mental apparatus, or apparatuses of the mind, etc. Thus, for example, they say: "According to the structural theory, those mental functions which are called the ego, which normally form a coherent and integrated whole, . . . develop from the apparatuses of the mind which have to do with an individual's response to the world about him. Thus the ego may be characterized in either of two ways. (1) It may be defined as a group of functions of the mind which are usually associated with one another in situations of mental conflict; or (2) it may be defined as the group of mental functions which in one way or another have to do with mediating between the demands of the id and those of the outer world" (p. 41).[2]

The terms apparatus or ego apparatus also do not appear in the index of Fenichel's *The Psychoanalytic Theory of Neurosis* (1945). An examination of the text shows a similar absence of the concept of ego apparatus in Hartmann's sense, though occasionally Fenichel employed the term apparatus in expressions such as "It [the ego] operates as an inhibiting apparatus" (p. 16), or "The mental functions represent a progressively more complicated apparatus for the mastery of stimuli" (p. 34).

---

2. The argument here seems to me to be weakened by the fact that the authors fail to specify what they mean by apparatuses of the mind and that they do not define their use of "mind" as a concept and its relation to the concept of ego.

A similar situation exists in Nunberg's *Principles of Psycho-analysis* (1932). Apparatus or ego apparatuses are not listed in the index of the book, though the bibliography includes references to Hartmann's work, including Hartmann's *Ego Psychology and the Problem of Adaptation* in its German edition.[3] In the text very few references to ego apparatuses are to be found, for example, the ego "possesses a receptive, defensive, and inhibitory apparatus for mastering ... " (p. 118). Occasionally instead of referring to the ego apparatus concerned with thought processes, he will refer to a "thinking organ" or instead of the *perceptive apparatus* he refers to "the system of perception" (p. 128).

Even in Waelder's more recent and very fine textbook, *Basic Theory of Psychoanalysis* (1960), the concept of ego apparatus is not discussed.

THE BIOLOGICAL MODEL AND ITS INFLUENCE ON THE PSYCHOLOGICAL MODEL

As we see, apparatus is a term that has a variety of connotations. These are derived from the fact that it is used in different sciences, such as physics, biology, and especially medicine. Gould's Medical Dictionary (fifth edition) defines apparatus as "1. A collection of instruments or devices used for a special purpose. 2. Anatomically the word is used to designate collectively the organs performing a certain function. ... "

Generally speaking, expressions such as the organ of vision or the apparatus of vision usually mean for the layman the eyes, while for the biologist or neurophysiologist a great deal more is included, that is, the optic nerve, the specific occipital brain areas to which the stimuli received in the eye are transmitted, the links with other areas of the brain, etc.

3. Fenichel, too, lists in the bibliography of his book the German edition of Hartmann's monograph (the English translation appeared in 1958). In Nunberg's case, the English version of his book (1955), though not representing a word-for-word translation, is based on his German text published in 1932, that is to say, before Hartmann's monograph appeared in German.

In medicine, an apparatus, such as the apparatus of vision or the respiratory apparatus, includes several anatomical entities, organs that combine in coordinated ways the functions they are capable of performing individually to accomplish some other, more elaborate, and specific set of functions. In other words, different organs perform a number of functions specifically assigned to them and simultaneously work as part of a more complex apparatus. Although these different apparatuses are complex anatomophysiological units in themselves with a number of specific functions, they keep at the same time the closest relationships with other somatic apparatuses, some of whose services and functions are essential for the performance of their own specific tasks. Thus, for example, the physiological processes carried out by the respiratory apparatus (i.e., the exchange of gases) are dependent on the normal activity of the circulatory apparatus which pumps the blood at different rates through the lungs, etc.

I wish to highlight here the interdependence between the different apparatuses and their functions because this type of model is implicit in our concept of ego apparatus. What we call an ego apparatus is an extremely complex organization, to which several physical organs or apparatuses may contribute their functional capabilities in different degrees and combinations. But we should note that in the case of the circulatory apparatus, for example, these functional capabilities are described as the physiological processes of which the corresponding anatomical structures are capable, while in the case of many of the somatic organs subserving the mind more directly, for example, the brain, some of the physiological processes have a concomitant psychological equivalent—a fact that is of the greatest significance.

We assume that to start with the "inborn apparatuses" (Hartmann 1939) which later form part of the ego organization are rather primitive in their functional possibilities. These are in any case essentially determined and closely linked to the physical organ or organs on which they are dependent. This rather obvious statement is made only to emphasize the very close connection that exists at the very beginning between function and specific organs. As ego development progresses, many other apparatuses and functions become integrated in the performance of the perfected form of the function. That is to say, the contribution of the somatic apparatus, say of visual perception, essential as it remains in terms of the reception of visual sensations, is nevertheless relative when contrasted with the contributions that are made to actual visual perception by other ego apparatuses and functions. In Hartmann's words (1939): "Ego development is a differentiation, in which these primitive regulating factors are increasingly replaced or supplemented by more effective ego regulations. . . . Differentiation progresses not only by the creation of new apparatuses to master new demands and new tasks, but also and mainly by new apparatuses taking over, on a higher level, functions which were originally performed by more primitive means" (p. 49f.).

As mentioned above, our conception of the ego apparatuses has striking similarities with the explanatory construct of the somatic apparatuses, but there are also striking differences that deserve some further consideration.

We have no conscious awareness of the many physiological processes that take place in the different apparatuses of our organism, for example, while we breathe or digest. Mostly silent and automatically regulated, these processes find no conscious expression in our minds unless something is at fault, in which case we perceive feelings along the unpleasure-pain series. In other words, the possibility of translating these physiological processes into psychological terms, into terms that the mind can manipulate, is extremely restricted.

A completely different situation exists with regard to the mental apparatus, as I have already suggested. We are of course not aware of the innumerable physiological processes in the brain that underlie our mental activities per se. Yet, many of these underlying physiological processes are retranslated—by means that escape us so far—into what I can describe only (lacking a better and more accurate expression) as the psychological language of the mind, the language of the ego organization. These are phenomena of which we frequently can become conscious, which have acquired a certain independence, which can be manipulated in different ways, which form part of our psychical processes. In other words, when certain physiological processes are retranslated, transformed, or raised to the level of the psychological, they are perceived in the mind, the mental apparatus (or rather that part of it which we call the ego), as ideas, thoughts, visual or auditory images, memories, feelings, etc.

SOMATIC APPARATUSES AND PSYCHOLOGICAL EGO APPARATUSES

Although we all have some notion of what is meant by ego apparatus, there remains a great deal of obscurity and ambiguity with respect to this concept. I shall use *visual perception* as a concrete example to illustrate the difference between somatic and psychic apparatus and to consider the distinct roles played by these ego apparatuses in the performance of this ego function. We agree, first of all, that the physical apparatuses, the somatic organs involved in the perception of visual stimuli, must reach an appropriate degree of maturation before they can appropriately perform the basic functions involved in visual perception. We agree, furthermore, that the mere fact of the physical apparatus having reached maturity and therefore being potentially ready to perform its function does not imply that this function will immediately be performed in all its complexity. Visual perception is an extremely complicated process that needs exercise and learning for its perfection. Such learning takes time and requires a coordinated interaction with several other apparatuses and mental processes that must themselves reach a certain maturational level and organization before they can contribute to the performance of visual perception as a perfected function.

At the beginning of life, the somatic organs concerned (the eye, the nervous pathways carrying the sensory impression to the appropriate areas in the occipital cortex, and the multiple links between these areas and other centers in the brain) are capable of receiving and carrying different types of visual stimuli (light, dark, color, shapes, etc.). However, the sensory impressions that these stimuli produce in the organism are devoid of specific meaning. Whatever sensation they create, it is not understood without an appropriate relation to a given context, in short, unless it is organized and integrated with other mental phenomena. As other apparatuses develop, as increased discrimination is possible, as memories are laid down, perceptions become integrated and processed in interaction with other mental processes that take into account previous experiences and knowledge. This is naturally a gradual process of development becoming more and more complex and refined.

In this way we learn to perceive not just primitive and simple sensory impressions, but impressions that can now be discriminated in terms of form, shapes, color, depth, spatial relations, causal connections, meanings, and the like. This not only allows for the identification of objects according to their different qualities, in the abstract so to say; but more important, by means of complicated processes of association with other memories of other objects, experiences, and things, all these impressions have for each person a special individual meaning that belongs in the life context of his own experiences and knowledge.

We have seen the role played by the somatic ego apparatus of vision in terms of receiving the stimuli and producing specific sensory impressions, but we could not have failed to notice that without the contribution of other physical apparatuses, of other mental functions and processes, without the organization of the stimuli perceived visually according to certain laws, without the necessary coordination and integration with the content of innumerable other experiences, past, present, and even future (through the function of imagination), perceptive processes would have remained at the level of *primitive sensory impressions* registered by the *somatic apparatus* concerned with vision. What raises visual perception from the level of primitive sensory impressions conveyed by the somatic organ to the sophisticated, invaluable process that we know as vision is the existence of the *psychological ego apparatus* of perception. By this I mean an intangible, nonmaterial organization, with a *functional structure* of its own, which regulates its own activities and those of the multiple somatic structures or organs it utilizes according to a well-established (though largely unknown) hierarchy of regulating principles and laws; a preordained set of processes that has structured itself slowly and gradually through development; a functional structuralization that has been earned, partly perhaps through trial and error (though not exclusively) and whose basic regulating principle during its organization (and perhaps afterward as well) was its adaptive value, even its survival value. Much of the development of the psychological ego apparatus of visual perception can be assumed to follow, at least in part, a preordained course determined by the genetically controlled maturational unfolding of the physical structures that will allow for a gradual and increasing complexity and integration of those mental processes that such maturational unfolding makes possible.

The quality of the psychological ego apparatus concerned with the function of perception will vary enormously from one individual to another. These variations are dependent, on the one hand, on the "quality" of the somatic ego apparatuses underlying some of these processes (the quality being itself determined by constitutional and hereditary factors in interaction with environmental influences insofar as their physical maturation is influenced by it) and, on the other hand, on all those factors that generally influence development and more specifically the development of the ego apparatuses concerned with the function of visual perception. Among these are suitable stimulation, accumulation of all sorts of experiences, opportunities to practice the skills involved in order to perfect them further—in short, factors that influence learning, in this particular case, learning to perceive and to organize percepts in a meaningful way.

What I have described for perception applies, I believe, to all other ego functions. Although at present we do not have as much knowledge about the physical structures underlying such mental activities as ideation, thinking, etc., as we have about visual perception and the physical structures and physiological processes underlying it, I have little doubt that the day will come when these relationships will be understood. Such an understanding will enrich psychoanalytic and psychological propositions dealing with these aspects of mental functioning. Nevertheless, in the absence of such knowledge, we are still forced to operate at a level of abstraction that occasionally seems to carry with it the danger that some of our working hypotheses might acquire metaphysical or mystical connotations, as it were, and these could hinder our scientific development.

I would like to end this section by applying to my discussion what Hartmann (1939) said: that many of these "lengthy—but still incomplete—considerations are not psychoanalytic in the narrow sense, and some of them seem to have taken us quite far from the core of psychoanalysis" (p. 108). Following him, I would add that psychoanalysis as a general psychology and as a developmental theory can no longer avoid branching out into different directions and borrowing from biology, neurophysiology, and other sciences whatever is necessary for its further development on its own independent lines.

THE DEVELOPMENTAL APPROACH TO THE EGO AND ITS SOMATIC ROOTS

Many analysts have attempted to describe and understand the developmental steps leading from the rudimentary ego at birth to the final ego organization. While a full description of these attempts is beyond the scope of this paper, these studies have made it quite clear that ego development is predicated on a number of factors interacting with one another. I single out the physical maturational processes taking place in the somatic structures whose functional capacities will at the appropriate time become integrated into the ego organization. I have mentioned earlier that physical maturation itself is not enough, that the performance of the function must be learned and perfected, and that experiencing and different forms of stimulation play essential contributory roles.

It is in relation to the *physical* maturation occurring simultaneously in various organs and in interaction with each other that we observe the beginning of certain psychological activities that I refer to as primitive or elementary ego functions. Further maturation, stimulation, learning, experiencing, and practice in the use of these physical apparatuses lead to greater efficiency of their functioning and to the slow and gradual development of the ego structure. This naturally includes an increasing and more efficient interaction and integration of the various functions and apparatuses which contribute to the building of the ego structure until we reach, at the appropriate time, the "final" ego organization. At this point the ego has acquired the capacity to use, control, and command all the resources available and functions with an amazing degree of complexity. Even then we have to qualify the statement, "the ego in its final form," because we know that the capacity of the mature ego structure in terms of learning, imagining, and functioning in ever more complex ways continues to increase for many years and in some fortunate individuals throughout their lives.

Among biologist, neurologists, and neurophysiologists there seems to be a measure of agreement that actual physical maturation of the brain structures and other elements of the central nervous system is more or less completed during the first year and a half of life.[4] Since the level of ego development reached at this stage is very limited, we appreciate the degree to which development in the human depends upon learning, on constant stimulation, on a great variety of experiences, and on the constant exercise of the ego organization dealing with new situations in more complex ways. These experiences are recorded and laid down, so that this storehouse of memories and knowledge can be used to deal with further new experiences in more purposeful and adaptive ways. In this manner, the ego widens its ability to understand and master the complexity of new situations and stimuli that reach it.

Two aspects deserve further discussion. The first one concerns the fact, referred to earlier, that in the physical maturation of

4. It is hardly necessary to remind the reader that the young of the human species is born with a degree of immaturity that has no equivalent in any other mammal species. To reach a degree of physical maturation equivalent to that of other species at birth, he takes a good year and a half of extrauterine life, a factor of the greatest psychological significance.

somatic structures appropriate stimulation by the mother or mother substitute seems to play an essential role. Many studies and observations have shown that, in the absence of such stimulation, the development of several somatic apparatuses, initially having a normal potential, is delayed to a point where they are quite incapable of performing certain functions (Provence and Lipton 1962). Since it is these functional capabilities that constitute the very essence of the ego structure (when a certain level of functioning and organization has been reached), we can see the close association between external stimulation, the development and maturation of the somatic apparatuses, and their final functional expression, that is, their ego dimension.

These functional capacities are qualitatively very different in different individuals because the constitutional givens as well as the quantity and type of stimulation received vary. The developmental continuum I have tried to describe highlights the dangers and oversimplification implicit in a conception in which the psychological ego organization is totally divorced from the somatic apparatuses on which it depends not only for its inception but also for its more mature functioning. In this respect, Hartmann (1939) stated: "It is obvious that these apparatuses, *somatic and mental,* influence the development and the functions of the ego which uses them; we maintain that these apparatuses constitute one of the roots of the ego" (p. 101; italics mine). In 1950, he added:

> The problem of maturation has a physiological aspect. Speaking of this aspect we may refer to the growth of whatever we assume to be the physiological basis of those functions which, looked at from the angle of psychology, we call the ego; or we may refer to the growth of such apparatus which sooner or later come to be specifically used by the ego (e.g., the motor apparatus used in action). However, the role of these apparatus for the ego is not limited to their function as tools which the ego at a given time finds at its disposal. We have to assume that differences in the timing or intensity of their growth enter into the picture of ego development as a partly independent variable; e.g., the timing of the appearance of grasping, of walking, of the motor aspect of speech (see also Hendrick 1943). Neither does it seem unlikely that the congenital motor equipment is among the factors

which right from birth on tend to modify certain attitudes of the developing ego (Fries and Lewis 1938). The presence of such factors in all aspects of the child's behavior makes them also an essential element in the development of his self-experience. We can assume that from the earliest stages on the corresponding experiences are preserved in his system of memory traces. We have also reasons to think that the reproduction of environmental data is very generally fused with and formed by elements of that kind, e.g., the reproduction of motor experiences. [p. 121]

By obscuring these links we deny ourselves a better understanding of what we call the ego organization, of how it is established, how it acquires the special qualities that characterize it as a finished product and distinguish it from all other ego organizations. Further, by depriving ourselves of understanding these processes of interaction throughout development, we place out of our reach the possibility of learning how we can favorably influence the processes, or at least prevent detrimental influences.

As long as psychoanalysis was primarily concerned with the neurotic conflicts of the adult personality (the finished product)—as was certainly the case in 1923, when Freud introduced the structural model of the mind—it could afford to conceive of the ego structure without expanding on the relationship between the ego's functions and the apparatuses.[5] At this point in the development of psychoanalysis it was sufficient to say that such apparatuses were at the service of the ego organization and under its control. But when psychoanalysis moved in the direction of a *psychoanalytic psychology* and more especially of a *developmental psychoanalytic psychology,* the situation changed; what had been a most useful set of formulations pertinent to the problems dealt with was no longer sufficient. Further study and elaboration of our propositions concerning the ego are necessary if we are to meet in a more systematic way the requirements of child development, normal as well as psychopathological.

We have only to think of some children with minimal brain damage whose egos are atypical because of the primary defects in

5. Hartmann also refers to this problem in 1939.

the somatic apparatuses on which the ego structure is based. These ego deviations cannot possibly be understood without reference to the organic structures that support it. Further, the indiscriminate extension of the formulations concerning the ego structure of normal or neurotic adults to this type of case may lead—and, I believe, has in fact occasionally led—to serious misconceptions about the true nature of these children's basic disturbances. They consist, in these brain-damaged children, of primary defects and abnormalities of the somatic apparatuses, which naturally enough produce atypical ego organizations lacking in certain functions and having defects in the integrative capacities. The same arguments apply to *some* so-called borderline, or autistic children, or children with atypical personalities. These terms are purely descriptive classifications based on behavioral manifestations; they are meaningless with regard to etiology because each such group can contain children whose disturbances were caused by very different factors. With such cases, too, no headway can be made without a better understanding of the close relationship between the final ego organization and the different somatic apparatuses that sustain it and make it possible. The symptomatology of some of these cases may in fact also be due to primary deficiencies in the apparatuses. (These primary deficiencies need not always be due to organic disturbances. They may be due to insufficient or excessive stimulation at the inappropriate stage, to overwhelming traumatic experiences which, if they occur at certain periods, may completely disrupt development.)

Another example may further clarify the issues involved. At the Hampstead Clinic we have had the opportunity to observe and study a number of children who were blind, some of them from birth. The lack of the organ of vision, one of the somatic apparatuses at the disposal of the ego at later stages, tends to distort the development of these children in practically every area of their functioning at least for some time. Most of these blind children lag behind sighted children in all their achievements. Their drive development deviates from the norm, and so does their ego and superego development. (For more detailed account of these deviations in the blind, see chapter 10.) It is particularly interesting to note, by means of the contrast with the sighted, the essential contribution that sight makes to the development of a multitude of other ego apparatuses and functions. Without this fundamental contribution from the organ of sight many of these functions do not develop, or are faulty and incomplete. Sometimes the ego handicap remains for life. In these cases we cannot fail to appreciate the intimate dependence between apparatus and function and, even more important, the essential contribution that the organ of vision makes to the development of other apparatuses and functions.

As I have tried to demonstrate with these examples, it will prove profitable for the further development of psychoanalysis as a developmental psychology to focus some of our interest on the close correlation between the physical and the psychological. Moreover, in this way we might succeed in further closing the artificial gap that still exists between the concepts of body and mind, of physical and psychological, and thus reestablish the natural continuum between them.

Obviously, there were many reasons why the formulations in *The Ego and the Id* were not aimed at closing this gap. I have already referred to the fact that they adequately dealt with the type of problem they were meant to deal with (neurotic conflicts, especially in the adult). They did not involve the type of problems and interactions that could not be escaped when analysis branched out in several new directions. Insufficient knowledge in other disciplines also did not favor attempts at integration.

Hartmann, Kris, and Loewenstein (1946) have pointed out that Freud was by no means unaware of these problems, quite the contrary. They stated: "In adopting the *functions* exercised in mental processes as the decisive criterion for defining the psychic systems Freud used physiology as his model in concept formation. However, this does not imply any correlation of any one of the systems to any specific physiological organization or group of organs, though Freud considered such a correlation as the ultimate goal of psychological research. Psychological terminology, he assumed, has to be maintained as long as it cannot be adequately substituted by physiological terminology" (p. 15). Yet, in my opinion, attempts to correlate psychological structures (id, ego, superego) and specific areas of the brain, anatomical structures, or physiological processes are ill-advised and bound to fail. They do not seem, at least to my mind, to take full account of the functional-psychological nature of our conceptualizations of these agencies or, for that matter, of the true significance of recent neurophysiological advances.

To equate or correlate, for example, the brain cortex with our ego agency may occasionally be quite tempting because many of the functions of the cortex and the physiological processes taking place there are usually accompanied by psychological experiences and functions that we attribute to the ego. However, these striking similarities are due only to the fact that all psychological phenomena have a physiological substratum, which in some cases can be located in one or another area of the brain. But our ego concept cannot be tied down to any area or areas of the central nervous system, nor can it be restricted to or identified with the functions performed by them. As a functional construct, the ego cannot be localized anywhere or made identical with any area (or group of areas) since what it utilizes for its performance is the psychological translation of a physiological process or group of physiological processes located in the central nervous system. What is important is not the location of the physiological processes underlying the psychological retranslation (which the ego uses for its operation), but the psychological laws that regulate the organization of these psychological processes, giving them distinct qualities[6] that characterize a given mental process as the product of the ego organization. As a psychological construct it deals only with psychological phenomena and not with the neurophysiological processes underlying it. As such and without in any way wanting to deny the close links with such processes, we can say that it has simultaneously acquired in conceptual terms, and otherwise, a marked independence from them.

I emphasize once more, to avoid misunderstanding, that the developmental approach to the ego and its somatic roots that I am

6. These were well defined by Freud (i.e., secondary processes, delay, binding of mental energy, etc.).

suggesting here does not have as its aim a correlation between the ego or any other psychic agency (id and superego) and specific anatomical or anatomophysiological localities of the central nervous system. But it does try to correlate (not equate), relatively and within limits, the interrelations between what psychoanalysis conceptualizes as "ego functions" and the underlying physical structures and physiological processes on which the former are dependent.

References

Brenner, C., and Arlow, J. A. (1964). *Psychoanalytic Concepts and the Structural Theory.* New York: International Universities Press.

Fenichel, O. (1945). *The Psychoanalytic Theory of Neurosis.* New York: Norton.

Freud, S. (1923). The ego and the id. *Standard Edition* 19:3-68.

——— (1937). Analysis terminable and interminable. *Standard Edition* 23:209-254.

Gill, M. M. (1963). *Topography and Systems in Psychoanalytic Theory. Psychological Issues,* Monograph 10. New York: International Universities Press.

Hartmann, H. (1939). *Ego Psychology and the Problem of Adaptation.* New York: International Universities Press, 1958.

——— (1950). Comments on the psychoanalytic theory of the ego. In *Essays on Ego Psychology* pp. 113-141. New York: International Universities Press, 1964.

——— (1952). The mutual influences in the development of ego and id. In *Essays on Ego Psychology* pp. 155-181. New York: International Universities Press, 1964.

——— (1959). Psychoanalysis as a scientific theory. In *Essays on Ego Psychology,* pp. 318-350. New York: International Universities Press, 1964.

——— (1964). *Essays on Ego Psychology.* New York: International Universities Press.

Hartmann, H., Kris, E., and Loewenstein, R. M. (1946). Comments on the formation of psychic structure. *Psychoanalytic Study of the Child,* 2:11-38.

Nunberg, H. (1932). *Principles of Psychoanalysis.* New York: International Universities Press, 1955.

Provence, S., and Lipton, R. C. (1962). *Infants in Institutions.* New York: International Universities Press.

Waelder, R. (1960). *Basic Theory of Psychoanalysis.* New York: International Universities Press.

Chapter Nine

STRUCTURE, STRUCTURALIZATION, AND CREATIVITY

The need for the conceptual clarification undertaken in this chapter arose from the application of the developmental profile (diagnostic profile) to a large number of children with a wide range of psychopathology studied and treated at the Hampstead Clinic. The ambiguity of some terms and assumptions of the structural theory as formulated for the adult personality hindered to some extent our progress in the understanding of the normal and psychopathological processes in the development of children. I believe that clarification of our conceptual tools and present theories in respect of so important an area of the personality as that represented by the ego structure cannot fail to help in furthering our understanding of the normal and the psychopathological processes of children at any given age. The significant role played by the ego in normal adaptation, in the solution of conflicts, in symptom formation, etc. justifies this attempt.

PSYCHOANALYTIC USAGE

The term *structure* derives from the Latin *structura*, meaning to build. Structure is defined in Webster's Third New International Dictionary as:

The action of building; something constructed or built; something made up of more or less interdependent parts or elements; the manner of construction; the arrangement of particles or parts in a substance or body; the arrangement and mode of particles or parts in a substance or body; the arrangement and mode of union of the atoms in a molecule; the interrelation of parts as dominated by the general character of the whole; the elements or parts of an entity or the position of such elements or parts in their external relationships to each other.

Structural [is defined as]: of or relating to structure or a structure; affecting structure.

Structuralization [is defined as]: the process of structuralizing.

Structuralizing [is defined as]: embodying in structural or material form.

All these different connotations seem to be implicit in psychoanalytic terminology.

Structure is defined by Lewis (1965) in the following terms: "By *structure* we mean an ordered arrangement of elements, which may be perceptions, events, thoughts, reactions, etcetera of sufficient stability to give some predictability. It is important to note that structure may refer to sequential, as well as to simultaneous, relations among elements" (p. 151).

Beres, discussing "Structure and Function in Psycho-Analysis" (1965, p. 55) states quite rightly I think, that a "distinction must be made between the 'structural theory' of psycho-analysis and the use of the term 'structure' by some authors in the attempt to set up a psycho-analytic psychology." He further pointed to three areas requiring clarification in this respect: first, the tendency to reify id, ego, and superego; secondly, the confusion that arises when the concept of structure is used in a sense that differs from Freud's limited structural formulations without defining such differences; and thirdly, the need to emphasize constantly the *functional basis of structure* in psychoanalysis.

We also talk of organic or physical structures and of psychological, philosophical, and social structures, etc. The main implication seems to be that a certain manner or order, a certain organization of the elements involved, is in existence. According to this definition, a mental mechanism can be considered a structure, mental processes of the most diverse kind can be considered structures too, an ego function is a structure, an idea is a structure, a memory trace is a structure, etc. At least on one occasion Freud (1915, p. 178) even referred to affective structures. Beres states that on the basis of these definitions, concepts, theories, and scientific laws are structures; at the same time he warns that these psychological structures are not physical entities and are not to be treated as such (p. 54). The last point is also stressed in Colby's definition of structure. He says: "By 'structure' we do not mean any material substance, but again a hypothetical ordering of psychic elements which must await further description" (1955, p. 16).

Schur (1966, p. 13) points out too that the "structural point of view has been the center of our interest to such an extent that we often encounter the term 'structural theory' as a substitute for 'the structural point of view of metapsychology,'" a situation that no doubt further contributes to the ambiguity of the terms and concepts used.

Viewing the difference between structures from one angle, I believe it can be said to consist in how many elements are involved in any given structure and in the complexity with which the different elements are organized. Some structures are simple because they contain few elements or because the elements they contain are organized in very simple ways. Others can be considered complex structures because they contain numerous elements and/or because the relationship between these elements is multidimensional and of great complexity.

As is well known, the topographical theory aimed at classifying mental processes into one of three systems according to their relationship to the phenomena of consciousness. These systems were named the unconscious, the preconscious, and the conscious. When this guideline proved unsatisfactory, Freud put forward a theory (later called the structural theory) that defines three mental agencies (now called id, ego, and superego) on the basis *of their different functions.* The characteristics of these functions or of the mental processes underlying them vary greatly according to the degree and quality of structuralization that is typical of each one of the agencies. It is for these reasons that Beres (1965, p. 12) has proposed to call the structural theory the "functional theory of psychoanalysis" since the different structures are to be understood in reference to their different functions.

The ambiguity of the term structure when utilized in psychoanalysis is partly due to the fact that in reality all things that can be said to exist have a structure of their own, no matter how primitive it may be. This applies to inorganic and organic matter on the one hand as well as to processes of all kinds on the other hand. Thus, in psychoanalysis, what we really mean when we speak of structuralization is the steps taken from relatively little or primitive structuralization to more complex forms of it, more complex functional organizations than those existing to start with. On the basis of these steps further structuralization can take place. Thus we are making a relative statement and not an absolute one. Strictly speaking, we do not move from nothing (no structuralization whatsoever) to structuralization. Perhaps the best example of this is the contrast between the id and the ego. It seems to me beyond question that the id is structured, since the processes that take place in its realm follow primary-process laws. These laws are themselves a form of organization of regulation of mental processes. Nevertheless, we generally speak of the id as a chaotic agency (ignoring that this is chaos with an order of its own) in contrast to the ego, which we consider as a highly organized agency. When Freud referred to these two agencies in those terms, he proceeds as if he had decided to call the degree of more primitive organization of the id the absolute zero (in terms of order, structure, and organization), with which he then compared the degree of organization and structuralization of the other agencies[1] (see Schur 1966).

---

1. Colby (1955) too has some objections in this respect. He said: "One theoretical drawback to the tripartite model concerns the concept of id. Freud conceived of this entity with its impersonal pronoun as being completely chaotic and unorganized. This does not seem theoretically possible if metapsychology is to remain logically consistent. A structure by definition is an organization, and each part of it must, therefore, also be organized. Organization within the parts of a structure may differ from system to system, but all the systems must possess some kind of order" (p. 76).

As useful as the concepts of structure and structuralization are, they inevitably carry with them some degree of ambiguity.

As we have seen, the different agencies of the mind are structures, although we speak most often of the ego structures.[2] The ego apparatuses are themselves structures; the ego functions are structures as well; even primary processes are structures, and so are secondary processes, according to a number of analysts whose views will be discussed later.

SURVEY OF THE LITERATURE

A cursory review of psychoanalytic writings shows that Rapaport was among those who made a more liberal use of the terms structure, structuralization, control structures etc.; moreover, there is much evidence of his influence on the writings of many of the so-called ego psychologists. For these reasons I shall discuss his monograph on *The Structure of Psychoanalytic Theory* (1960c) in detail.

According to Rapaport, it was the realization of the contrast between "the drive processes, whose rate of change is fast and whose course is paroxysmal, [and these forces] which conflict with them and . . . appeared to be invariant, or at least of a slower rate of change," that laid the foundation on which the concept of structure was built, the latter relatively abiding elements being the prototype of it (p. 53). Rapaport considered that the study of the forces that opposed or delayed drive discharge (the defenses) with their permanent deployment of countercathexis marked the beginning of the structural conception. He added that "An explicit formulation of the structural conception became necessary when it was realized that not only the drives but also most of these invariant factors which interfere with drives are unconscious" (p. 53f.).

The recognition of the structure building and structural role

2. Occasionally the term substructure is applied to this agency; for example, Hartmann (1950, p. 114) stated that the ego "is a substructure of personality and is defined by its functions."

played by the process of identification (Freud 1923) was soon followed by the recognition of the ego's defensive *substructures*. In addition, psychoanalytic ego psychology came to recognize other substructures such as orienting (perceptual), processing (conceptual), and executive (motor) substructures that are ready-made tools available to ego processes (Hartmann 1939, Rapaport 1951b). Rapaport refers to Hartmann's concept of inborn ego apparatuses (such as memory, perception, motility) as *structural givens*. By this term he means neither the muscular apparatuses of motility, nor the end organs used for perception, "but rather their psychological regulations: for instance, those psychological structures through which the control and triggering of the motor apparatus is effected" (p. 53, n. 13).[3]

As I have already noted, Rapaport refers to the defenses as "structures": "they are the most extensively studied structures," and for this reason many analysts may have gained the incorrect impression "that all structures are conflict-born and all controls are defenses" (p. 56).[4] He further states that, to begin with, psychoanalysis assumed that all psychologically relevant structures arise in ontogeny and are conflict-born; today, however, we accept that some of these structures are inborn givens, for example, Hartmann's ego apparatuses of primary autonomy. Rapaport contrasts these with the group of functions or structures that were born out of conflict or subserved drive gratification but later underwent what Hartmann called a "change of function," thus becoming means of adaptation in the service of the ego. Quoting Hartmann (1939) Rapaport refers to this group as *structures of secondary autonomy*. Hartmann, however, uses the term *functions* and not *structures* of secondary autonomy.

Rapaport summarizes this section of his discussion by stating

3. Rapaport's formulations could be misleading or misunderstood. The existence of the inborn ego apparatuses is perhaps self-evident, but this must not be taken to imply that the psychological structures that control them (and it is to these that Rapaport is referring) are inborn as well and present in their final form from the beginning. All evidence demonstrates that they are only primitive to start with and have to be built up, acquired later on, and that this happens only very gradually.

4. A fuller account of defenses as stable structures playing a number of different roles in the mental economy is to be found in his paper. "On the Psychoanalytic Theory of Motivation" (1960a). See also Gill (1963).

that "inborn structures and acquired structures are apparatuses of primary and secondary autonomy. Structure-building transforms motivations and thus gives rise to new (more neutralized) motivations" (p. 56).

Rapaport concluded that "The concepts of structure and relative autonomy (Hartmann) are indispensable to the theory, and at present it is not possible to foresee changes in the theory which could eliminate them. But the concepts of id, ego, superego, and the differentiation of the ego into defense-, control-, and means-structures are neither as indispensable to nor as independent from the theory. However, a variety of subordinate structural concepts (e.g., specific primary-process and defense mechanisms, like displacement, condensation, substitution, symbolization, repression, isolation, reaction formation, projection) which are more directly related to observations and of a lesser generality, are likely to survive" (p. 128).

Some further understanding of Rapaport's ideas about structure can be gained by his considerations concerning cognitive structures. He defines them as "those quasipermanent means which cognitive processes use and do not have to create *de novo* each time and those quasipermanent organizations of such means that are the framework for the individual cognitive processes" (1957, p. 157).

He thinks of memory organizations as possibly the most common cognitive structures, which are organized in terms of spatial and temporal contiguity, in terms of the drives, interest, and affects, as well as conceptually. He describes other forms of cognitive organizations such as cognitive styles, styles of perceiving, conversing, dreaming, etc., which show striking interindividual differences. According to him, all these cognitive organizations or structures do no constitute a random assembly but are closely interrelated in a multiple complex hierarchy.

He believes that "A distinction between cognitive processes on the one hand and the structured (patterned and persisting) tools of cognition and their organizations on the other can probably be made by the criterion of rates of change; the processes may be defined as showing a high rate of change, the tools and their organization as showing a low one. In other words, the processes are temporary and unique, the tools and their organizations permanent and typical" (1957, p. 161):

As Rapaport himself remarks, he focused on the relatively enduring forms in contrast to passing processes, because "we need concepts of organization- or structure-character to account for all these quasistable enduring forms" existing in the personality. His stress upon this relatively enduring organization parallels, as he says, a change of emphasis in psychoanalysis, that is, the development of psychoanalytic ego psychology, a development that added to the earlier emphasis on motivation and gratification processes an equal stress upon the study of defensive organizations, controls, and structures. "It seems that with this stress on relatively enduring controlling- and means-organizations, psychoanalytic psychology finds itself again in a pioneering role" (p. 194).

Rapaport concludes this 1957 paper with a clear statement of his views of the concept of structures and the conceptual difficulties involved: "The specific cognitive organizations or structures that I discussed were meant only as illustrations. My study of these is still in the intial stage and I hold no brief for them, except insofar as they illustrate my general point. Nor for that matter do I hold a brief for any specific psychoanalytic concept that refers to relatively enduring structures. Further study may well replace these concepts. But it cannot abolish the phenomena to which the present structure-concepts refer. So far psychoanalysis is the only theory that has attempted to take account of these phenomena" (p. 194).

In his paper "On the Psychoanalytic Theory of Motivation" (1960a), Rapaport makes a number of interesting points in relation to structures and their maintenance. He thinks that sufficiently consolidated structures are self-sustaining, but he acknowledges that evidence to show actual instances where this is the case is difficult to come by. In an earlier publication (1958) he had suggested, and he repeats the suggestion here (1960a), that structures do not stand in isolation but are in fact integrated with other structures and are nourished and maintained through their relations to one another. He further suggested that activation by external stimuli makes a contribution to the maintenance of the structures (including the defensive structures and other types). It is the environment that provides structures with "stimulus nutriment," a term that according to Holt (1965, p. 158) Rapaport has taken and adapted from Piaget's concept aliment.[5] Rapaport categorically stated that there is "independent evidence available indicating that it is the development and maintenance of structures rather than a special kind of motivation which prompts the organism to reach out for stimulation" (1960a, p. 223f.). Thus Rapaport's concept of stimulus nutriment includes nutriment both from without and from within. According to Miller (1962, p. 8), Rapaport's "stimulus-nutriment from the environment includes all that is perceived in the external world, while nutriment from within is provided by ego- and superego-structures and ultimately by drives."

Although I cannot include an extensive discussion of Rapaport's concept of ego autonomy (see 1951b, 1958), it is necessary to refer to it briefly because it is closely related to his ideas about ego structures and their maintenance. He conceived of an autonomy of the ego from the id (as seen in the ego's capacity to postpone drive discharge, modify it, etc.), and of a relative autonomy of the ego from external reality (as seen in the ego's capacity to adapt in different ways or to postpone its reactions to external stimuli). Since on the one hand this autonomy of the ego is dependent on the ego structures and their stability and on the other hand the latter depends on the reception of appropriate quantities of stimulus nutriment, the interference with stimulus nutriment or the lack of stimulus nutriment disrupts—by affecting the structure's stability—the autonomy of the ego, especially that from the id.

As Holt (1965, p. 155) points out, Rapaport cited sensory deprivation and hypnosis as examples of instances in which the stability of structures can be seen to suffer. Further, Rapaport conceived of a complementary relationship between these two types of autonomy; that is, the ego's relations to reality guarantee

---

5. Cf. Rapaport (1960a, p. 221ff.) where he makes this link.

autonomy from the id; consequently, excessive autonomy from reality impairs the autonomy from the id; and, similarly, an excessive autonomy from the id (since the drives are the ultimate guarantee of autonomy from the environment) may impair the autonomy from the environment (1958, p. 24).

According to Holt (1965, p. 154), Rapaport does not distinguish clearly between the role of stimuli in *structure building* in contrast to their role in *structure maintenance*. Holt does not agree with Rapaport that all structures are in need of stimulus nutriment "lest they wither away," giving as examples memory-trace structures, disused for many years, which are found intact and recovered by means of hypnotic suggestion, brain stimulation, and psychoanalytic treatment. He also refers to psychic structures involved in seasonal activities (i.e., ice skating) which after months of lack of nutriment show no sign of decompensation. He nevertheless concedes that Rapaport's point of view applies to a limited number of structures, describing as an example the disruption of perceptual structures in experiments of isolation. Holt adds an interesting qualification: if there is a change in the type of stimulus input, the perceptual structure not only is disrupted after some time but starts to rebuild itself on the basis of the new conditions. This type of structure if deprived of input lies quietly in storage and remains relatively unchanged; however, if it is fed the wrong or an insufficient diet of stimuli it begins to rebuild itself on a new plan.

Holt says:

> The psychic apparatus is capable of re-writing its programmes continuously and automatically to take account of changes in the information fed to it. Introduce any kind of systematic distortion, and, soon, or later, a new programme is written that makes the old sense out of the new information. . . . The fact that we have such structures requiring nutriment is one reason that organisms become so profoundly incapacitated when they are brought up during the critical early stages of development in impoverished environments; the psychic apparatus that develops may get a built-in rigidity and inability to cope with stimuli as chaotic as the average expectable environment if it is fed highly simplified information for a long enough time. [p. 162]

Holt concludes that the "principal role of structures is to widen the tolerable range of inputs (whether of urge, press, inner and outer information, or tonic support)," while pointing at the same time to the existence of what he calls *maladaptive structures*, such as those involved in a phobia, which "may narrow the range of inputs, as do inhibitory structures generally" (p. 164).

It should be noted that Rapaport stated that Piaget's structure concept, "just like the psychoanalytic, assumes a hierarchic layering of progressively differentiating structures" (1960a, p. 222).

He also described some of the economic factors involved in the building of structures, using memory traces as an example. He thus explained how an excitation capable of attracting a sufficient amount of attention for a sufficient length of time gives rise to a structure such as a memory trace. Structures so built retain only a small quantity of the attention cathexis that was necessary in their formation process (the energy becoming bound in the structure), while the rest becomes available again to deal with other excitations (1960a, p. 229).

Rapaport also refers to learning as a process of structure formation (1960a, p. 231), a point to which I shall come back later.

A comparison between Rapaport's and Hartmann's uses of the terms structure and apparatus (ego structures or ego apparatuses) seems to me to show clearly that Rapaport greatly favors the term *structure*. He uses it, generally speaking, as synonymous with ego apparatuses. In fact, in quoting Hartmann, Rapaport occasionally substitutes structure for apparatus. Hartmann, on the other hand, favors the term *apparatuses*, most certainly so in his book *Ego Psychology and the Problem of Adaptation* (1939), in which the term *structure* appears only rarely.[6]

Nevertheless, it is in most cases feasible (in the writings of both Hartmann and Rapaport) to use these terms interchangeably without greatly altering the meaning of the statements. Indeed, on page 26 (of the above-mentioned book) Hartmann uses the terms interchangeably. He writes: "An attitude which arose originally in the service of defense against an instinctual drive may, in the

---

6. The index of this book contains only two references, one to structure on page 26 and one to structural development on page 52. There are, nevertheless, throughout the book, two or three other places where it can be found.

course of time, become an *independent structure,* in which case the instinctual drive merely triggers this *automatized apparatus.* . . .*Such an apparatus* may, as a relatively *independent structure,* come to serve . . . " (italics mine).

Further, Hartmann (1964, p. xii) stated that the "differential study of the ego suggests also a broadening of the concept of structure, and it has become meaningful to speak of 'structures in the ego' and of 'structures in the superego.' This refers, in contrast to 'flexibility,' to a relative 'stability' of functions, as it is clearly observable, e.g., in the automatisms." Rapaport (1951a, p. 692f.), on the other hand, while talking of structural givens (existing from the beginning) such as the apparatuses that lay down memory traces, thresholds of tension tolerance, etc., and how these structures are later on embodied in the superorganization that we call the ego, states clearly that "These structures are also referred to as *ego-apparatuses."*

This difference in the usage of or preference for certain terms is characterisitic of other authors as well. Arlow and Brenner, for example, in their book *Psychoanalytic Concepts and the Structural Theory* (1964) mostly manage with the use of terms such as ego apparatus or functions where Rapaport would have used structure. The index of their book does not include the term structure (in Rapaport's more specific sense), though there are a large number of entries listed under structural theory. It is quite interesting that Rapaport appears neither in the index nor in their bibliography. Spitz, in his *A Genetic Field Theory of Ego Formation* (1959), uses the term *structure* in the more general sense implied by terms such as *psychic structure,* although there is no lack of occasional references to structure in Rapaport's more concrete sense (as I shall show below).

It should also be noted that it is not clear how the term *structural theory* came to be coined and generally accepted. References to "structure" are rather sparse even in Freud's *The Ego and the Id* (1923), and the term "structural theory" does not appear there at all.[7]

7. Anna Freud has suggested to me that it was probably Ernst Kris who coined the term. Others commented that the term they heard Ernst Kris use most often was "structural hypothesis," and since such terms were generally used in discussions of "theory," they believe the two were wedded.

With regard to structures Gill (1963, p. 113) says that once one "has been formed it constitutes a fixed organization, so that neither the structure nor the function it regulates undergoes any change." This rigidity of the structures was rightly questioned by Beres (1965, p. 58), but it seems as an unhappy form of expression, since Gill explained in a discussion with Beres that he really means to imply a "slow rate of change." Beres quotes Brierley (1944) whose formulation he prefers: "first, mental organization involves continual reorganization and second, . . . although mental life is conditioned by organization, it is also emergent or new from moment to moment." On this subject Colby (1955) remarks, "One of our great metapsychological problems is how to conceptualize this constancy of change within a constancy of order" (p. 86).

In his monograph Gill (1963) is careful in stating that he will not attempt to discuss what is meant by psychic structures as such (p. 3) and is similarly careful in maintaining a distinction between "mode of function" and "mode of organization." The former refers to a process, the latter to a structure (p. 2 n.).

He introduces two variations of the term structure when he designates id, ego, and superego as *macrostructures* while utilizing the term *microstructures* to refer to relatively stable organizations within the macrostructures, such as memories and ideas (p. 135).[8]

Gill describes what he calls ad hoc functioning, which may take place according to either primary or secondary process. He adds: "When a particular form of discharge becomes regular and habitual, a structure has been formed which regulates discharge of what was at first either primary- or secondary-process *ad hoc* discharge" (p. 113).[9] When a pattern is formed that repeats the pattern of the ad hoc primary- or secondary-process event, a structure has developed that can be referred to as primary- or secondary-process structure. He was explicit in stating that analysts fail to distinguish clearly between functioning regulated by a structure and the ad hoc

8. The term *microstructures* was introduced by Glover in 1948.
9. As I shall discuss later, I regard ad hoc functioning as a result of ad hoc structures, the further vicissitudes of which vary according to circumstances.

psychic functioning (just mentioned) not thus regulated, Beres (1965, p. 57) took exception to this statement because it implies, among other things, that function can take place without structure.[10] Beres asked "whether one can conceive of human psychic function without structure?" Although I believe Beres's objection to be valid, he seems to have overlooked that Gill retraced his steps on the next page of his monograph where the following appears: "It is conceivable that even *ad hoc* discharges are regulated by structures and that what we are accustomed to call the primary-process mechanisms are structures which regulate *ad hoc* primary-process functioning" (p. 114). A similar argument applies, he believes, to secondary-process functioning. Beres similarly objects to mechanisms and processes such as primary and secondary processes being conceptualized as structures because all they really are is a mode of discharge of psychic energy (p. 60).

Gill makes clear that by using the terms primary- and secondary-process structures he does not mean to imply that the structures themselves are thus organized. He means only to refer to the structures that regulate such functioning.

Gill probably takes his lead from Rapaport who also referred to primary-process mechanisms as "structures." In his paper "Psychoanalysis as a Developmental Psychology" (1960b, p. 243), Rapaport, discussing how secondary processes integrate and use primary-process mechanisms, speaks of the difference existing between *structuralized* and *nonstructuralized* primary-process mechanisms. According to him, the essential difference between them is that the structuralized primary-process mechanisms can be integrated by secondary processes, in which case they are energized by more neutralized cathexis than the nonstructuralized primary-process mechanisms. Further he stated: "the primary-process mechanisms (displacement, condensation, substitution) are basically means of immediate drive discharge. In this role they have a structural characteristic, since the discharge attained through them is slower than a discharge which can take place without them. Nevertheless, they are at best *ad hoc*, short-lived

10. This lack of clear distinction between the two possibilities is blamed for the failure to distinguish between a structure and the process or function it regulates.

structures. When they appear in a form which is integrated into the secondary process, their lifetime is increased: they have become further structuralized" (1960b, p. 243, n. 24). One area in which Rapaport believed one can observe structured primary-process mechanisms is in the primitive thought processes of children (p. 245). He maintained to the end that primary-process mechanisms are structures (see, for example, 1960c, p. 128, n. 5).

Spitz (1959) makes a number of interesting links between structural development, the development of specific structures, and his concepts of developmental imbalance and mental organizers such as the smiling response in the third month, or the anxiety response of the eighth month. He says: "When a developmental imbalance is firmly established at one level, then it will modify the pattern of the next major organizer, in conformity with the law of dependent development. Structures which now should emerge may remain absent or emerge in a distorted form. In either case the intra-systemic and the intersystemic relations will be severely impaired or at least modified. Ego apparatuses, ego functions, ego systems will be out of balance, some inhibited, some emphasized. . . . But the process does not end there. If each successive organizer is dependent on the establishment of the structures integrated under normal circumstances through the preceding organizer, then the distortion of the structure pattern of the preceding organizer must lead to a distortion of the subsequent organizing process, whether this distortion be one of delay in time or a compensatory reshuffling of the structures themselves" (p. 93f.).

In referring to the smiling response as the third month organizer he states: "It is as if a number of functions had been brought into relation with each other and linked into a coherent unit. A structural pattern emerges which did not exist before in the psyche. After the establishment of this integration, the response to experience will no longer be in terms of unrelated, discrete components, but in terms of the integrated operation of the unit as a whole" (p. 27). He further clarifies the organizer and its role in terms of psychic structures when he states: "The organizer is a modification of the psychic structure, be that from an undifferentiated to a structured state, or, at the next step, a restructuration of already existing structure on a higher level of complexity" (p. 75).

I have referred earlier to Spitz's more flexible use of the term structure. A good example of it is the following passage when he discusses the many changes in the ego that have taken place by the eighth month of life in relation to the second organizer (eight-month anxiety): "It [the ego] has developed a series of systems [Rapaport probably would have said structures controlling the functions of . . .], like memory, perception, the thought process, the faculty of judgment . . . and ego apparatuses [Rapaport might have used the term structure here too] like the understanding of space, the social gesture, a little later the capacity for locomotion, all of which make the ego a more effective, but also a more complex structure" (p. 42).

Lustman, in his paper on "Impulse Control, Structure, and the Synthetic Function" (1966), makes a number of interesting points concerning the acquisition or failure of acquiring appropriate *controlling structures* (impulse control) during development and, perhaps more important, in the course of therapy. He says: "There can . . . be no doubt that primitive identification processes played a dominant role in the failure of *controlling structures* to emerge . . . and that, in addition to insight, identification processes with the analyst likewise played a part in the subsequent emergence of such *structures* via internalization during the treatment" (p. 200; italics mine). He makes clear that by structuralization of control he means the acquisition of a "stable function highly resistant to change via regression or reinstinctualization" (p. 201), a formulation that I believe can be extended and applied to all structures and not only to those in charge of impulse control. Lustman states that structuralization of a function is linked with stability: "as soon as a function becomes structuralized, i.e., as soon as it begins to function with a degree of stability, its further differentiation will tend to be modified by its own activity, in addition to other forces. . . . Further, this functional differentiation of one structure may very well act as an inducer to other structural development" (p. 203). (Cf. Spitz's views cited above.) In the case Lustman uses to illustrate his propositions, the deficiency in the child's ego structure "was apparent in little or no internalized delaying or controlling substructures, and a fragmentation of other ego functions such as thinking" (p. 202). He clearly suggests how deficient structures or substructures, such as those concerning impulse control, will affect the performance of many ego functions that are dependent on such structures or ego apparatuses.

Although the id is considered one of the "structures" of the personality, there are few references to be found to structures in its realm, unless one includes the primary-process mechanisms as structures (which were mentioned above). Schur (1966) is something of an exception when he says: "The application of the genetic point of view and of the concept of a continuum has also led me to the assumption that the id is structural and has 'content.' Moreover, as we saw earlier, . . . my discussion postulates the maturation and development of the id, a development which was described by Freud after his exposition of the various phases of psychosexual development" (p. 118).[11]

Naturally enough, the structural theory did not escape criticism. As Arlow and Brenner (1964, p. 2) point out, these criticisms may apply only to specific aspects of the structural formulations or, in some cases, may go as far as a preference for the "topographical theory;" and in still others, the need is felt for a completely new formulation that will take the place of both the topographical and structural models of the mind.

Among the more recent exponents of such criticisms are Apfelbaum (1962, 1965, 1966), Loewald (1952, 1960), Colby (1955),[12] Kubie (1958), White (1963), and even Glover (1961). A discussion of their criticism of the structural theory as a whole (such as that of Kubie) or of specific aspects of it, either in Freud's formulation or in those of Hartmann, Kris, Loewenstein, Gill, Brenner, Arlow, Anna Freud, Rapaport, and many others would be beyond the scope of this chapter.

My own view is closer to that of Hartmann, Gill and even that of

11. Colby (1955) too has argued against the idea of lack of structure in the id, as I have mentioned earlier.

12. Colby has in fact proposed an alternative model of the psychic apparatus that he has named a cyclic-circular model. He does not deny the usefulness of the structural theory in a clinical setting but considers it insufficient from the theorist point of view. According to the author, his model is particularly useful in terms of the interrelation of the basic postulates of psychic energy and structure.

Arlow and Brenner, without going as far as proposing a complete and total abandonment of the topographical theory as the last two authors do. To my mind there is much in that earlier model that can be retranslated into the structural one and thereby enrich it.

If we speak in terms of structures rather than apparatuses or functions, it is necessary to postulate the existence from the very beginning of life of a number of ready-made primitive structures or organizations in charge of primitive mental processes that deal with the regulation of early perceptual activities, the laying down of memory traces, and certain motoric activities, etc. This is completely in line with Hartmann's assumptions of inborn ego apparatuses belonging to the conflict-free sphere. In fact, it is only another way of stating exactly the same set of problems. These structures exist at birth, while most other structures have to be created during development; that is, further structuralization is taking place all the time as development proceeds.

SOME IMPLICATIONS FOR A THEORY OF LEARNING AND CREATIVITY

In these processes of further structuralization[13] a number of factors are involved. There is, first of all, the ongoing physical maturation of the physical structures or somatic apparatuses on the basis of which ego functions will become possible. In humans, however, an equally important role is played by experience and learning. Physical maturation per se will allow only a certain (unknown) level of performance in terms of the ego, a level that is then raised by the essential contribution made to the development of ego functions by the processes of learning and experiencing. Thus, for example, we have to learn to perceive or to organize percepts in a meaningful way before we are capable of exercising the function of perception (in the sense of apperception) as we know that function in the adult. "Experiments of nature" involving persons born blind with congenital cataracts or corneal lesions, later remedied by grafts of the cornea, have shown that when

13. One could also say: acquisition of new apparatuses or functions.

sight is restored, the reception of visual stimuli coming from the different objects does not allow for the recognition (apperception) of such objects. The sensations produced by the objects are registered but remain meaningless until the person learns to perceive them, that is, to organize the perception according to a system that makes apperception possible. Clearly, this requires a multiplicity of interaction of ego functions and apparatuses in specific hierarchical orders, an ability that is normally acquired in the early years of life through experimentation, trial and error, experiencing, and learning. What applies to perception persumably applies to most other complex ego functions. It is possible to assume that in the absence of experiencing and learning opportunities (a completely hypothetical situation) the somatic apparatuses would only be able to register the stimuli in ways that are not completely clear to us but that include in many cases an awareness of an impression or sensation and the laying down of a memory trace.

Learning, as used by me here, refers not only to learning facts about the environment and its objects, or learning about the subject; but, even more important, it includes learning to use the mental apparatus as it develops, learning to combine in an infinite number of ways the different functions of which it is capable. The combination of various functions in specific ways (that have to be learned) enables the mental apparatus to perform any number of new functions, suitable for the solution of ever more difficult problems confronting the organism. When such a combination of functions in a predetermined sequence or hierarchical functional order proves a suitable tool to deal with specific problems, or specific aspects of external or internal reality that frequently confront the human being, a new ego apparatus (to use Hartmann's term), a new psychological structure (to use Rapaport's term) has been acquired, one that is capable of dealing with the specific aspects of internal or external reality.[14] It is to be

14. Hartmann (1939) has expressed a similar view: "Ego development is a differentiation, in which these primitive regulating factors are increasingly replaced or supplemented by more effective ego regulations. . . . Differentiation progresses not only by the creation of new apparatuses to master new demands and new tasks but also and mainly by new apparatuses taking over, on a higher level, functions which were originally performed by more primitive means" (p. 49f.).

presumed that such processes of structuralization of creating new ego apparatuses, are never-ending processes, although their rate of development is of course by far the greatest in the early years of life.

Three factors seem to be relevant as determinants of the rate and extent of structuralization that is acquired. First, there are innate limitations which account to some extent for interindividual differences in general, and for differences in the individual's abilities in certain specific areas. There can be little doubt that differences in the inborn qualities of the different somatic structures play some role. Secondly, human needs and human nature partly determine the degree of structuralization required. Our instinctual equipment is not such that we can satisfy our needs according to rigid "instinctual patterns"; rather, we are in most cases dependent on intelligent behavior for their satisfaction; moreover, our mental apparatus is itself sufficiently complex to allow for such learning and intelligent responses. Thirdly, there is the question of the environment into which we happen to be born. The demands of a highly civilized society are much greater in these respects than those of a primitive one. The adaptation to a high degree of civilization demands a greater extent in ego structuralization.

In describing the performance of the mental apparatus of an adult or child, we ought to distinguish between ad hoc performances activated to deal with a single new problem just once and more automatized performances utilized to deal with problems which we encounter regularly and for the solution of which we have developed specific ad hoc psychological structures or ad hoc psychological ego apparatuses. This is not a purely academic question but seems to me to be relevant in terms of our conceptualization of structures, intelligence, learning processes, and preconscious automatisms.

Let us imagine the hypothetical situation of a child of three or four years who is for the first time confronted with the task of learning to add and who is presented, for example, with the problem that 1+1=2. He has to master a new situation and faces for the first time the task of mastering a number of new conceptual propositions and abstractions (I am assuming that the child is not just memorizing the figures but attempting to master the conceptual problems involved and posed to him). The child at that age has available a large number of structures (or ego apparatuses) capable of performing a variety of functions. What he has to do to master the new situation is to combine the function of several such structures (or ego apparatuses) until he hits on a combination that produces the desired result in terms of insight, i.e., one allowing him to understand and master the conceptual problems involved. The combination of the structures thus selected (in whatever hierarchical functional order) constitutes a new and ad hoc structure. Before the right combination of structures is produced for the solution of the specific new problem, several unsuitable combinations presumably are tried out until partly through trial and error, partly perhaps through intelligent selection, the correct combination is produced.[15] In any case the scanning process performed by the ego for the selection of the most suitable of the available structures or ego apparatuses (and in what combinations) is one of the most important functions of which it is capable. I suggest calling it the *functional-coordinative function of the ego*.[16]

The situation I have described above applies whenever a human being, child or adult, is presented with a completely new task, with a new set of problems requiring solution. Further, since intel-

15. The older child has a greater variety of structures at his command. The more experience the child has acquired in the solution of problems, the more intelligent selection by the ego of the suitable structures becomes possible, but trial and error can always be restored to when intelligent selection fails.

16. The *functional-coordinative function* of the ego must not be confused with Nunberg's synthetic function (1930) or with the *organizing function* of the ego, a term that Hartmann considers more appropriate (1947, p. 62). Hartmann has described the synthetic or organizing function as "the constant balancing of these three systems [id, ego, superego] against each other as well as the checking of demands of the outer world against those of the psychic systems" (p. 62f.). See also Hartmann (1948, p. 86; 1950, pp. 115 and 138; 1959, p. 329). The functional-coordinative function only scans for the right combination of *the resources available within the system ego*, in terms of the appropriate structures or ego apparatuses (and their possible combinations), so as to find the best combination for the solution of the problem posed. But this is a solution in ego terms only and need not have taken into consideration the demands of the other two systems, id and superego. It is conceivable that in many cases the synthetic function—whose task it is to take these demands into account—works over the results of the functional-coordinative function once they have been put forward, while in many others both functions operate simultaneously.

ligence is frequently defined as the capacity to solve new problems, it follows that the quality of this special function of the ego is an essential aspect of it, as are the number and quality of structures available to this functional-coordinative function.

When the child has produced the suitable combination for the mastery of the new conceptual problems and their solution, he has created, as I said above, a new and ad hoc structure. The fate of such ad hoc structures is variable. Once they have served their particular purpose they may never be required again, unless the same or related conceptual problems arise again. Thus, they can be transitory in nature, although the ego now has the potential ability to re-create such a structure if necessity arises; that is, the ego has enriched itself, its functional possibilities. If, as in the case of the mathematical problem referred to earlier, the conceptual problems involved are frequently met by the child's ego, the structure becomes perfected and a permanent feature of the ego organization.[17] Adding up, the solution of this and related types of mathematical problems is a task that confronts the ego frequently. The permanent structure that is thus established within the ego organization is the appropriate tool or instrument (in fact, a new ego apparatus) for the solution of a group of related problems. But the establishment of such a new structure or ego apparatus performs another important role, that is, its existence enables the ego to develop further and to solve problems of increasing complexity, since the newly acquired structure can be taken as a fresh point of departure and reference for other more sophisticated ones. A "permanent structure" of this type soon becomes, functionally speaking, automatized to a high degree insofar as it is constantly used for the solution fo the specific problems it is meant to deal with. On the other hand, it can still be used when required to contribute to the building up of ad hoc structures for the solution of new specific problems presented to the ego in new ad hoc combinations. What I wish to highlight in all this is the sharp contrast between the ego's extreme flexibility and freedom to

17. This is perhaps a good example of Rapaport's "stimulus-nutriment" referred to above; that is, a case in which environmental stimulation of a sort contributes if not to the maintenance of a permanent psychological structure at least to its perfection and readiness.

recombine the available structures to produce ad hoc solutions to new problems by means of ad hoc structures having only a temporary character, and the ego's simultaneous use of the same structures for its specific aims in more rigid, automatized fashion. Intelligent behavior and all learning processes are naturally highly dependent on the former ability.[18]

There are, speaking relatively, no limits to the number of new problems that can be presented to the human mind, especially if we take into account that the solution of a scientific problem or question simultaneously raises a number of other problems and questions that in turn require more answers. Just as there seems to be no limit (for all practical purposes) to the number of problems that can be presented to the ego, there seems to be no limit (again for all practical purposes) to the number of structures, or *functional combinations,* that the ego can produce in order to deal with them.

The role that the process of adaptation (of the individual and of the species) plays in this must not be underestimated. As I said, we are constantly confronted with new problems as we go along in the solution of old ones. Moreover, man is capable of modifying his environment, and these modifications frequently carry with them the need to adapt to new changed conditions and the solution of sometimes new and unsuspected problems. The modifications I have in mind here refer not only to the physical conditions of his milieu and their multiple derivations but to those in our social, political, philosophical, and even religious systems.

It is in the nature of physical conditions to change constantly and it is precisely the nature of the human mind (or mental apparatuses)—its flexibility and man's ability to produce adaptive solutions—that partly guarantee survival. Thus, there is no limit to the potential number of ego functions, just as there is no limit to the number of *psychological ego apparatuses*—or, if we prefer it, to the number of structures—that can be created within the ego organization to deal with new problems.

18. I believe it is abundantly clear from the discussion so far that terms such as "psychological ego apparatus" and "psychological structures" can be, and frequently are, used synonymously in the psychoanalytic literature.

In the course of civilization the human species has developed a number of functional structures (psychological ego apparatuses) that were required to deal with the new changing conditions. As civilization progresses and is itself structured first by tradition, later by education and organized transmission of knowledge, the establishment of political, social, and religious institutions, in short, as civilization becomes more complex, it makes further demands on the ego's capabilities to deal with the ever-increasing complexity of propositions of the new order of things. (Freud's statement about the child having to achieve in a brief period of time what took civilization thousands of years to accomplish is relevant here.) From this point of view education as we know it today is, among other things, the system devised to teach children in a condensed and simplified manner the means by which they can build complex psychological ego apparatuses capable of dealing with the complexities created in our world. All education does is to exercise a number of mental capabilities in special directions and combinations until the ego learns to perform a number of complicated functions in interaction.

The multiple interacting functions required to achieve the ego's aims follow a logical system, an order, a sequence. There is a hierarchy in the functional order and interaction. Slowly, we teach the child how to establish a *functional structure,* which, once learned, has an independence of its own and enables him to deal with a particular aspect of reality in an economic and systematic fashion. In fact, we have by this means established a new *psychological ego apparatus* to deal with specific problems. This process is repeated ad infinitum by education (including formal schooling and informal general education of the young by society in general, and parents in particular) and covers a mulitplicity of areas in human development. Nevertheless, it will be true to say that, in most cases and with respect to what I have referred to here as informal education, we have no explicit awareness of having such aims (of furthering the development of certain psychological ego apparatuses) since these aims are implicit in the social order we have developed.

If we take the training of a physicist, a mathematician, an

engineer, etc., a similar process is in action. In fact, we are teaching him an abbreviated form of what took thousands of years to develop and required the minds of innumerable outstanding men. We are trying to develop in him specialized ego apparatuses capable of performing the complex activities required for the solution of a number of specific types of problems. This is, of course, a special case; but adaptation to the conditions of our special environment requires the development of a number of educated men in the community are quite capable of assimilating individuals) if we are to function within normal limits in that environment.

The nature and the quality of such structures or ego apparatuses will vary greatly according to the level of civilization and the specific requirements of a given milieu. The ego function and apparatus of perception of a primitive savage living in the jungle will obviously be inadequate to cope with stimuli in the streets of London, while those of the Londoner will be similarly poorly adapted to the conditions of the jungle.

Finally, I want to call attention to a significant difference between human beings that is highlighted by my form of presentation. I refer now to the difference between those with highly creative minds and the ordinary members of the community, as well as to the significance of the creative process itself. Most educated men in the community are quite capable of assimilating and mastering the complexities involved in a new scientific advance, but few of them possess the capacity to unravel the secrets that have to be unraveled for scientific progress to take place. Only a limited number of people seem to have this ability developed to an exceptional degree, and they are the pioneers of scientific progress.

Thus, once a new and revolutionary step forward is taken, for example, in science, due to the efforts of a particular scientist, we are in a postion to impart that new knowledge to many members of our community. We can teach them, so to say, the steps that are necessary to organize the different psychological structures in the right hierarchical functional order for the mastery of the new discovery. There is indeed little difficulty in doing this; and yet, as

I pointed out, very few, if any of those able to learn it, would have been capable of solving the riddle themselves, however hard they may have tried. Thus it seems (leaving aside "chance discoveries," if such a thing does exist) that exceptional creative capacity is in part related to the special qualities and flexibility of that function of the ego that scans, combines, and recombines the functions of any number of psychological structures in the search for the solution of a problem, a capacity that presumably is associated with special sets of motivations.

References

Apfelbaum, B. (1962). Some problems in contemporary ego psychology. *Journal of the American Psychoanalytic Association* 10:526-537.

——— (1965). Ego psychology, psychic energy, and the hazards of the quantative explanation in psycho-analytic theory. *International Journal of Psychoanalysis* 46:168-182.

——— (1966). On ego psychology: a critique of the structural approach to psycho-analytic theory. *International Journal of Psychoanalysis* 47:451-475.

Arlow, J. A. and Brenner, C. (1964). *Psychoanalytic Concepts and the Structural Theory*. New York: International Universities Press.

Beres, D. (1965). Structure and function in psycho-analysis. *International Journal of Psychoanalysis* 46:53-63.

Colby, K. M. (1955). *Energy and Structure in Psychoanalysis*. New York: Ronald Press.

Freud, S. (1915). The unconscious. *Standard Edition* 14:159-218.

——— (1923). The ego and the id. *Standard Edition* 19:3-68.

Gill, M. M. (1963). *Topography and Systems in Psychoanalytic Theory* [*Psychological Issues, Monograph 10*]. New York: International Universities Press.

Glover, E. (1948). The future development of psychoanalysis. In *On the Early Development of Mind*, pp. 333-351. New York: International Universities Press, 1956.

——— (1961). Some recent trends in psychoanalytic theory. *Psychoanalytic Quarterly* 30:86-107.

Hartmann, H. (1939). *Ego Psychology and the Problem of Adaptation*. New York: International Universities Press, 1958.

——— (1947). On rational and irrational action. In *Essays on Ego*

Psychology. pp. 37-68. New York: International Universities Press, 1964.

——— (1948). Comments on the psychoanalytic theory of instinctual drives. In *Essays on Ego Psychology,* pp. 69-89. New York: International Universities Press, 1964.

——— (1950). Comments on the psychoanalytic theory of the ego. In *Essays on Ego Psychology,* pp. 113-141. New York: International Universities Press, 1964.

——— (1959). Psychoanalysis as a scientific theory. In *Essays on Ego Psychology,* pp. 318-350.

——— (1964). *Essays on Ego Psychology: Selected Problems in Psychoanalytic Theory.* New York: International Universities Press.

Holt, R. R. (1965). Ego autonomy re-evaluated. *International Journal of Psychoanalysis* 46:151-167.

Kubie, L. S. (1958). *Neurotic Distortion of the Creative Process.* Lawrence, Kansas: University of Kansas Press.

Lewis, W. C. (1965). Structural aspects of the psychoanalytic theory of instinctual drives, affects, and time. In *Psychoanalysis and Current Biological Thought,* ed. N. S. Greenfield and W. C. Lewis, pp. 151-180. Madison and Milwaukee: University of Wisconsin Press.

Loewald, H. W. (1952). The problem of defence and the neurotic interpretation of reality. *International Journal of Psychoanalysis* 33:444-449.

——— (1960). On the therapeutic action of psycho-analysis. *International Journal of Psychoanalysis* 41:16-33.

Lustman, S. L. (1966). Impulse control, structure, and the synthetic function. In *Psychoanalysis—A General Psychology: Essays in Honor of Heinz Hartmann,* ed. R. M. Loewenstein, L. M. Newman, M. Schur, and A. J. Solnit, pp. 190-221. New York: International Universities Press.

Miller, G. C. (1962). Ego-autonomy in sensory deprivation, isolation and stress. *International Journal of Psychiatry* 43:1-20.

Nunberg, H. (1930). The synthetic function of the ego. In *Practice and Theory of Psychoanalysis,* 1:120-136. New York: International Universities Press, 1960.

Rapaport, D. (1951a). *Organization and Pathology of Thought.* New York: Columbia University Press.

——— (1951b). The autonomy of the ego. *Bulletin of the Menninger Clinic* 15:113-123.

——— (1957). Cognitive Structures. In *Contemporary Approaches to Cognition,* pp. 157-200. Cambridge: Harvard University Press.

——— (1958). The theory of ego autonomy: a generalization. *Bulletin of the Menninger Clinic* 22:13-25.

——— (1960a). On the psychoanalytic theory of motivation. In *Nebraska Symposium on Motivation*, ed. M. R. Jones, pp. 173-247. Lincoln: University of Nebraska Press.

——— (1960b). Psychoanalysis as a developmental psychology. In *Perspectives in Psychological Theory*, ed. B. Kaplan and S. Wapner, pp. 210-256. New York: International Universities Press.

——— (1960c). *The Structure of Psychoanalytic Theory Psychological Issues*, Monograph 6. New York: International Universities Press.

Schur, M. (1966). *The Id and the Regulatory Principles of Mental Functioning*. New York: International Universities Press.

Spitz, R. A. (1959). *A Genetic Field Theory of Ego Formation*. New York: International Universities Press.

White, R. W. (1963). *Ego and Reality in Psychoanalytic Theory, Psychological Issues*, Monograph 11. New York: International Universities Press.

Chapter Ten

THE CONTRIBUTION OF SIGHT TO EGO AND DRIVE DEVELOPMENT

This study is based on six blind children observed in our Unit for the Blind. It is an attempt to organize and describe by means of the Profile headings what was learned during "periods of observation," analytic treatment, and diagnostic profiles about this group of children. For each of the children a developmental profile (see chapter 1) was prepared and discussed in the Profile Research Group at the Hampstead Clinic.

At the time of the assessment the children ranged in age from four to eight and a half years; four of them were between five and six years; one was four, and the other was eight and a half years.

A brief description of the children's history of blindness follows:

George (5;3 years). Pregnancy was normal, born in hospital. Nothing was said to the parents about eyes at this time, though, according to the father, there was no pupil present in the left eye from birth. First seen at Moorfields in December, 1957 at age 2 months, when examination under anesthesia showed that he had a mass in the right fundus and the left eye was large and prominent with a raised intraocular tension and hazy cornea. It was thought that the right fundus picture was not that of a neoplasm but probably of developmental or inflammatory pathology. The tension of the left eye remained high and the globe increased;

Written in collaboration with Alice B. Colonna

therefore, in March, 1958, the left eye was enucleated. Histology of the eye showed a chronic endophthalmitis. Since then, the right eye has been kept under observation regularly; the mass in the right eye showed no change in size and tension was normal. It is difficult to assess accurately George's visual acuity at present.

Joan (4;6 years). Totally blind as a result of high concentration of oxygen. Born prematurely (30 weeks). Retrolental fibroplasia.

Gillian (4;6 years). Retrolental fibroplasia, blind from birth. Born by Caesarian section. Mother very ill during pregnancy, child's weight at birth 3 lbs.; spent 9 weeks in oxygen tent. When the child was 10 weeks old the mother was told that Gillian was blind.

Helen (4;6 years). Helen was born prematurely (at 20 weeks), had little sight afterwards, remaining sight was lost when she had measles, at age of 3. Mother had three miscarriages, but Helen was the first pregnancy. Weight 2 lbs. at birth in an incubator for 102 days, at which time she weighed 5 lbs. and was taken home. When she came home her mother went to a home for a week.

Winnie 7 years). Congenital cataract. Born 1 month premature (weight 6 lbs. 1 oz.) (not in oxygen tent).

Janet (8;6 years). Blind from birth, pseudoglioma, eyes removed at 4 months.

Speaking very generally, we have had the opportunity to observe two very different possibilities of development among children who are born blind and we include here as well children who may have become blind very early in life, perhaps soon after birth). In a small number of such cases their development, in spite of their blindness, does not seem to lag much behind the development of sighted children. Their ego processes, their drive development, their object relationships are not too far behind those of the sighted of similar ages. In another very distinct group, one finds blind children whose developmental processes are atypical. They lag behind in different degrees in the different areas, giving in some extreme cases the impression of a marked mental retardation. These two types are the two extremes on a scale with all sorts of possible combinations in between.

The cases we are referring to here belong mostly in the second group; they show a specific clinical and developmental picture which they have in common with many other blind-born[1] but which is by no means representative of the developmental possibilities of all blind-born children.

We further believe that the study of these two different groups of children born blind may teach us a great deal about how some overcome their handicap to a degree that brings them closer to the level of the sighted. Even when the blind grow up under the most favorable circumstances (which are rarely encountered) in terms of ego endowment, good early mothering, reasonable environmental conditions, favorable object relations, etc., there is a point at which the development of one or another ego function clearly requires a contribution from the side of vision. When that contribution is not available, a disruption in the development of a specific function ensues. In turn, the insufficiency of these functions or of other aspects of the ego leads to further developmental interferences in all areas in which such functions are a necessary prerequisite. A somewhat similar point of view was expressed by A.-M. Sandler (1963) and by Fraiberg and Freedman (1964). It seems to us that this state of affairs can be somewhat alleviated by the environment, its handling of and attitude to the blind and their problems. It can make a postitive contribution to the blind child's development by teaching him directly and at the right points the suitable alternative means of compensating for the lack of sight. Left to itself the ego of the blind may never achieve this, or only do so through long and painful detours and at much later stages. It may well be that some of the differences in development of the two groups of blind we are describing are related to these very factors.[2] Thus, the observation of the means by which the blind child's ego finds alternative solutions can give us clues to the

1. See, for example, some of the cases reported in the recent literature by Omwake and Solnit (1961), Segal and Stone (1961).

2. We are planning a close study of the group of blind children that develops more like the normal in the hope of clarifying some of the problems here posed.

kind of teaching and handling required at the different development points at which help may be needed to stimulate further
development.

In our study we have made special efforts to single out those
aspects of development and personality which are specific to blind
children—in which they differ from sighted children. In this way
we hope in time to be able to understand the nature of the
contribution sight makes to normal ego development and how
much blindness can distort it. Though our study is based primarily on the six children described above, we have also checked
relevant material of a large group of other blind children to verify
certain aspects of our formulations. These formulations are nevertheless to be considered as tentative. The study of more cases will
either confirm or modify them. With growing insight into the
developmental processes of the blind new formulations may become necessary.

As previously stated, we shall present our formulations in terms
of the relevant headings of the developmental profile introduced
by Anna Freud (1962).

THE DRIVE DEVELOPMENT OF THE BLIND

Libidinal Development

All the cases studied show that the blind develop in this area at a
much slower pace than the sighted child.

Helen's profile at five years eight months showed that even at that age
there were no significant signs of her being in the phallic phase and no
indication of oedipal development. There is a great deal of oral activity
that finds direct expression in the sucking of objects and in the way she
devours food and drink. She sometimes spits them out. Drooling is still
observable. Anal messy behavior is noted in her intense enjoyment in
pouring water or powder on the floor in a provocative manner.

Janet, at eight and a half, showed no signs of latency. The material
contained only tenuous indications of her having reached the phallic

phase, but oral and anal activities are still very prominent, including rinsing of her mouth and spitting; she does a great deal of mouthing (which is partly an ego exploratory activity); anal masturbation was noted during her analytic sessions. She pulls at her knickers and skirt and places her index finger in her anus. She comments on smells and noises, frequently passes wind and once soiled herself in doing so. There are endless and repetitive games and fantasies of other children soiling and wetting themselves and having to clean up the mess. Water play is accompanied by fantasies of mother forcing her to defecate and of other children soiling and wetting and being smacked.

Even more striking perhaps is the fact that this group of blind children in marked contrast to the sighted children, seems incapable of leaving behind the previous phases when a new developmental move occurs. The move into the phallic-oedipal phase does not at all imply that drive gratification and autoerotic activities pertaining to the anal and oral phase will tend to disappear or even to recede notably into the background. On the contrary, marked activity of the anal and oral stages is always observed simultaneously with the newly found phallic-oedipal forms of drive gratification. This can best be illustrated in the case of Winnie.

At the time she came into analytic treatment (at the age of three) there were clear manifestations of active libidinal interests on the anal and oral levels of libidinal development. After five months of treatment, Winnie progressed into the phallic-oedipal phase, as the following material illustrates. Envy of little boys made its appearance and began to be openly expressed. She made clear what she wanted to do to them by attempts at dismembering dolls with much giggling. The dolls previously called "girl doll" were now "boy dolls." On one occasion when her envy of boys was verbalized, she strutted around the room with a boy doll held between her legs, saying, "Look what I got stuck up my fanny." She expressed wishes to sleep with her brother-in-law, Martin. Nevertheless, and in spite of this move, there remained a great deal of anal and oral concerns which were expressed in her fear of messing, her discomfort due to constipation, her use of anal swearwords, and her attempts to seduce her therapist to "smell" her fanny. Similarly noticeable were her strong ambivalent (anal-sadistic) feelings toward objects.

It may perhaps be concluded that blindness can so much interfere with finding new means of gratification both in drive discharge and ego activities that any form of gratification once
experienced is not easily abandoned or left behind, even when
further developmental steps are taken by the blind child; all earlier
forms of gratification remain ego syntonic. We shall come back to
this point.

Cathexis of Self

Self-esteem regulation. In this area our group of blind differs
from normally sighted children in that the blind have a more
marked and presumably longer period of dependence on the
external world in order to maintain the cathexis of themselves at a
level compatible with well-being. In many of the children we have
studied and observed in our Nursery for the Blind, this extreme
dependence upon the object world is further shown in an inability
to maintain their own self-esteem and cathexis of the self when the
object world withdraws cathexis from them.

When Winnie's mother was depressed, Winnie suffered a loss of the
feeling of well-being and tended to become immobilized, particularly so
at the nursery, where she also retreated from interaction with the other
children. However, she showed very different behavior in the treatment
situation, where she was able to enjoy a one-to-one relationship with the
full attention of the therapist concentrated on herself. Thus, she was
often verbal and active in treatment, while in school she appeared
withdrawn and involved in manneristic gestures.

Cathexis of object. It seems clear from our observations that
even apparently retarded blind children can reach object constancy and can relate to the object world on that level. On the other
hand, they may not completely leave behind the other phases and
will sometimes relate to and use the objects on a need-fulfilling
basis. Indeed, they tend to move forward and backward from the
one to the other phase quite frequently.

They sometimes give the impression that they readily and easily
exchange objects, even for unfamiliar ones, as if object constancy
had not been properly established.

A more careful examination of the facts will support the view that, owing to the lack of sight, the blind child experiences extreme anxiety when someone is not nearby to protect him. The blind child, fully aware through experience of the very many dangers around and of his inability to care for himself in the absence of a protective object, tends to cling to anyone present when the familiar or dearest objects are, for wharerver reason, not available. It is presumably this attitude, which in fact serves self-presevation, that leads to the false impression that some blind children are not attached to their objects on the level of object constancy. We have noted that the blind group we studied shows a strong tendency to comply with the wishes of their important objects and especially with those of the mother. This is carried to extremes that are hardly observable in sighted children of the same age.

Aggression

We have formed the impression that these blind children show a tendency to inhibit any form of overt expression of aggression against those objects on whom they are dependent. The fact that they do inhibit aggression in this specific way may not be apparent to the casual observer who may easily gain the impression that the children's behavior is quite aggressive. This misunderstanding of the real circumstances is due to two factors.

First, many of these blind children are still largely at the anal-sadistic stage of libido development. Winnie, for example, was fully at the anal-sadistic stage and behaved accordingly; it is true that descriptively, i.e., to an observer, behavior of this type may seem extremely aggressive, but it is in fact the phase-adequate expression and type of relationship of children in that phase. The extreme ambivalence of the anal-sadistic phase allows us to see, for example, the child's expressions of love followed by violent biting. It may be profitable to distinguish this type of phase-adequate expression of the aggressive drive from aggressive behavior as a more organized type of response which is phase independent; the blind child's inhibition is of the second type.

The second factor concerns the child's relationship with other children. In Winnie's case one must take into consideration that on the line of development "from egocentricity to companionship" (A. Freud 1963) she has not yet developed any empathy for other children's feelings; consequently they can be used freely for the expression of her strong ambivalence. This type of aggressive behavior must be distinguished from the later forms where the aggressive act is carried out with full awareness of its effect on the other child.

Although Winnie was able to express open aggression to the therapist in the "permissive situation" of the treatment, it was not quite the same in relation to other objects or in other environments. In the nursery, for example, Winnie rarely made aggressive assaults; during a period in which she was unusually destructive in her sessions (throwing bottles, breaking glass, lashing out at the therapist, etc.), she was described at the nursery school as moving less freely, with a bad posture, "as though she were carrying the cares of the world on her shoulders," and indeed she presented the picture of a depressed child. Similarly, she rarely expressed openly aggressive, hostile impulses toward her mother. On one occasion when she did, after playing out having been nagged by her mother for making too much noise, she said, "What have you done with your mummy, did you throw her in the muck bin?" The next day, she snuggled up to the therapist and said, "But I wouldn't really do that; I'm a helpful girl, I help mummy."

In this way, she behaved very much as other blind children do, that is, with a marked inhibition of the expression of aggression. This is due partly to the fear of losing the favor and love of the object, a fear that is immediately transformed into a fear of annihilation caused by the extreme dependence on objects for reasons of safety.

In Winnie's case we noted that it was important for her "to hear" the result of her aggressive actions (breaking objects, glass, etc.), but we have not been able to confirm that this applies generally to other blind children. Some instances of very disturbed behavior which takes place in moments of regression provoked by current difficulties at home, in school, etc., may be wrongly interpreted as object-directed aggression. In fact, some of these manifestations are the panic reactions of an overwhelmed ego; they lead to disorganized behavior and other primitive expressions of the infant stage such as crying, throwing things at random, etc.

THE EGO OF THE BLIND

The consistent and systematic study of the personality of a number of blind children, by means of the application of the developmental profile, has forced us to conclude that there is an unwarranted readiness to interpret their peculiarities of behavior, fantasies, symptoms, etc., in the same light and on the same basis as those of sighted, normal, or neurotic children.

Thus, we proceed in our assessments as if the blind were ordinary children except for their lack of sight. This may be so when the loss of sight has taken place late in the child's life, when his development in every direction may have been fairly well advanced. Clearly, when the child's lack of sight dates from birth or early babyhood, drive and ego development proceeds in atypical and distorted ways. The correlations valid for the sighted between surface (behavioral material) and depth (unconscious determinants and meaning) are not directly applicable to the blind. Many of the pointers, indicators, clinical evaluations, etc., on which we can rely with a fair degree of certainty in assessing the sighted child's personality and neurotic conflicts are unreliable instruments in the evaluation of the blind.

Many of the blind children we have studied tend to show a marked fear of animals and noises. Helen feared dogs, horses, birds, and noises. Janet feared thunder, rain, wind, trains, drilling machines, dogs, etc. When these fears occur in sighted children of a comparable age, they can be taken as a sure indication of an area of disturbance, of specific conflicts, of clear defense activity, and symptom formation. In the sighted child of a given age, the presence of fear or phobic avoidance of certain animals such as birds, horses, dogs, etc., entitles us to assume that the animal stands for the oedipal rival and that the fear of being attacked by it is the result of the child's projecting his own aggressive feelings onto the hated rival.

In the case of the blind it is frequently very difficult to determine how much of the above behavior or symptomatology is the result of defense activity against the drives, i.e., the result of conflict, and how much is in fact appropriate adaptive behavior (in terms of survival) in a child who lacks vision. Here one has to remind oneself that when a blind child hears a barking dog he cannot see whether the dog is big or small, whether it is playful or hostile, whether it intends to bite or not.

The same viewpoint applies to the blind child's unusual degree of clinging to and dependence on the object at an age when he would normally be expected to have outgrown this type of relationship. In the sighted of the same age such clinging constitutes a clear indication either of important fixation points at the oral level or of defense activity directed against certain specific conflict situations. In the blind this extreme clinging and dependence, as already mentioned, are characteristic for a long period of life. Rather than being the result of defense activity, they may be another sign of the complex pattern of ego adaptation to a sighted world.

Other pieces of behavior characteristic of the blind, like their withdrawal (into fantasy or otherwise), their passivity, etc., can be understood in a similar way.

The sighted adult who has learned to cope with the ordinary conditions of his immediate environment experiences "fear of reality" only in the face of true danger situations. For him, it is practically impossible to imagine the state of extreme helplessness and anxiety of the blind child, for whom a great deal of the external world represents dangers that he is ill equipped to master. The blind child is swamped by constant waves of anxiety derived from an unending variety of occurrences which are incompletely understood or wrongly interpreted.

This state of permanent alertness to external dangers which have to be mastered seems to occupy the child's mind to a degree which outweighs the importance of the internal dangers, represented by the impulses and other drive representatives. Compared with the dreaded hazards of the environment, the inner world is a source of safety and gratification to the blind child. It is this combination of factors (fear of the external, retreat to the internal world) which may explain the marked delay in the mastery and control of drive activity which we observe in our blind children.

On the other hand, the children's fantasy life seemed extremely limited in comparison with the richness of imagination and fantasy production of the sighted (either normal or neurotic) of similar ages, a fact which may be due, of course, to the comparatively low level of ego development of the group of children studied. Fantasy production, as a well-known prestage of neurotic symptom formation in children and adults, usually represents the withdrawl from an unpleasant external reality which interferes with processes of drive gratification. The blind children, in spite of their most unpleasant external reality, cannot afford to withdraw from it. Only constant surveillance, with the alternative senses at their disposal, will avoid unpleasant, hurtful experiences. Consequently many of their mental activities consist of attempts to master through repetition and in imagination the many painful situations which they have experienced.[3] No less important is the fact, mentioned above, that the blind child allows himself a great deal of direct drive gratification which may make the function of fantasy less vital for him.

As regards the development of certain ego functions in the blind, it is important to note that their ego performance can be extremely unreliable even in cases of reasonably well-established functions. Most important in this respect is the ease with which anxiety can become overwhelming and traumatic and result in the temporary collapse of otherwise well-established functions.

Thus it was frequently observed than when in distress, danger, or in extreme anxiety, many of the children would become immobile. Winnie, for example, became immobile to the extreme of being rigid. This immobility may well be a response learned very

3. D. Burlingham (1964) has pointed to a piece of behavior that is often misleading. To the casual observer the blind children frequently appear to be fully withdrawn into passivity when in fact behind this facade there is an extremely active listening and a close attention to what goes on in the environment.

early in order to protect themselves from further pain, damage, or dangers.

Immobility in blind children was observed as well when they were introduced to a new environment. For a short while they tended to remain still in order to orient themselves, perceiving and collecting as much information as possible through the appropriate sense organs, especially the ear.

In the cases studied, walking started at any time between thirteen months and three years, the parental attitude to the child being a significant factor in connection with this function. Winnie started walking at thirteen months. She did not crawl but used to turn round and round on her behind, then pulling herself up. The father used to help her by walking alongside. Helen began walking at eighteen months without previous crawling. She was given a large doll to push and in this way began to walk. George walked by twenty months; Joan at two years without having ever crawled before; while Janet did not sit up until she was two years, crawled at two and half years, and walked at three years of age.

The following examples illustrate the blind child's use of ego functions in the service of adaptation to the world around him.[4]

Winnie relied on other sensory modalities to orient herself in and explore the environment, and for her own stimulation. Her reliance on tactile sensations was great (e.g., feeling the bumps on the windowpane, stroking a new object with her cheek). She also used her head as a drum knocking an object against her temples, which would seem to involve both tactile and auditory sensations. She enjoyed being barefooted and explored her environment in this way. Her awareness of surfaces was seen in her recognition of certain streets with cobblestones. Her hearing was most acute: she would aim objects correctly at the therapist when she wanted to throw them; she felt more at ease when she heard the therapist knitting and thus was assured of her awake presence; she derived much pleasure from hearing the sound of glass breaking; she would knock two objects together and listen for their sound. Smell was also important to her: she could locate the local bakery by means of the smells. Smell was at

---

4. D. Burlingham's paper (1964) contains an interesting account of the development of hearing in the blind and the role of the relationship to the mother. See also D. Burlingham (1961).

the same time sexualized as can be seen in her request to the therapist, "Come, smell my fanny." Throughout the treatment, she often sought close physical contact by sitting on the therapist's lap and asking for love, which suggests that the total surface of her body was a major receptor of stimulation.

Helen showed and made use of a very well-developed sense of hearing. She was able to tell when the paper boy was coming down the road long before her mother could hear him. She was also clearly attracted to her mother's powder and scent.

George compensated for his lack of vision mainly by means of auditory and tactile senses. In addition, testing, mouthing, and licking (very frequent in blind children) were used by him when he was five years old, in a manner similar to the ways of a sighted toddler.

Memory seems to serve the blind well. In practically all the cases studied and in many others observed, this function showed itself as adequate and helpful. Not infrequently it served purposes of orientation, as shown in Winnie's trips with her therapist to the local shops. Things recalled for such purposes were memories of smells experienced, of noises herard, of texture of surfaces felt (cobblestone surfaces, etc.).

Contact with the object world through words plays a particularly important role in the blind. In the cases here studied the acquisition of speech was not precociously developed and the timetable for the beginning of talking ranged roughly from eighteen months to three years of age. George began talking at eighteen months; Helen was fairly fluent by two and a half years; Winnie was talking by two years; Janet talked when she was three years.

It is a well-established fact that certain forms of thinking and the development of several other ego functions are dependent largely on the acquisition of a proper imagery, and of adequate symbols, on the basis of which thought processes of an ever-increasing complexity and quality are possible.

The synthetic and integrative functions of the ego are very dependent on the intactness of these processes, which are essential for the proper understanding and mastery of the world around us, making further ego development possible on that basis.

It is likewise well established that words are the essential units, the required symbols, on the basis of which the above-mentioned processes can take place. Quite clearly, whatever interferes with the child's ability to acquire such symbols may bring aspects of his ego development to a near standstill and be responsible for sometimes creating the impression of extreme backwardness. Extreme examples of such cases can be observed in children with congenital deafness. When they are taught to lip-read and to talk, dramatic improvements often take place in their ego development, and with it in their object relationships, in their understanding and mastery of the world. This happens because words as symbols have become available for thought processes and for the performance of functions which are contingent upon secondary-process thinking of a certain quality.

Although the blind child's disadvantages in this area are not on a par with that of the deaf, there is some evidence that lack of vision interferes with the ability to acquire and make use of words as symbols. Many essential elements of these "word symbols" can be contributed only by sight. For this reason the concepts abstracted by these words have no real meaning for children blind from birth. "Dark," "light," and the whole range covered by words describing "color," etc., belong in this category. No other sense can convey suitable alternative information to clarify these concepts and abstractions. It is not difficult to imagine how many limitations are thus imposed on the mental processes of the blind. A few observations from our Nursery for the Blind can exemplify some of these problems.

> Gillian (six years) was in the lavatory. "Put the light on, it's dark."
> Teacher: "What do you mean?"
> Gillian: "You know, it is cold and horrible."

> Matthew (age four), playing hide and seek in the cupboard, called out, "It's all dark in here." When asked what he meant, he answered, "Well you know, all cold and rainy."

In a still larger group of words the contribution of sight may not be as fundamental but nevertheless important enough to render these symbols somewhat insufficient when compared with the equivalent symbols of the sighted.[5]

Whatever ego functions are dependent on the availability of the right kind of imagery or symbols are thus limited in a proportional degree. The imagery of the world of sighted people is of necessity in many ways inappropriate for the blind. Nevertheless, it seems that in spite of the absence of the visual contribution to many of these "word symbols," alternative compensatory means are finally found so that these symbols become useful elements in the performance of the complex mental processes for which these basic units are required. This need not imply that they finally become identical with the same "word presentation" of the sighted. Experiments on blind adults (from birth) who have recovered sight in adulthood through certain operations have shown that they are unable to pick out objects by sight, to recognize or even name them, even though they know all about them and their names by touch. As Young (1960) points out:

> At first he only experiences a mass of colour, but gradually he learns to distinguish shapes. When shown a patch of one colour he will quickly see that there is a difference between the patch and its surroundings. What he will not do is to recognize that he has seen that particular shape before, nor will he be able to give it its proper name. For example, one man when shown an orange a week after beginning to see, said that it was gold. When asked, 'What shape is it?' he said, 'Let me touch it and I will tell you'. After doing so, he said that it was an orange, when he looked again at it he said: 'Yes I can see that it is round'. Shown next a blue square, he said it was blue and round. A triangle he also described as round. When the angles were pointed out to him he said, 'Ah, Yes, I understand now, one can *see* how they feel'.

5. "A word is thus a complex presentation; . . . or, to put it in another way, there corresponds to the word a complicated associateive process into which the elements of visual, acoustic, and kinaesthetic origin enumerated above enter together. A word, however, acquires its *meaning* by being linked with an 'object-presentation,' at all events if we restrict ourselves to a consideration of substantives. The object-presentation itself is once again a complex of associations made up of the greatest variety of visual, acoustic, tactile, kinaesthetic and other presentations" (Freud 1891). The quotation appears as part of Appendix C, Words and Things, attached to Freud's paper "The Unconscious" (1915, p. 209), because the last section of that paper is based on these views expressed in *On Aphasia*.

Further evidence supporting the limitations we are describing is presented by the indiscriminate use of words that can be observed in many blind children. They use words in a "parroting fashion" without having a proper understanding of their true and complete meaning.

For example, when Janet was nine she frequently used words such as "contradict" and "nuisance," without knowing their meaning, obviously having taken them over from her mother. Mathew (four and a half) was washing the stuffed bunny and said that at home in the bath when soap gets into his eyes it stings. "They are delicate," he said, adding, "I wonder what delicate means?"

The occurrence of word parroting long before the child grasps the corresponding abstract meaning of the words shows how much longer it takes the blind to assimilate many of the concepts symbolized by words.

Not all words represent the same level of abstraction; many are more concrete than others. The blind learn the concrete first and more easily than the abstract. Though there exist noticeable individual differences in this respect, in general the blind children show a certain tendency to concreteness in their verbalized thoughts and some difficulty in the formation of abstract concepts. Similarly, abstract concepts are readily concretized.

Wendy, for example, shows concern with the meanings of "wearing out" and "worn-out" as used with regard to people, objects such as toys, feelings, etc. She worried whether worn-out people are discarded like worn-out music boxes.

Peter at around five years of age was gingerly fingering dough. He said, "Squeeze it; can he squeeze it? Will it hurt?" On another occasion he tried to open a peanut, saying, "That hurts it." He then stopped the activity.

Matthew (at around six years of age) heard at home the story of *Pinocchio*. He asked at the nursery what "conscience" is. "Can you really hear a little voice when you do something naughty? He decided to try it out and with a serious expression tore up a paper napkin. He then pushed over a chair and said, "I still can't hear it."

These limitations help to explain why, in many cases, the blind children are not able to master and fully understand the world outside; large areas of it remain sources of intense fear and anxiety.

Nevertheless, at some point of development, some of these limitations disappear or are reduced to a minimum compatible with performances on the ego side more similar to the level of performance of the sighted. We have no doubt concerning the usefulness of the close study of how, when, and through what means the ego finds alternatives and compensatory ways that finally to some degree help overcome its original limitations. Such a study will throw abundant light on many developmental processes undergone by the ego. It will also clarify and establish the essential elements that must combine to bring about the performance of more complex ego functions.

It is our belief that the ego of the blind must first find alternative means of coping with some of the problems described in this chapter before it can turn to the rather primitive drive organization and establish appropriate controls over drive activity. In many blind children this seems to happen at a much later stage than in the sighted. At this later point the ego can make use of alternative sources of gratification and find sublimatory outlets. Exactly when this happens should be determined by detailed study and analyses of blind adolescents and adults.

THE SUPEREGO STRUCTURE

The whole question of how the superego structure as a controlling agency develops in the blind deserves a study in its own right. We are limiting ourselves to highlighting some striking differences between sighted and blind.

First of all, in the group we have studied, it is very difficult to find signs of guilt when specific transgressions occur, even at ages when such signs are plentiful in the sighted. For example, the blind children engage freely in a great deal of autoerotic activity and drive gratification corresponding to all sorts of levels, as pointed out above. These activities are performed openly in the presence of adults; on the whole they seem to be ego syntonic and free of guilt.

It is also important to point to an apparent contradiction in these children's superego development. In the sighted child the process of internalization of external demands (leading to super-ego precursors and in due course to the final establishment of the superego structure) is assumed to start when the child's awareness of the importance of the object forces him to give up drive gratification, out of concern and fear of the loss of the love of the object. The blind children, in spite of their extreme dependence on their objects, do not seem forced (by fear of loss of the object's love when his disapproval is incurred) to internalize prohibitions and commands or to give up the multiple and primitive forms of autoerotic activities and drive gratifications to which they cling so tenaciously.

DEVELOPMENT OF THE TOTAL PERSONALITY (LINES OF DEVELOPMENT AND MASTERY OF TASKS)

A marked retardation and unevenness in the development of the total personality as shown on the lines of development seems to be the normal picture in this group of blind children. This is in part due to the lack of sight which implies interference with develop-ment in every area and in part to environmental interferences such as pity and overprotection. We anticipate that the study of the blind in terms of the lines of development (A. Freud 1963) estab-lished for sighted children will throw some light on certain aspects of ego development, especially on the contribution made to that development by the organ and the function of vision.

It is also possible that for an independent assessment of their development we shall have to set up entirely new standards permitting us to explore the possibility of different interactions between the expressions of drives and the severely handicapped ego and superego structures.

REGRESSION AND FIXATION POINTS

This is another area where we have become aware of the fact that the behavior and symptomatic manifestations of sighted children, usually taken as indicators and pointers to the levels at which they may be fixated, are not always applicable to the blind.

Thus, the intense mouthing observed in most blind children up to a very late age cannot be taken as a sure indicator of a fixation on the oral level. Mouthing in the blind, quite apart from the oral drive gratification, must in some of its aspects be considered as an auxiliary exploratory ego function. A very similar situation exists with regard to the prominent use of the sense of smell. It is, of course, not an easy matter to distinguish between drive and ego activity in this respect.

We suggest that one should try to note whether an organ is used by the ego in a limited way to compensate for the lack of vision (as in the exploration of objects through mouthing). In this case the activity will cease when this purpose has been accomplished; otherwise it will continue well past the exploratory phase and show an impulsive, instinctual quality.

Another example is the frequent touching inhibition of the blind. As an indicator of fixation to the anal phase it does not have the same value it has in the sighted.

There are many other important differences between blind and sighted children with regard to fixation and regression. For example, it is very difficult to establish where phase dominance lies in the blind, since drive activity remains spread through all levels of development and the ego acquiesces in this state of affairs. The picture is further complicated by the extreme readiness of the blind children to regress temporarily from higher to lower levels of gratification as soon as any difficulties arise. In fact, the group we observe gives the impression of moving backward and forward far more readily than sighted children would in similar circumstances.

On the other hand, it is not quite correct to refer to what we have been describing as "fixations" proper, since it may well be that the reluctance to give up earlier forms of gratification is due to the immense and constant frustrations experienced by the blind; these make the ego more tolerant of obtaining gratification by whatever means possible. In fact, we have the impression that if sight could be restored (which would lead at once to a better balance between pleasure and frustration, etc.), very many of these earlier forms of gratification would disappear, a development which could, of course, never occur in the case of true fixations.

The constant shift in functioning from the one level to another (with backward and forward moves), for example, in relation to external events, tends to support this view.

DYNAMIC AND STRUCTURAL ASSESSMENT
(CONFLICTS)

External Conflicts

Owing to the extreme and very prolonged dependence of the blind child on his objects, the "external type" of conflict is perhaps more prominent than it is in the sighted. The blind need a longer period of time for internalization to take place and even then they seem to remain to some extent dependent on the approval of the outside world. They are more likely to have conflicts between the wish for independence and self-assertion and the ever-present realistic need for continuous support and protection from the objects. The outcome of such conflicts frequently seems to be extreme passivitiy and a readiness to comply with the demands of the object out of the fear of loss of love or fear of annihilation.

Internalized Conflicts

Blind children of the age group we have studied may show some superego precursors. They have internalized some environmental demands. For example, they may take over from the environment the command to become clean and dry, and make it into an internal concern. On the other hand, it has been noted that in blind children it is not easy to come across clear examples of "guilt" when transgressions of these or other commands do occur.

Although at the present time we cannot be more specific, there is no doubt that there are important differences between this group of blind and the sighted in the process of internalization as well as in the ego and the superego (or its precursors), as shown by the apparent "lack of guilt." On the whole internalization probably starts later and takes longer in the blind than in the sighted.

ASSESSMENT OF SOME GENERAL CHARACTERISTICS

Frustration Tolerance

It is very difficult to evaluate the blind child's reaction to frustration. On the one hand, a great deal of direct drive gratification occurs all the time, a circumstance that would indicate low frustration tolerance; on the other, there is little doubt that in their dealings with the external world they are constantly exposed to and must tolerate excessive frustrations owing to their blindness and the resultant helplessness.

Sublimation Potential

It seems that the tendency to cling to any form of gratification that has been experienced previously, the general tolerance of the ego in this respect, etc., are factors working against whatever capacity or potential these children may have for sublimation. Moreover, the need for close bodily contact with the objects may further interfere with the blind child's capaicty to sublimate or to accept substitute gratification.

These statements are true only up to a given age. Random observations of blind adults seem to point to the fact that at some stage there occur important economic and structural developments and rearrangements in the personality of the blind (partly described under the Ego section), which sometimes allow satisfactory sublimations to take place.

Overall Attitude to Anxiety

This is an area of special interest in blind children (see under Ego Development).

Because of their readiness to develop anxiety to a traumatic degree in times of stress, the function of anxiety as a signal is frequently overruled. At such moments the children tend to look for very close bodily contact with the object. It seems that up to a comparatively late age the children's anxiety, as observed in our group, is aroused mainly by their inability to deal with, understand, and master external dangers and the external world.

Progressive Developmental Forces
versus Regressive Tendencies

In this group of blind children the material seems to point to a very marked backward pull exerted by the regressive tendencies. We have already mentioned the need to cling to old forms of satisfaction which does not make it any easier to take progressive steps into new phases. Although progressive tendencies are seen, development on the whole takes place at a slower and rather retarded pace; certain environmental attitudes, such as overprotection, etc., may further obscure the true state of affairs concerning the blind child's potentialities in this area.

References

Burlingham, D. (1961). Some notes on the development of the blind. *Psychoanalytic Study of the Child* 16:121-145.

——— (1964). Hearing and its role in the development of the blind. *Psychoanalytic Study of the Child* 19:95-112.

Fraiberg, S., and Freedman, D.A. (1964). Studies in the ego development of the congenitally blind child. *Psychoanalytic Study of the Child* 19:113-170.

Freud, A. (1962). Assessment of childhood disturbances. *Psychoanalytic Study of the Child* 17:149-158.

——— (1963). The concept of developmental lines. *Psychoanalytic Study of the Child* 18:245-265.

Freud, S. (1892). *On Aphasia.* New York: International Universities Press, 1953.

——— (1915). The unconscious. *Standard Edition* 14:159-218.

Omwake, E.G., and Solnit, A.J. (1961) "It isn't fair": the treatment of a blind child. *Psychoanalytic Study of the Child* 16:352-404.

Sandler, A.-M. (1963). Aspects of passivity and ego development in the blind infant. *Psychoanalytic Study of the Child* 18:343-360.

Segal, A., and Stone, F.H. (1961). The six-year-old who began to see: emotional sequelae of operation for congenital bilateral cataracts. *Psychoanalytic Study of the Child* 16:481-509.

Young, J.Z. (1960). *Doubt and Certainty in Science: A Biologist's Reflections on the Brain.* New York: Oxford University Press.

PART III

ADOLESCENT DEVELOPMENT

Chapter Eleven

DIAGNOSTIC, PROGNOSTIC, AND DEVELOPMENTAL CONSIDERATIONS

Most observers of adolescents will probably agree that the usual and developmentally normal adolescent revolt has acquired in recent times forms of expression that are in many cases, to say the least, distressing and frequently totally maladaptive and destructive, both in the personal and the social sense. Naturally, this does not apply to all adolescents. It does, however, seem in this country to apply to a constantly increasing number of young people. Further, though some casualties have always resulted from attempts to master the developmental tasks of adolescence, it seems to me that the number of such casualties has grown significantly in our time. Even more, such failures as take place have a degree of "malignancy" that is alarming. Take for example drug addiction with its nefarious results, or the many varieties of "dropping out" from college, society and life, or organized destruction and quasi-warfare, increased numbers of suicides, etc. Obviously, no sensible society can afford this wastage of human talent and lives, nor tolerate the amount of individual suffering created by such maladaptive results. Furthermore, since the percentage of adolescents and children, in terms of our total population, has recently reached new heights and will continue to do so, there can be no question that we can ignore these problems much longer without concomitant disastrous results.

CAUSES OF BEHAVIORAL DISORDERS

I consider it essential for the diagnostician of adolescent disturbances to differentiate among five different kinds of phenomena
that can lead to symptom formation and/or behavioral disorders.
First, there are those symptoms, character traits, or behavioral
disorders observed in the clinical picture of the adolescent that are
left over from the conflicts of developmental phases previous to
adolescence and that have led to psychopathology of various
kinds, including the establishment of fixation points. As such,
they have been manifested all the way through childhood and
latency and continue to be apparent during the adolescent stage.
Properly speaking they are not derived from the adolescent revolt.
Nevertheless, they will contaminate and to various degrees influence the form taken by the adolescent revolt itself.

Second, some symptoms or behavioral disorders are derived
from the intrapsychic conflicts and typical developmental conflicts of the adolescent stage. These different types of manifestations have been widely described in the literature and we are well
acquainted with them. They are based on internal imbalances
between the different agencies of the mind, imbalances that are
typical of this stage of development. As such they are to some
extent independent of what is happening outside.

Third, there are those symptoms and behavior which are derived
from the impact that special environmental conditions have on
the internal problems of the adolescent during this stage. They can
be considered in the nature of developmental interferences of
which two types deserve consideration. The first type can best be
described as parental or familial developmental interferences such
as take place when either the parents or the immediate family of
the adolescent does or does not do something that is required for
the developmental process of the adolescent to evolve normally. A
sexually exhibitionistic or bodily seductive mother will be such an
example, complicating by this behavior the strength of the incestuous phantasies, wishes, etc. of the adolescent and the concomitant guilt and defensive maneuvers required to cope with
such heightened feelings. The second type can be described as

social or environmental developmental interferences, that is, social or environmental conditions that hinder the adolescent developmental processes. Since one set of factors, the environmental conditions, are constantly changing, the responses may change from generation to generation.

Fourth, there are some symptoms and behavior which are not derived from the individual intrapsychic conflicts but are due specifically to peer group pressure. Here we are in the realm of group psychology, not of individual psychology. There is no doubt that the impact of the peer group will be frequently modified by the personality characteristics of the recipient. For example, large numbers of adolescents are introduced to a variety of drugs. Among the young people exposed to the use of drugs by their peers, a certain number seem to become drug addicts while a substantial number, after a few experiences, stop taking them. It seems possible that those adolescents that are "hooked" after being exposed to drugs have reached this stage with significant weaknesses in the personality. Such weak spots as important oral fixations acquired early in life may favor the establishment of a long-term and sometimes irreversible addiction.

Fifth, it seems to me that a substantial number of the behavior disorders and symptoms produced during this stage have a completely different mechanism. I believe that the conditions operating here are similar and somewhat akin to those observed and described for the traumatic neuroses. The conflict here is between opposite ego ideals and superego ideals. These contradictory ego ideals or superego ideals may have been acquired simultaneously, or they may have been acquired in the course of many years; some in early infancy, some during the resolution of the oedipus complex, some in the latency period, or some during the adolescent stage. These conflicts, for some adolescents, seem insurmountable and lead to a kind of paralysis of the constructive and adaptive capacities of the ego. We are accustomed to thinking of traumatic neuroses in terms of the individual. What I have in mind now is a kind of "collective" traumatic neuroses. Large numbers of adolescents are exposed simultaneously to the sudden realization that they carry within themselves contradictory and irreconcilable ego and superego ideals. This appears to overwhelm their egos and, in some cases, since it has been acquired collectively, it leads to collective attempts at solution. I believe that such phenomena as "dropping out" from college, the organization of communities of "hippies," "flower children" and the like may occasionally be the result of the mechanisms described. I believe too that this state of collective traumatic neuroses to which some adolescents succumb is a phenomena that is on the increase and in good measure determined by current social conditions.

In addition, many adolescents of the present generation find it difficult to maintain certain forms of splits in their introjects—splits which seem to have been quite common for earlier generations. In the past, it was possible, for some reason, for these splits (in terms of introjects) to coexist without necessarily leading to conflict. Past generations, just like the current generation of adolescents, were given as ideals: brotherhood among mankind, and equality among all men. They too were told that we are all children of God; they were told to behave well, not to abuse their neighbors or to exploit them. They were told not to discriminate, etc. All such moral ideals have long been embodied in the teachings of religion, school, and furthermore, have long been an intrinsic part of the constitution of this country. Nevertheless, though at a conscious level these were the explicit ego and superego ideals that were offered for assimilation, there was a second more subtle message concomitant with it which allowed many people to behave in any manner that suited their interest while consciously professing these high ideals. Such people are quite capable of discrimination and abuse without of necessity finding themselves in conflict. Thus, two sets of introjects were actually acquired, one as it were for external consumption and the other one for internal consumption. It seems as if adolescents today find it difficult to live with such a split. For some reason the second and more subtle message "do as you please as long as it suits your purposes" becomes conflictive and the clash between these two opposite introjects leads to unrest, shame, guilt, and anxiety. Not infrequently, it seems to reach such proportions that the ego becomes paralyzed and offers no constructive solutions.

The final result is a maladaptive compromise for large numbers of adolescents.

The parallel drawn earlier with the traumatic neuroses is in need of some further elaboration. In a traumatic neurosis the ego becomes overwhelmed and is largely put out of action. It is not capable of producing an adaptive solution to the traumatic event. Further, it frequently remains incapable (to different degrees) of coping with ordinary events due to the high tenor of unbound anxiety present. For as long as this is the case the ego remains disrupted. Two significant factors in the development of the ordinary traumatic neuroses are: first, the element of surprise, the lack of preparation on the ego side to cope with the suddenly overwhelming event and second, the dramatic, overwhelming nature of the event that becomes traumatic.

Although the mechanism I have in mind in the case of the adolescent is in some ways similar to what I have described above, it is in other ways different. First, it lacks the sudden, dramatic nature of those traumatic neuroses that result from a car accident or natural catastrophe. *The trauma is more subtle, continuous, has retrospective elements and its effect is cumulative,* to use Masud Kahn's term. An example may clarify this. The present generations of adolescents have been exposed through the different communication media (press, radio, and TV) to the effects of human aggression and destructiveness through war. Their exposure started many years ago with the Korean war. It continued shortly afterwards with exposure to the atrocities of the Vietnam war. It is likely that such prolonged exposure had some influence in the development of their ideals and in the process of identification. Anybody observing children's reactions, to the TV news showing cities being bombed and destroyed, mutilated bodies, wounded civilians (children and adults), and dead bodies would have noticed their fear, horror, and simultaneous fascination. Not infrequently their sleep may be disrupted directly or through nightmares, or they are clinging for awhile, etc. We have here the continuous exposure to frightening events, including the threat of nuclear war. We must wonder about the possible cumulative effects. Naturally, the younger the child the more confusing and frightening these observations are. Similarly, though the events are real and in some form or another assimilated, for most children they have simultaneously an air of unreality, at least for some time. In later years when better understanding and fuller awareness of what has been observed becomes possible they have a retroactive traumatic effect. More especially so when such events become an actual narcissistic threat and are seen in reference to the self. The adolescent, more so the late adolescent, becomes suddenly aware that he is destined to be an actor in the tragedy. He knows he may be drafted, he may be asked to kill and destroy (without being motivated for it), and furthermore his own personal destruction becomes a serious consideration. The confluence of all these factors, the cumulative effects of the exposure, acquire a retroactive traumatic effect which for many is of overwhelming proportions—hence the trauma. By the time this happens the adolescent belongs to a community of peers and much of his insight, awareness, and anxiety are brought about through group and peer interaction. Solutions to these basic anxieties are frequently brought about collectively too. Naturally, the solutions may be either adaptive or maladaptive.

The diagnostician should always take the trouble to dissect from the symptomatic and behavioral picture offered by the adolescent which of the manifestations observed corresponds to which one of the five groups of mechanisms outlined above. It is clear that the five groups of mechanisms described are not identical. It is clear too that there are significant diagnostic and prognostic differences and considerations to be taken into account. Similarly from the therapeutic and corrective point of view different measures will be required to deal with these different types of conflicts and their results. Attempts at understanding what I can only describe as the "adolescent revolution" are, to say the least, daring and frequently bound to fail. Whatever approach one takes, whatever point of view one decides to adopt can only be a very simplistic, pale, and partial reflection of what in reality is a multidimensional and extremely complex phenomenon. Nevertheless, I shall discuss a number of factors concerning changes in child-rearing practices, sociocultural changes, and their possible influence in structure formation and development. After all, development is in good measure a function of the interaction between internal and environmental forces.

SOCIAL CHANGE

In considering what factors may be influencing the clinical pictures presented by adolescents nowadays or what factors may have determined or influenced some of the present forms of the adolescent revolt, I think we can assume that the nature of the drives (instinctual-impulses) has not changed nor have the tasks the adolescent must accomplish before reaching adulthood. Other factors must be held responsible for what we observe.

It may be that certain changes in our society and in child-rearing practices can account for some of the problems. Thus for example, the role played by the family organization in development has been gradually undermined, distorted, and disrupted. Many factors are influential here. Sometimes they act in isolation, at other times they are reinforced by a number of other variables. Consider for example the significant increases in the number of broken marriages and divorces. We are all familiar with the disruptive results that growing up under these conditions has for many children, as well as with the numerous complications introduced in the development of children under such circumstances. Naturally, the impact is variable according to age and stage of development.

The very affluence of present day society may be a significant and subtle factor capable of influencing human development in negative directions. We seem to live more and more according to the pleasure principle. This is an attitude that seems to be influencing all sectors of our social organization as slogans such as "buy now, pay later," and "enjoy your vacation today, worry about payments afterwards," clearly illustrate. By a similar token we have become very tolerant in child rearing, perhaps excessively so. As a result we not only encourage living according to the pleasure principle but we may unintentionally interfere with the sound development of the reality principle, and as such with the ability to postpone gratification, the capacity to accept substitutes, the tolerance and handling of tension, the development of the capacity to establish controls, etc. To give but one example we need only think of the question of masturbation in children. We have turned around from earlier attitudes, taking a much more lenient and tolerant view of such practices in early childhood. Many people in the field, including child psychoanalysts, take the view that masturbation need not be discouraged. In fact, it is frequently encouraged (if only indirectly) as long as the child does it privately. We hear such things as, "it's alright to play with yourself to get the nice feelings but we do not do that in front of other people, only when we are alone." It seems to me that we tend to forget that masturbation is a composite, consisting of both the actual manipulation of the genitals (in different ways) and the fantasies that accompany it. It is the latter that are particularly troublesome in terms of psychopathological development. When we say to the child to go ahead and masturbate as long as he does it privately, we are obviously not taking into account the nature of the fantasies that accompany the masturbatory act. Since, for example, the masturbatory practices of the phallic-oedipal child are frequently accompanied by highly conflictual incestuous fantasies, one cannot but wonder how sound this attitude is. As early as 1897, Freud established a connection between addictions, of whatever type, including of course drug addiction, and masturbation.

He wrote in a letter to Fliess (letter 79): "It has dawned on me that masturbation is the one major habit, the 'primal addiction' and that it is only as a substitute and replacement for it that the other addictions—for alcohol, morphine, tobacco, etc.—come into existence" (Freud 1892-1877, p. 272). Years later, in a letter to Reik (1929) concerning "Dostoevsky and Parricide" (1928), he established a connection between those neuroses accompanied by a severe sense of guilt and the struggles against masturbation. Further he linked masturbation and addictions to gambling such as that shown by Dostoevsky (Freud 1928, pp. 183, 196). In his view excessive masturbation was both biologically and psychologically damaging. Thus he thought that excessive masturbation predisposes to various neuroses "which are conditional on an involution of sexual life to its infantile forms." He thought too that it vitiates the character in several ways through indulgence . . . "it teaches people to achieve important aims without taking trouble and by easy paths, instead of through an energetic exertion of force—that is, it follows the principle that *sexuality lays down the pattern* of behaviour; secondly, in the phantasies that accompany satisfaction the sexual object is raised to a degree of excellence which is not easily found again in reality." Later on in the same publication he stated that men given to masturbatory practices go into marriage with diminished sexual potency (1908, pp. 199-201).

In "Contributions to a Discussion of Masturbation" (1912), Freud objected to Stekel's position. The latter claimed that there was no real damage produced by masturbation, only prejudices associated with it. Freud argued: "We are therefore brought back once more from arguments to clinical observation, and we are warned by it not to strike out the heading 'Injurious Effects of Masturbation.' We are at all events confronted in the neuroses with cases in which masturbation has done damage" (p. 201).

Similarly, there has been a marked change in the attitude of many parents regarding the setting of limits and controls in respect of their children. Many parents have gone to extremes that seem to me highly questionable. Frequently, they have chosen to abandon many of their obligations and prerogatives as parents, and since they are hesitant in setting the necessary controls and limits they finally pass much of the responsibility for this to the teenager. In my experience this frequently happens far too early and in areas where the teenager and young adolescent are neither ready nor able to assume such responsibilities. Such areas include the control of sexual and aggressive impulses. Teenagers are allowed to come and go freely without any supervision, either of hours, individuals, or groups with which they mix. In so doing many are exposed to intolerable stresses and seductions of a sexual and aggressive character by the environment and peers. It is possible that those children reaching adolescence with important weak spots in their personality development—and given the fur-

ther upset created by the typical adolescent developmental processes and revolt—are an easy prey to the negative influences of a
sick environment and especially to their most disturbed peers.
Some support, even some sheltering against such influences seems
to me essential. Furthermore, I consider it advisable for parents to
continue to play the role of ego and superego auxiliaries when and
where required. Naturally, such a parental stand may well increase the clashes with the adolescent in revolt. Naturally too, it
should be done sensibly and with due awareness of legitimate
adolescent developmental needs and rights. Briefly, in my view,
parents should continue to play their parental roles with the
necessary modifications during their children's adolescent revolt.
A total abandonment of the young adolescent to his internal and
external struggles for the sake of peace is at best a disservice to him
or her, and may occasionally lead to undesirable consequences.
Indifference is always worse than legitimate concern, even when
the parental concern is frequently interpreted by the adolescent as
an interference with "his freedom and rights."

The parents' confusion regarding their parental roles may be
partly related to the fact that many among them were subjected to
similar upbringings. One can not avoid being concerned with the
fate of the children of substantial numbers of the present adolescent generation. The capacity of this problem to be geometrically
compounded seems to me a realistic risk and a serious consideration.

Other potential dangers in sight concern the increasing demand, especially by feminist activists for day-care services for their
babies and infants. Children are somewhat burdensome to some in
the new generation of parents, perhaps especially to college and
graduate students. Hence there is the demand for day-care services.
Unfortunately, many such services are bound to become dumping
places for babies and toddlers with little consideration given to the
best interests of the child and his future emotional health. Many
young mothers are unaware of the potentially damaging effects of
such practices on their children's emotional growth; but they are
led in that direction by the feminist demand for equal rights and
opportunities for young student mothers on campus. Though I

have no objection to equal opportunities and rights for men and women, I do have objections to children's rights being neglected, especially the right to the best chance to be emotionally healthy. Such babies and toddlers as will grow up under inappropriate conditions in the new day-care services will in due time become adolescents. I fear that many of them will be damaged to the point of becoming irretrievable casualties during their own adolescent revolt. Clearly, serious thought and consideration will have to be given to the conflictual needs of different generations, parents and children, if we are to avoid major catastrophies a few years hence.

It is also important to refer to the manipulation techniques that our teenagers are exposed to. Because of our country's affluence, adolescents have become an important market of many billions of dollars. They get bombarded by stimulation and seductive techniques of all kinds. Still worse, they have become an excellent target and market for drug peddlers and the like. We have a social obligation to examine such problems and to develop solutions—perhaps some form of regulation of present day assaults on the teenage generation. This situation is an example of collective or social developmental interferences. Forces in society have been organized to exploit this new market without any consideration of the results that such techniques may produce in the child or the adolescent's development.

Our last example illustrates how a specific change in societal conditions may interfere with one of the fundamental developmental tasks of adolescence: the task of acquiring a final and definitive degree of independence from the primary objects. This task is complicated by the revival and recathexis of oedipal figures during adolescence. It is further complicated by the fact that at this point adolescents experience the full strength of their sexual drives as the result of their recently acquired sexual maturity. Yet, with the constantly increasing length in the time required for education, we have significantly extended the adolescent dependence on parental support well into the years of young adulthood. It is common enough in a university setting to come across young men and women anywhere from twenty to twenty-five years of age, in the senior year of (for example) their medical studies, who not infrequently, are married, with one or two children, own a car, etc. But these young families and couples are economically supported by their parents. Naturally, this has many implications in terms of the dependence-independence conflicts.

Consider too, another fundamental task of adolescence. That is, the search for an identity, by which I mean not only a sexual identity but a professional identity as well, and even more important, a personal, individual identity.

All these developmental tasks and the inner turmoil that accompanies them are well known to all of us. To master such turmoil and such tasks has been traditionally, I believe, one of the developmental obligations of that age group. Since these are processes that come from inside and are related to the instinctual nature of human beings there is no new factor here. Yet these same tasks have to be accomplished against constantly changing environmental circumstances. These changes take place at such a rate of speed that adaptation to them is becoming an extremely difficult task. Since internal developmental processes take place in interaction with the specific environmental circumstances and life experiences of any individual, it is conceivable that such constantly changing external conditions may at times favor and at times hinder the accomplishment and mastery of the internal developmental processes needed for adolescence and then adulthood and maturity.

SUPEREGO DEVELOPMENT

In the sociocultural sense (up to relatively recently) superego development was for the most part and in the great majority of individuals based on a process of introjection of standards, behavior, and ideals that were handed down from generation to generation with only slight modifications. These standards and ideals (imposed from the outside) were not as generally or as widely questioned earlier as it seems to be the case today. It thus seems to me that a fruitful line of inquiry and speculation may lie in the direction of asking why there is so much questioning today of our traditions, codes of behavior, moral standards, and ideals. Similarly, why was this not so to the same degree, in the case of earlier generations?

Developmentally and structurally speaking I think that there are two essential mechanisms involved in the process of developing the superego structure and the ego and superego ideals. The first one is based in the process of introjection of those standards, morals, behavior codes, and ideals that are passed down to children by their progenitors, teachers, cultural environment, etc. These are, as it were, blind introjects, mostly accepted at their face value and without questioning by their recipients. In this way, at least that part of our cultural heritage concerning our norms of behavior is passed on. This was and still is a very efficient procedure in terms of the acceptance and maintenance of the established order of values of any given society. Though efficient, it is a rather primitive mechanism since it does not involve in most cases much ego participation, questioning, or rational examination of what is being introjected. The rules are accepted and obeyed just because they come from the elders and their wisdom is not open to examination, nor is such examination encouraged or promoted. On the contrary, anyone attempting to do so is, to say the least, discouraged, frequently reprimanded, and in extreme cases severely punished.

The second mechanism in superego development and in the establishment of ego ideals is totally different. It is not based on the introjection of standards imposed from outside or on identifications with special figures in the environment, but in introjects and ego ideals resulting from (among other things) subjective introspection, inner awareness and convictions, knowledge, rational processes of thinking, and empathy.

It seems plausible that in the last thirty years there has been a substantial shift from the first type of ego and superego ideal formation described above to the second type, or at least that there has been an increased contribution from the latter. In my view several factors may have contributed to this hypothetical change. Let us consider for example the whole area of education. While formerly higher education was the privilege of the few, nowadays

in many countries it is available to all. Higher education obviously means that more individuals are in possession of more
information, more knowledge, a better capacity to think, en-
lightened understanding—many more young human beings can
judge by themselves the merits or lack of them of all sort of
problems and propositions. It certainly does not favor blind
obedience to our traditions or to the opinion of our elders, but
leads to examination and questioning. Further, this increased
capacity for independent critical judgment is coupled with the
fantastic developments in the communication media. Together,
they have created a situation where we are in possession of the facts
(we not only hear about them but can indeed see the actual events)
practically at the same time they occur. Thanks to their increased
knowledge, information, and education, the young are quite
capable of drawing their own independent and frequently quite
legitimate conclusions. It is on this basis that many more young
people are building up their own idiosyncratic ego and superego
ideals.

These factors are contributing to the development of more and
more human beings, and doing so earlier and earlier. And yet,
though all the above seems to me highly desirable and welcome,
something must be wrong since some of the results are coun-
terproductive. These social developments do not always lead, at
least not initially, to constructive solutions, to more order and
better relations among members of any given community or
among nations. On the contrary, they frequently misfire, producing disruption, chaos, and destruction. Is this to be considered a
transitory unbalance between the results of the earlier order and
the new one, an unbalance that will correct itself at some point? Or
are we overlooking something fundamental to human nature in
this new order of things? If so, what?

By the same token the role played in the past by religion, the
church, the police, and the courts as auxiliary external superegos
is no longer as effective as it used to be and in many cases has
totally broken down. Though some of this is desirable it seems
that in the new order of things many individual's egos and

superegos are unable to take over the controls previously exercised by these institutions.

The police, for example are ridiculed, and not feared but provoked (frequently not without good reasons). The armies are no longer a source of strength and admiration but are despised. The courts do not inspire respect but contempt, often with good reason. The question is whether religion, the church, the police, the army and the courts were any better or fairer in the past than they are at present? I think the answer is an emphatic no.

If anything they were more abusive, conceited, oppressive, and discriminatory than they are nowadays. These factors have not changed. Our attitudes to all these superego auxiliaries has changed. Again, the question is why this should be so. Perhaps our increased education, information, etc. makes us—and certainly the younger generation—question their roles, their honesty, their inherent contradictions, and with some of them their very validity. Yet, the lesser influence of such social organizations (with their behavior control functions) is not always supplemented by a concomitant increase in internal and individual controls among the members of society. This naturally tends to undermine to some degree the previously established social order without introducing corrective measures that, while allowing for desirable social and political changes, will keep the minimum of structure and order required for the survival of an organized society.

In this chapter I have concentrated on the negative or maladaptive aspects of the adolescent revolt as it affects large numbers of adolescents. This coin has another side represented by similarly large number of adolescents who successfully sail through these turbulent waters. They emerge as mature adults quite capable of positive and constructive solutions. Our hopes for the future lies at their door.

References

Freud, S. (1892-1899). Extracts from the Fliess papers. *Standard Edition* 1:173-282.

——— (1908). Civilized sexual morality and modern nervous illness. *Standard Edition* 9:177-204.

——— (1912). Contributions to a discussion on masturbation. *Standard Edition* 12:239-254.

——— (1928). Dostoevsky and parricide. *Standard Edition* 21:175-198.

Chapter Twelve

FEMALE ADOLESCENCE, SEXUAL IDENTITY, AND HOMOSEXUALITY

A review of the literature on female adolescence produces rather scanty results. There are very few publications on the subject, regardless of the content matter. Nevertheless, the theme of adolescent female delinquency (including sexual promiscuity) appears most often within the general scarcity.

For example, in the first 25 volumes of the *Psychoanalytic Study of the Child* (covering 26 years up to 1970), there are to be found only four papers that specifically address female adolescents and their problems. One of them, incidentally, is by Peter Blos (1957), entitled "Preoedipal factors in the etiology of female delinquency. "More recently, as if to remedy this situation, Max Sugar has a volume entitled *Female Adolescent Development* (1979).

How are we to explain this paucity, at least in years past? Impressionistically, one may be tempered to think that in those years fewer female than male adolescents were referred for treatment. That is a possible factor, and would be important in terms of the limited number of publications. Is one then to assume that the actual incidence of psychopathology was less in female than in male adolescents, or perhaps that it was less severe and so went unattended? But if that is true, how are we to reconcile it with the fact that female development is considerably more complex than that of the male? For example, the oedipus complex of the female is much more complicated than the male's. She goes through two stages, while the boy goes through only one. She must, to achieve a mature adult position sexually and otherwise, exchange mother for the object father and then choose a nonincestuous displaced male object, while the boy needs no such exchange of object. All he made in terms of erotogenic zones. His phalius was, and will (mother), to an appropriately displaced nonincestuous female object. The female must give up her active-masculine identifications, which are quite normal during the first stage of the oedipus complex (phallic-oedipal stage), for the passive-feminine one, that would be more chacteristic of her sexual position as an adult. The male can retain the active-masculine strivings from his oedipal stance at three to five years of age into adulthood.

During adolescence and adulthood, the girl has to combine her genital erotogenic zones, so that the early (and practically exclusive) clitoridal activity becomes integrated with the complementary role played by her vagina and uterus, especially from the menarche onwards, in the achievement of her genital primacy. The boy has of course no such complicated arrangements to be made in terms of erotogenic zones. His phallus was, and will remain, the instrument of his genital primacy.

We know that in adolescence all these conflictual situations, and many others, are not only reactivated but are suddenly backed up by physical sexual maturity, making the intensity of the conflicts all the more severe. How can we then understand the smaller representation of female adolescents in terms of referrals, treatment, etc. in the near past?[1]

Could it perhaps be related to cultural patterns and expectations in our "male dominated" society, that forces women into submission generally, and condemn them to suffer and endure passively a lack of fulfillment as a sexual being, as a human being? Consider for example, that a sexual dysfunction in a male such as impotence or lack or orgastic capacity constitutes a major unacceptable catastrophe, while frigidity or other sexual dysfunctions and

1. Even during latency the ratio of referrals for evaluation and treatment is nuch higher for boys than it is for girls, though there has been noticeable increase for the latter in recent years.

dissatisfactions in the female were, and still are, frequently ignored and endured passively as women's fate and lot. Clearly, of late there have been significant changes for the better in society's and women's attitudes to these problems, so that at times, there is now an excessive swing of the pendulum with a reification of orgasms. But be that as it may, there can be no question that women have now quite a different attitude and quite rightly expect to fulfill themselves sexually and otherwise. They are no longer contented with the passive sufferer, sacrificial, uncomplaining position vis-a-vis the male. Thus, that societal roles, as assigned until recently, played a significant part cannot, in my judgement, be denied.

But are there other factors beyond social and cultural mores that could help to explain the discrepancies we are here confronted with? In the mind of many, that is the case. Freud (1925) himself postulated that given the special characteristics of the oedipus complex and particularly of its resolution in the female, they developed a final superego structure that was less severe, less demanding, less strict—in other words, more benign and more corruptible in the good sense of the word (p. 257). Indeed, if that assumption is correct, it may well help to explain in some measure the fact, that though female development is a more complex, sensitive, and delicate matter than male psychological development, the former escape conflict more frequently and more successfully than the latter. But this view has become very unpopular nowadays, specifically among feminists, women's liberationists and fellow travelers. Personally, I think there is some truth to it. This is no derogatory comment on my side; I believe it makes women more flexible, adaptable and tolerant than males tend to be.

There are also differences, we are told, in the level and balance between activity and passivity in males and females, just as some claim that there are differences between the sexes in the their respective endowment with aggression, and in their physical endurance.

Some have tried to account for the differences in the crime rates, its violent nature, its type, etc. on the basis of these factors. I believe, that any one of these factors may play a significant role in explaining some of these discrepancies. Yet, on the whole, it is a combination in various proportions of many internal and external variables that may offer us the best handle in understanding some of the problems we are concerned with here.

Thus far we have been talking of differences between male and female adolescents (and by implication even children and adults) in terms of incidence of illness, frequency of referral, severity of pathology, behavioral disorders, and as the result of all the above, frequency of publications.

But we have been referring mostly to the experience of the past. Looking at the present certain things seem, at least impressionistically, to be changing (though this is not yet reflected in the number of publications). Human nature has not basically changed. Therefore, one is forced to look at societal changes, attitudinal changes, changes in child-rearing practices, and the interaction between these factors and the basic human endowment as it determines psychological development, to try to understand the increases in incidence and new behavioral manifestations that are nowadays observed.

Consider the question of female homosexuality briefly. Is it correct to assume that the number of female homosexuals has greatly increased in recent years? If so, how do we explain the increase? Or could we say that their numbers have not really changed, but that given a more "permissive" environment many female homosexuals are coming out of the closet? (The same questions and arguments apply of course to male homosexuality.)

This is a difficult question to answer, but if I were to make a guess, I would have to say that probably it's a bit of both. It might be somewhat more difficult, though by no means impossible, to pinpoint the reasons for the increase in female homosexuality.

Let us examine now what factors determine the outcome during adolescence of a heterosexual or a homosexual identity. It should be understood that I am not at this point making any distinctions between comfortable and nonconflictual heterosexual or homosexual outcomes and those that may be riddled by conflict, anxiety, guilt, or shame in variable degrees, and for a variety of different reasons.

What happens in adolescence, in a manner of speaking, is that there is a decisive confrontation between the role or identity assigned very early on in life, based on biological factors, and the identity our developmental processes and experiences, innate givens, and environmental factors (favorable or unfavorable) force us to acquire.

We know from Money's work (1955, 1955, 1957) with hermaphrodites that gender role (being male or female) depends essentially on the sex assigned to them, at a very early age, either by parents or by doctors. Since such assignments were and are still not always easy to make, we have become aware of the enormous importance of the psychological and developmental factors in this regard. Thus, if mistakes are made, they tend to have catastrophic results since once the sex is assigned it is difficult if not impossible to change that assignment.

Stoller's work (1974) has further confirmed and clarified this situation.

But the fact that we are assigned an early sexual identity, only means, that in the end we might find ourselves enjoying that identity in a reasonably conflict free manner, or in case of developmental failure, in conflict if not at complete odds with it in extreme cases.

As we know, during the adolescent stage all oedipal and pre-oedipal conflicts are reactivated and telescoped. They are so to say reexamined and open (within limits) to a new revision on the light of the adolescent phase. That revision implies a participation not only of the drives, but of the ego and superego as well. As Helen Deutsch (1944) remarked, "in adolescence just as in previous phases of development, the ego manifests powerful developmental thrusts that do not depend directly and exclusively on sexual processes" (p. 94). Consequently, all the above, combined with the developmental forces that typify adolescence, will be determinant in the final outcome of the new revision.

OEDIPAL PHASE AND SEXUAL IDENTITY

Thus, in order to understand what happens in adolescence and why it is happening, we must consider those aspects of child

↑↓ FIRST STAGE Phallic-oedipal		↓↑ SECOND STAGE Oedipal	
↑ POSITIVE +++MOTHER ———FATHER	↑↓ INVERTED ++++FATHER ————MOTHER	↑ POSITIVE +++FATHER ———MOTHER	↓↑ INVERTED ++++MOTHER ————FATHER
a	c	d	f
↑ NEGATIVE + father — mother		↑ NEGATIVE + mother — father	
b		e	

Figure 12-1. Stages in a girl's oedipal development, occurring between the ages of two and a half and five years.

development, starting with the oedipal phase, that are central to the sexual identity outcome in adolescence.

Figure 12-1 depicts the various steps in development that the little girl must traverse during her oedipus complex, a process that takes place between the ages of two and a half and five years of age. It is to be noted that this developmental stage is much more complex in the case of the girl than the boy. To start with, as already mentioned, her oedipal development has two distinct stages, as can be seen in the schema. But beyond this she has to accomplish a variety of significant changes in at least four lines of development. She must exchange the object mother for the object father. She must reorganize her infantile genital erotogenic zone so that the vagina comes to play the fundamental and complimentory role to the clitoris to which it is destined. Her early ego phantasies must be modified so that she can come to terms with the sexual differences between boys and girls. In this way her castration anxiety, penis envy, etc. will not become a severe interference with her sexual functions as a mature female, or with her mothering functions. She must exchange the active-masculine position of the first stage of her oedipus complex for a passive-feminine stance (in intercourse) during the second stage of her oedipus complex. (For a more detailed account of all the above, see Nagera 1975.)

The boy is spared all of these developmental tasks.

If the girl's resolution of her oedipus complex is accomplished essentially on the basis of the oedipal constellations represented by squares d and e in the schema, as should be the case in normal development, all that remains is for her to produce a displacement from the incestuous object father, to a suitable and neutralized one. This of course, will lead in adolescence to an interest in and a capacity to relate to boys of her own adolescent peer group. She would have acquired an "effective" superego and the necessary basic feminine identifications for her future role as a female, and— if she so wishes—possibly a wife and a mother. I should make clear though, that this identification, fundamental as it is if the path of normality is to remain open, is not as yet totally finalized, nor can it be said that it cannot be undone. Indeed, this first feminine identification must continue to build itself up during latency, prepuberty, puberty and adolescence, in a favorable manner for a normal outcome, and innumerable factors are capable at any of these points of interfering with it. Think for example of the role that the menarche will have, and how much hangs on the girl's attitude to it. As Kestenberg (1961) says: "The positive aspect of the menarche as a turning point in the acceptance of femininity has been greatly overshadowed by the emphasis placed on the 'traumas' of the first and even subsequent menses" (p. 19). Naturally, the girl's attitude is affected by her mother's feelings to her own menses and femininity. This cannot fail to influence the processes of identification, and of valuing the function of menstruation for what it represents. The same of course applies to the father's response and reaction to his daughter's menstruation, as well as to that of any female and male siblings; but this latter phenomena is not well understood.

Similarly, in this developing feminine identification, a very significant part is played by the body changes that take place during prepuberty and puberty. The development of the breasts, hair, the rounding of the figure, etc. can be a welcome confirmation and growth of the early feminine identification. In that case, they are viewed with enormus pride and excitement as the harbingers of their final and very desired feminine development.

Kestenbaum (1979) rightly says in this regard: "Breast development is one of the more prized achievements of female puberty. Girls will compare breast size, order training bras, and in general derive great pleasure from the comments of classmates about the new protuberances in their T-shirts" (p. 150).

But these changes might be frightening (beyond proportion), unwelcomed, and felt as shameful and undesirable. The latter may be due to current events and circumstances that may have turned unfavorable. Alternatively, they may be due to earlier conflicts making femininity or growing up a highly conflictual and frightening proposition, especially at the point that the external signs and evidence of it become manifest, and cannot be postponed or denied any longer. An extreme example of this is a grossly seductive father, with manifest incestuous wishes at unconscious or conscious levels. Another would be the marked envy and hostility of the mother at the budding femininity of her daughter.

But let us go back to the little girl at the point of the resolution of her oedipus complex. If she was unfortunate enough to remain fixated at the first stage (squares a and b), she would move into what ought to have been her latency period with a significant handicap. Because of her fixation she would not have laid the foundation, for the developments that are needed to complete feminine identification through the contributions of latency, prepuberty and puberty. This little girl, having retained the active-masculine posture of the first stage of her oedipal complex, will not at all welcome the events that are follow developmentally, and that should, under normal conditions, further her femininity and female identification. Indeed, she would very likely become the hard-core tomboyish girl who refuses being a girl, dresses like a boy, plays like a boy, and is riddled with fantasies of being a boy. She will feel resentful of the fate that made her a girl, of the development of her breasts, and other secondary sexual characteristics, and of course of her menses. She may either overtly or covertly express her anger about all of this, and in extreme cases later on will become a transvestite, possibly a lesbian playing the male role, and may or may not demand a transexual operation. This behavior, that is clearly observable during the latency period, will continue into the actual adolescent stage, where it is bound to create havoc. This is so because the phantasies and potentials of latency can, and on occasion do, become the reality of adolescence, thanks to sexual maturation, the tendency to act out and actualize, and other factors. It is thus feasible that what the latency girl fantasized, the adolescent will act out and live in reality. As Peter Blos (1957) has written, "the age of instinctual tension-rise is puberty. At this time the individual normally reenacts his personal drama on the wider stage of society, and it is of course at this juncture of maturational stress that the inadequacy of the ego becomes apparent" (p. 230).

Whether the above will be directly expressed in the behavior and verbalization of the adolescent (and earlier in the latency child) depends on the amount and severity of the conflicts which arise between such fixations and the instinctual impulses derived from them, the ego and the superego. If the latter structures strenuously object to such wishes and impose defensive measures against them, the outcome will be severe neurotic conflicts, restrictions, inhibitions, anxiety, guilt, shame, etc. In this case, these impulses and wishes are not acted out, but are driven underground by various defensive means, so that they are only manifested in fantasy at the unconscious or perhaps partly conscious level. Yet, the symptoms and inhibitions present, the disturbances in object relationships with members of the opposite sex, including the lack of sexual interest and excitement with them, or overt fear and revulsion about sex, will be manifest enough. The difference between the adolescent and the latency girl, in this respect, is that the former is under the tremendous pressure of the now "mature" sexual drive and sudden violent upsurges of it, while the latter is enjoying the relative calm introduced in the drive activity by the period of latency. It is for these reasons, that in the case of the adolescent girl one is liable to see occasional breakthroughs of the impulses, followed by intense guilt and ruminations, except for those exceptional cases where the defenses are so massive and effective that this is not possible. But this is more often the exception than the rule. Obviously these breakthroughs will tend to show, in a rather clear and direct light, the nature of the impulses and conflicts that are being defended against.

In those cases where such feelings are ego syntonic and the superego raises no particular objection, the behavior then is manifest and overt, with the extreme cases leading into perverted organizations such as lesbianism, transvestitism, etc. A less malignant situation, that is more spontaneously correctible by later positive events of cetain types, such as strong positive feedback from the environment, and even the self, in relation to breast development, menses, and other body changes, is seen in other cases. I refer to those girls where the fixation at the first stage of the oedipus complex is not as massive, decisive, and encompassing. That is, when in spite of fixation sufficient libidinal moves to the second stage have taken place, thus favorably balancing the stance of femininity versus masculinity (see schema, squares a and b versus d and e).

Yet, it must not be concluded that all tomboyish behavior in latency girls will have an ominous outcome in adolescence or later life. If you observe the schema, you will notice that even those girls who satisfactorily negotiate the second stage and are well oriented in the direction of femininity, still have to contend with the "negative aspects" of the complex, given the bisexuality of human nature. Thus, some tomboyish behavior will be observable for a time, on the basis of the constellation in square e. It follows that whatever reinforces the "negative" side of the complex (conflicts, defenses, unfavorable environmental circumstances) will temporarily increase this tendency. But its manifestations will be much more benign and temporary, and the further advances in feminine identification during latency, prepuberty, puberty, and adolescence may dispose of it altogether. That is why Helene Deutsch (1932), who has studied female homosexuality extensively, could state that many tomboys develop into sweet feminine women (pp. 484-510).

Thus far we have discussed these developmental elements, which prepare the ground for the events that will influence the sexual outcome at adolescence, in terms of sexual identity and feminine identifications. But we have done so only in terms of what happens during the oedipal stage and onwards. Yet we have to be aware that the pregenital phases—that is, the oral and anal stages—contribute markedly to the sexual identity outcome in adolescence.

We have already mentioned that sexual assignment is a very early phenomenon that is well established precisely during these phases. Beyond this, in my opinion, the oral and anal stages make two distinct kinds of contributions. First, they will be most influential on the form taken by the oedipus complex, its resolution, and the expression of the symptoms typical for the conflicts of that developmental stage. On the one hand, important fixations at these early levels may not only determine the form taken by the oedipus complex but may make the normal traversing of it more or less difficult, or even at times impossible. Given that one of the most important foundation stones of a masculine or feminine identification is acquired during the oedipal phase and through its resolution, we can understand the significance of these earlier developmental vicissitudes. For example, an important oral fixation may help to explain cases where adult sexuality is heavily weighted to its oral components, at the expense of the genital ones. In extreme cases, such as some perversions, the genitals will be replaced by the mouth as the dominant erotogenic zone. Similarly, with some women the main source of pleasure, comfort, and reassurance comes not from the genital activity itself but from the foreplay activities, or perhaps from being embraced and held. Other more benign types show for example in the form taken by certain symptoms. Think of castration anxiety, where the fear of body damage may be expressed by means of a phobia of "biting" animals. This clearly pinpoints the oral aggressive conflicts that have contaminated and underlie the form of expression taken by the castration anxiety, an anxiety that itself comes from a much higher level of development, the phallic-oedipal one.

Second, I want to highlight an aspect closely related to the adolescent process (and perhaps one of its greatest dangers) that is, the tendency to act-out, to actualize and enact things in reality. Think again of an oral fixation point, one that is not significant enough to interfere with the move to the oedipal phase and onward. Given the present drug scene, it is conceivable that this weak spot in the personality may become particularly troublesome in adolescence. In fact, this is the way in which some young adolescents (both males and females) get started in a career of drug addiction leading to a final destruction of the personality if not the self. Their oral needs lead them to experiment with drugs, on which they may become dependent to an unusual degree. Once addicted, the addiction itself, as well as other destructive forces acting on the ego, such as increased interaction and identification with other severly disturbed adolescents, with its deleterious effects on their ego ideals, lead finally to delinquient and promiscuous behaviors, for the sake of obtaining the drug. This behavior would not have occurred, except fo the intervening addiction. These girls become delinquent and fall frequently into promiscuity or prostitution, and occasionally into lesbianism, sinking further and further into any activity that becomes the means to procure the drugs. I am trying to emphasize that in many of these girls the original basic faults in their personalities would not have led by themselves to these various outcomes. Yet the intervening drug addiction does.

Of course, anal fixations of various types may play similar disruptive and distorting roles in development. I will only repeat here as an example what I have stated elsewhere. A major anal-sadistic fixation to the preoedipal mother may, and frequently does, interfere with the move in girls from the first to the second stage of the oedipus complex. That move, which implies changing the object mother for the father, can be rendered impossible by the fact that it, of necessity, turns the mother into a hated rival. That situation would reinforce the hostility due to the anal-sadistic fixation, thus creating a highly conflictual situation. Many such girls avoid the conflict by not moving away from the first stage (squares a and b) or phallic-oedipal stage, which is at this point the less conflictual situation. This is because the phallic-oedipal strivings for the mother have somewhat softened the sting of the earlier and purely anal-sadistic interaction (see chapter 3; see also Nagera 1975). These earlier events are relevant for adolescence because they have laid down the blueprint on which the adolescent is forced to work with whatever specific assets and handicaps the adolescent stage brings. But no less important is the fact that all these conflicts come alive again during this stage.

ADOLESCENCE AND SEXUAL IDENTITY

Let us now briefly examine all that has been described so far, in terms of how this looks in the boiling "melting pot" of adolescence itself. It is out of this "melting pot" that a number of final statements about the personality will have to be made. These principally relate, of course, to developmental tasks that must be accomplished at this stage, in order to proceed into adulthood, particularly to the consolidation of a sexual and personal identity. Krohn and Binder (1974), Kaufman, Makkay, and Filbach (1959), Ritvo (1977), Moore (1974), and many others have referred to one aspect or another of these issues from different points of view and in different types of female adolescent cases.

I will, for my purposes, highlight the following tasks:

Some resolution, or attempt at resolution, of the conflicts of dependence-independence, adult-child, active-passive and masculine-feminine.

A better control of pregenital impulses by means of repression, sublimation, reaction formation, etc. This task, may be facilitated somewhat at this time, but the strong and rather sudden presence of genital impulses that may, in favorable circumstances, help to supersede the pregenital ones.

The acquisition of reasonable controls over the genital impulses themselves.

The establishment of more definite and firm ego boundaries, a more complete body and psychological self, now to include breasts, vagina, and uterus, with their accompanying sensations and feelings. Such developments will give a home, so to speak, to the wish for a child, as seen in the fantasies of the oedipal girl. This wish becomes now more intense and real, precisely because of the body changes, menses and the like.

A final and more definitive emotional separation from the parental figures, with a new binding of loving feelings and sexual yearnings, to nonincestuous and sex-appropriate objects. But, as we know, this is a gradual process with many intermediary steps. Kestenbaum (1979) quite rightly points out that in early adolescence heterosexual exploration may function less to establish an intimate tie than to explore new sensations (p. 150).

As a result of the various processes described, the acquisition of a good sexual identity.

Finally, significant steps toward the consolidation of a personal identity.

As we can see, this is quite a tall order, one that requires several years and many intermediary steps. I should add that environmental circumstances and societal changes may favor or hinder such processes. For example, as Kestenbaum (1979) remarks: "Now that the culture surrounding the young adolescent girl is providing her with so few limits, she often feels torn between desire and prudence in a manner seldom encountered in her mother's generation" (p. 155).

Clearly, some such changes can be seen not only from the sociological point of view, but seem capable of exercizing important influences in the developmental processes—in the contents of what is internalized, in the setting up of ego ideals, in superego standards, to name just a few.

Nowadays there are many more models available to female adolescents beyond marriage and motherhood, including a professional life and job opportunities at all levels. As Ritvo (1977) points out, these considerations serve as a transition to the social side of the ego ideal. He continues: "The total psychological significance of motherhood is also influenced by the value, recognition, and prestige society places on motherhood. In a time when a woman's fertility and childbearing functions had high economic value, her prestige and her worth depended very much on her fertility. Woman's fertility does not have that value in our society today. Bearing children is necessary for human survival in an ultimate sense, but in our society it is not necessary for immediate survival or economic well-being as it was in the past. Instead, children are an economic burden. This is an important factor in the reassessment of woman's view of herself and her place in society. If these conditions prevail for an extended time, we may have an opportunity to observe the impact of such external reality factors on unconscious wishes and phantasies" (p. 134).

One thing seems clear in relation to some of these changes. The new roles and greater participation of women in jobs, politics, and business may partly explain (on the basis of more opportunity) the findings of Simon (1975), who showed that there has been an increase in female arrests (1972 FBI report) in the areas of embezzlement, fraud, counterfeiting, and forgery. Sutherland and Cressey (1960) have indicated that the crime rates for females tend to be closer to that of males in those countries where they enjoy more opportunity, freedom, and equality with men. This is true for example of the U.S., Australia, and Western Europe. The opposite is true in countries such as Algiers and Japan, where women have a more subservient and controlled role.

Rosenthal (1979) described the situation well by saying: "The internal and external conflict, generated by the usual disruption of puberty, plus the ambiguity of new roles, creates complex identity problems for girls, perhaps more intense than for boys at present" (p. 504).

Let us now look at some of the conflicts that have traditionally been described as playing an important role in the development of some cases of female homosexuality, because of their interference with achieving a normal sexual identity:

1. Important unconscious fantasies of possessing a penis; with the variations that though not visible now it will grow later on, or that it is hidden in the vagina. This may lead to various sexual disfunctions: fear of intercourse, vaginismus, or in more extreme cases, a total denial of femininity, and possibly homosexuality, and tranvestitism.

2. A continuation and unmodified persistence of a preoedipal fixation to the mother.

3. A massive or traumatic rejection of the girl's femininity by the father.

4. An overt, traumatic and/or hostile reaction to any signs of feminiity in the daughter by the mother, who feels her as a competitor for the husband/father's love.

5. Identifications during the phallic-oedipal phase with a terrifying, sadistic, violent father. This is in many cases a form of

identification with the aggressor, and helps the girl to master her terror of her feared father and other males. Keiser and Schaffer (1949) made the interesting observation, in an institution for delinquent adolescents, that homosexual adolescents with this type of identification are referred to by other girls as "daddies" (p. 287).

6. A strong wish for a boy, by either or both parents.

7. Absence of a father or suitable father figure.

8. Absence of the mother or suitable mother figure.

I refer to these conflicts here so that we can examine how they may interfere with or influence the outcome of sexual identity. I further want to call your attention to the fact that important diagnostic and prognostic elements of judgment are to be gained, by contrasting and examining them, via-a-vis the basic oedipal constellation (and its resolution) at the time of the oedipal phase, but even more important during the adolescent stage. If the conflict is supported, or rather, finds a fertile ground because it runs on the same lines as the basic oedipal constellation, we have both diagnostically and prognostically a much more severe and pathological situation. But if this is not the case, we may well have a much less severe problem, one that is more flexible and fluid, and more liable to correction. For example, let us assume that the female adolescent shows a fixation to the first stage of her oedipus complex (squares a and b). This signifies that her predilection for the object is a homosexual one, and that she has remained in an active-masculine position vis-a-vis that object. Let us further assume, that for unknown reasons she has retained in an intense manner the quasi-universal fantasy from early infancy, that she too has a penis like the little brother. Only that it is inside (in the hole) and will grow later. We can understand her aversion or even horror at having a penis introduced into her vagina. According to her unconscious fantasy her own penis is there, and nothing can go in without her suffering damage. But notice how this ego unconscious fantasy is supported by the fact that because of her oedipal constellation, she is bound to see herself as a boy, an "active penetrator" and not a "passive receiver." Thus, they reinforce each other.

Yet, if this same fantasy had remained as active (for whatever reasons) in a girl or adolescent whose oedipal constellation is that of the second stage (squares d and e), they do not complement or reinforce each other. On the contrary, they are mutually contradictory, in conflict with one another. It is true that the unconscious fantasy may interfere "functionally" with the exercise of her genital function and her feminiity. It is true too, that it may force her to avoid the company of males, but the fact remains that there is a contradiction, a conflict between the fantasy and her basic feminine position and as such no reinforcement of the one by the other is taking place. Indeed, each one of them is on the opposite side of the conflict.

Finally, let me make a few comments about the value of the schema of the female oedipus complex that I have presented, when used in coordination with the other four lines of development mentioned earlier and when taking into consideration those relevant developmental mechanisms that precede and follow it. The latter are the result of internal processes on the one hand and of favorable or unfavorable influences on the other.

Keiser and Schaffer (1949), on the basis of their observations in a psychiatric ward, divided the homosexual adolescent girls into three types (pp. 283-295).[2]

1. Aggressive, fighting, masculine girls who carry knives.
2. Outwardly passive girls.
3. Completely maladjusted girls who refuse the feminine role from infancy.

The first type became aggressive, violent, and in every way the counterpart of a rapacious male, at adolescence or before. Their behavior, according to these authors, was meant to disprove femininity, which they regarded with loathing and fear. In juxtaposition to the above, there was a tremendous drive to live as if they really possessed a penis, forcing other girls into the role of a passive subject, and literally raping them with the threat of a knife. They walked, dressed, and spoke with masculine manner-

2. Many of these girls had other forms of pathology, including truancy, associated with their homosexuality. Some had been arrested for assaults, robbery, or mugging or forcing sexual relations upon other girls.

isms. The authors further remarked that these girls had vicious fathers, who abused their mothers, and had seen their mothers abused by other males.

In terms of the schema, the first type of adolescent girl could be said to be fixated at the first stage (phallic-oedipal), squares a and b. This is based on consideration of the homosexual object choice, and the fact that this type *seems* to behave from an active-masculine position. I say she *seems* to do it from an active-masculine position because that is what her behavior suggests, but as we know, overt behavior by itself can be a dangerous and misleading indication in many cases. Consider for example the Don Juan syndrome, where the overt behavior is super- or extra-heterosexual to defend against latent homosexual impulses. The only way to be more certain would be to find out the nature of the sexual fantasies used by these girls during masturbation, or during erotic reveries. They will reveal the true nature of the sexual position as active-masculine or passive-feminine. The same is true, if we can accurately determine which sexual activities actually give the patient the most satisfaction and fulfillment.

Without that knowledge, we would have to consider an alternative possibility that exists in spite of these gross clinical manifestations. This behavior could be a defensive reinforcement, because of conflict, of the negative aspects of the oedipal constellation, for a girl that has reached the second stage (oedipal), squares d and e. This is of course a much higher level of ego and drive development than the earlier stage. But if this is the case, sooner or later we will come across the evidence of that higher level of organization and development. For example, if we could get hold of this adolescent's sexual fantasies (during masturbation or reveries), we should not be surprised to find that she plays a passive-feminine role to a male, in spite of the fact that her overt behavior is just in the opposite direction.

As to the aggressive, violent, vicious, sadistic nature of her behavior toward the girls that she chooses as objects, the developmental history, in the limited way that is available, suggests strongly the possibility of an identification with the aggressor, the sadistic father, at the phallic-oedipal stage. Another possibility, that would have facilitated that identification, would be the existence of an anal-sadistic fixation in the preoedipal relationship to the mother; but in this respect the history as presented by the authors is vague, though somewhat suggestive.

The second type described by Keiser and Schaffer, that of the sweet, gentle, passive-feminine homosexual adolescent, will of necessity fall into the second stage (oedipal), square f. Her problem lies in not having been able to exchange the mother as an object for that of the father. Yet, her basic position is a normal passive-feminine one, only that she wants to play that role to a woman not to a male.

The developmental history will quite easily explain why, regardless of her advanced development in other areas, she could not accomplish the exchange of the object. A father rejecting the feminine overtures of the little girl, but otherwise a good father, may loom somewhere in the background. Or perhaps a mother that resented the daughter's competition for the father and other male figures, but that was otherwise a good mother may have played a role, or even a combination of both factors. Or, a mother who is unconsciously seductive to the girl but wants her daughter to achieve a passive-feminine position, at which point she retains her as her love object.

The third type Keiser and Schaffer encountered was that group that militantly refused to accept their status as female, and though not psychotic, demanded, at times vociferously, to be accepted as men. They had wanted to be boys since their earliest memories, enjoying boy's clothing and refusing feminine apparel. Not infrequently as late adolescents, they were arrested for transvestitism. They want to be treated as males and make no bones of expressing the fantasy of living their lives as men. They do not become caricatures of masculine mannerisms but walk, talk, and gesture as men, with no traces of femininity. Many among them are transsexuals and would like to be provided with male genitalia. Some describe their condition as that of a male imprisoned in a female body.[3] The fixation here is most likely to be at the first stage

3. Indeed, a few among the latter goes as far as to reject overt homosexuality, on the basis that anatomically they are girls and consider homosexual relationships inappropriate and vulgar. This sort of subtype does not want to be a homosexual girl playing a masculine role. She wants to become a man and then satisfy a girl.

(phallic-oedipal) positions a and b, and the vicissitudes of their developmental histories will explain the multiplicity of variations and manifest clinical forms observed.

Let me insist that these assessments be made on the basis of both the schema and the four lines of development closely associated with it. It is necessary to determine where in each line the patient is and the reasons for their being there. And beyond this, one must look at the relevant developmental processes before and after the oedipal phase that may affect sexual identity and its outcome.

I will finish with a relevant quote of Keiser and Schaffer (1949): "The study of the development of the girl is particularly fruitful during the adolescent period. The wild surges that are engendered by the biological growth into a mature woman lead to many disturbances. Deep unconscious mechanisms are readily activated and observed more easily during this period. In the more normal girl it appears that the ego is readjusting itself to the new demands placed upon it. There is a certain amount of trial and error method until healthy maturity is established. For the types of girls studied here, [by them], the adolescent period seems to be more the final expression of an ego that has already adopted a method of behavior" (p. 290). I will only add that for other cases, as distinct from their very disturbed population, adolescence itself may and does contribute very significantly to the methods of behavior the ego will adopt from there onward.

References

Blos, P. (1957). Preoedipal factors in the etiology of female delinquency. *Psychoanalytic Study of the Child* 12:229-249.

Deutsch, H. (1932). Female homosexuality. *Psychoanalytic Quarterly* 7:484-510.

——— (1944). *The Psychology of Women*. New York: Grune and Stratton.

Freud, S. (1925). Some psychological consequences of the anatomical distinction between the sexes. *Standard Edition* 19:243-260.

Kaufman, I., Makkay, E.S., and Zilbach, J. (1959). The impact of adolescence on girls with delinquent character formation. *American Journal of Orthopsychiatry* 39:130-143.

Keiser, S., and Schaffer, D. (1949). Environmental factors in homosexuality in adolescent girls. *Psychoanalytic Review* 36:283-295.

Kestenbaum, C.J. (1979). Current sexual attitudes, societal pressure, and the middle class adolescent girl. In *Adolescent Psychiatry: Developmental and Clinical Studies,* vol. 7 pp. 147-156; ed. S. Feinstein and P. Giovacchini, Chicago: pp. 147-156. The University of Chicago Press.

Kestenberg, J.S. (1961). Menarche. In *Adolescents, Psychoanalytic Approach to Problems and Therapy,* ed. Sandor Lorand. New York: Paul B. Hoever, Inc.

Krohn, A., and Binder, J. (1974). Sexual acting out as an aborting mourning process in adolescents. *Psychiatric Quarterly* 48:193-208.

Money, J., Hampson, J.C., and Hampson, J.L. (1955). An examination of some basic sexual concepts—the evidence of human hermaphroditism. *Bulletin of Johns Hopkins Hospital* 97:301-319.

——— (1955). Hermaphroditism—recommendations concerning assignment of sex, change of sex, and psychological management. *Bulletin of Johns Hopkins Hospital* 97:284-300.

——— (1956). Sexual incongruities and psychopathology—the evidence of human hermaphroditism" *Bulletin of Johns Hopkins Hospital* 98:43-57.

Moore, W.T. (1974). Promiscuity in a thirteen-year-old girl. *Psychoanalytic Study of the Child* 29:301-318.

Nagera, H., (1975). *On Female Sexuality and the Oedipus Complex,* New York: Jason Aronson.

Ritvo, S. (1977). Adolescent to woman. In *Female Psychology: Contemporary Psychoanalytic Views,* ed. H. Blum, New York: International Universities Press.

Rosenthal, P.A. (1979). Delinquency in adolescent girls: developmental aspects. In *Adolescent Psychiatry: Developmental and Clinical Studies,* vol. 7, ed. Feinstein and Giovacchini. Chicago: The University of Chicago Press

Simon, R. (1975). *Women and Crime.* Lexington: Heath.

Stoller, R.J. (1974). *Sex and Gender.* New York: Jason Aronson.

Sugar, M., ed. (1979). *Female Adolescent Development,* New York: Brunner/Mazel.

Sutherland, E.H., and Cressey, D.R. (1960). *Principles of Criminology,* Chicago: Lippincott.

Part IV

THE DEVELOPMENTAL APPROACH IN CLINICAL PRACTICE

Chapter Thirteen

SLEEP DISTURBANCES

THE FIRST YEAR OF LIFE

In 1955 Margaret S. Mahler introduced a panel on sleep disturbances in children with the statement "that research in child
development and child analysis, just as in physiology, affords
little knowledge of the normal patterns of the sleep cycle or of its
individual variations at various ages. She emphasized that except
for pavor nocturnus and sleep phobias we do not know . . . whether
we are dealing with *disturbances* of sleep or variations of the sleep
pattern" (see Friend 1956, pp. 514-515).

Although the amount of research on sleep has vastly increased
since this statement was made, the study of the sleep patterns of
infants has remained a comparatively neglected field. As a consequence we still know relatively little about the sleep disturbances
of children, especially in the first year of life.

In the same panel Samual A. Guttman noted the difficulties in
establishing whether or not an infant is asleep because the criteria
such as responsiveness to noise or vibration as well as movement
and posture are exceedingly complex. Gregory Rochlin made the
same point and mentioned the existence of similar observational
difficulties even in the case of older children.

Recent advances in our knowledge of sleep have solved some of these problems. With the help of EEG studies, it is now possible to establish accurately and quickly not only whether a child or adult is sleeping but also at which stage of the sleep cycle the person is. Nevertheless, more information is needed about the earliest periods of life. At that time the infant's nervous system is far from a finished product and still requires a long extrauterine period for its maturation. In view of this immaturity, it is not possible to draw too many inferences from the work on adults, whose central nervous system is a fully developed organ.

These early developmental stages are, for analysts, a particularly obscure period about which we can talk only in rather general terms. The different conceptualizations of these early phases are not only patchy and incomplete but frequently contradictory and sometimes even untenable. I believe that this state of affairs is a necessary stage in the development of our knowledge. I mention it here for two reasons: first, to highlight the difficulties involved in the study of sleep and its disturbances during the first year of life. Since we assume that development proceeds on the basis of a complex interaction between specific innate givens and environmental, experiential factors, we must evaluate not only the child but also the role of the mother and other specific environmental influences. Secondly, I believe that analysts in order to gain a better understanding of these stages must continue to give due weight to the many valuable contributions made by scientists in related disciplines. This coordination of findings[1] is essential, especially in view of the fact that direct observation and reconstruction—the only tools available to the analyst—have obvious limitations in their application to the earliest phases of development.

With regard to the infant's sleep pattern many authors agree that significant changes occur in the third month of life, but there is no agreement on whether this change is due partly to "learning" or fully determined by biological factors. In view of these changes and their relation to physical and psychological maturational

1. A good example of this procedure is Sanford Gifford's (1960) investigation of the infant's sleep-wakefulness pattern, which is viewed in terms of analytic theory, observational material, and Kleitman and Engelmann's findings (1953).

advances taking place at different points during the first year of life, I shall present the relevant material in chronological order.

The First Three Months

Analysts differ somewhat in their assumptions concerning the degree of ego development present at birth, the newborn's capacity to experience stimuli of an external or internal nature, his ability to process and integrate them, and the level at which bio-psychological integration and meaningful experiences take place. Yet these are essential considerations for a better understanding of the influences which the mother's handling and other environmental factors have on the normal or abnormal development of the child. In order to characterize the functional state of the mental apparatus of the newborn it is important to refer to Kleitman's very significant statement (1939): "We are accustomed to think of ourselves as being awake and something must be done to make us sleep. It is actually the other way round. We begin asleep and thereafter have interruptions of sleep by wakefulness" (p. 212). This statemet has been corroborated by a number of electroencephalographic studies. For example, Walter's EEG studies (1953) revealed that infancy is characterized by a pattern of delta waves, which in the adult are found only in states of somnolence. The delta waves become less prominent on some occasions, e.g., when the child is attentive, usually around the second or third month of life. This state of alertness coincides with the appearance of alpha waves in the electroencephalographic record; that is, when the "twilight state" of the newborn (Ribble 1943) begins to give way to a sharper demarcation between sleep and mental activity. These findings are relevant to any formulations of the mental processes taking place in the first few weeks and later stages of life. (I shall later formulate some tentative hypotheses based on these findings.)

In the panel previously referred to Rochlin stated that many "inferences drawn from observed behavior of the infant do have a natural tendency to be anthropomorphic and homuncular. The highly organized performance of the baby at the breast may not be so much an index of its cerebral-cortical activity as has been supposed, but may be that avenue of behavior through which a primitive, psychic, homeostatic state is arrived at by gratification of relatively simple visceral needs which have a distinctly temporal character" (see Friend 1956, p. 517).

Whatever view of the early stages one is inclined to hold, all authors agree on the fact that there is constant maturation and development of a physical and psychological nature and that this process reaches, in terms of the sleep-wakefulness rhythm, an acme around the third month of life. The newborn starts with a polycyclic type of existence, in which sleep is punctuated by irregular periods of wakefulness determined or regulated by his basic needs, especially by hunger. From this pattern the newborn moves into what Kleitman (1939) calls the "monocyclic type of existence" seen in older children and adults. He says: "one of the first *learned* performances is sleeping through the night by skipping one feeding, and the gradual lengthening of the daytime period of wakefulness" (quoted in Gifford 1960, p. 32).

Sanford Gifford (1960) utilized Kleitman and Engelmann's observations of the sleep characteristics of a group of nineteen normal infants from the third to the twenty-sixth week of life. He interpreted their statistical data "as indicating three developmental phases, approximately corresponding to hypothetical phases of ego development" (p. 38). These three developmental phases are: (1) an undifferentiated phase (from birth to the third week); (2) precursors of ego functioning (from the third to the twelfth or fourteenth week); (3) the beginning of object relations (from the twelfth or fourteenth to the twenty-sixth week).

Gifford states that "the development of the ego and the sleep-wakefulness pattern are both determined by an interrelationship between the infant's genetic pattern of neurophysiological maturation and his mother's characteristic mode of response to his biological and emotional needs. This continuous interaction between constitutional equipment and maternal responsiveness is a unitary process of psychophysiological adaptation, at a time when the infant's manifest behavior, homeostatic patterns, and precursors of ego structure are still undifferentiated" (p. 34).

From birth to the third week. Gifford (1960) characterizes the sleeping patterns of the "undifferentiated phase" (from birth to the third week) as "Seemingly random, irregular intervals of sleep and waking that follow an innate rhythm of hunger, awakening, motor excitation, feeding and sleep, unrelated to external events or the 24-hour calendar day" (p. 21). Toward the end of the third week, one can observe an adaptation of the sleep-wakefulness pattern to the periodicity of day and night. Gifford considers this adaptation to be one of the earliest precursors of ego functioning; it appears earlier than, for example, the smiling response and purposeful finger sucking. His view is that "an innate biological tendency [is being] progressively influenced by the environment as the infant's perceptual apparatus matures. A random, disorganized pattern undergoes a systematic modification that is mediated through the infant's relationship with his mother, beginning before the development of accurate distance perception or awareness of the mother as a differentiated object" (p. 13). In support of his thesis Gifford quotes Brazelton, a pediatrician who in a personal communication expressed the opinion "that after the third week the infant's innate tendencies, his activity level, responsiveness to the environment or ease in being satisfied by feeding, begin to reflect his mother's attitudes, to show the influence of her fears and anxieties, as when a relatively stable and easily satisfied baby becomes discontented and overactive" (p. 23).

This statement raises the question of how early the influence of the mother, in emotional and psychological terms, shows itself in the child's specific reactions. It is clear that babies react to their mothers' handling in one way or another from the very beginning of life, but what remains unclear is the level at which that response occurs. In this context, it is important to remind ourselves of Rochlin's statement that our observations of babies often are anthropomorphic and homuncular so that we tend to interpret the baby's reactions to environmental stimuli and maternal handling as taking place on a much higher level of complexity and integration than is possible in the early stages.

Although I agree with Gifford's view that the sleep pattern undergoes a systematic modification through the relationship

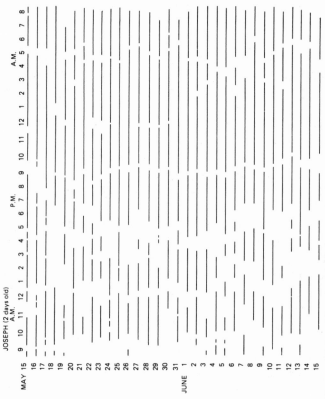

Figure 13-1. Sleep-wakefulness pattern of baby Joseph from the second to the thirtieth day of life. (Prepared at the Hampstead War Nurseries by Sophie and Gertrude Dann.)

with the mother, I have some doubts about considering the sleep pattern as disorganized and random as he describes it during the first three weeks of life. These doubts are based on observations made over twenty years ago in the Hampstead War Nurseries where charts on the sleeping patterns of a number of children of different ages were kept. One of them is a record of the sleep-wakefulness pattern of baby Joseph from the second to the thirtieth day of life. This graph shows from the very beginning a clearly defined pattern which subsequently developed in the directions outlined by Gifford and others From the third day onward there is a clear and consistent pattern of more prolonged and continuous sleep during the night period than during the daytime. Joseph slept approximately between the periods of 6 P.M. and 7:30 A.M., although during that period of time he used to wake up spontaneously three times for the first nine days. He was usually awake less than an half hour at a time. Beginning on the eleventh and twelfth day of his life he woke up two or three times during the evening period, usually for a short while, until nearly the end of the thirty-day period of observation, when in the last four evenings he started to wake only twice each evening. The daytime pattern of sleep during the whole month shows three sleeping periods, two generally of longer duration and the third a brief one. Toward the second half of the first month of observation the periods of wakefulness in the daytime noticeably increased.

As can be seen from Figure 13-1, the child slept almost continuously day and night only during the second, third, and fourth day of his life, but even then the evening periods of sleep were longer and less broken than those during the day. Since there was a very significant change in the general rhythm of almost continuous sleep on the fifth day, I wonder whether the pattern observed during the initial three to five days is not an artifact introduced by the trauma of birth.

It can be argued that at the Hampstead War Nurseries Joseph was living in a group and that his pattern of sleep-wakefulness clearly shows the influence of this condition. This is of course quite possible. For this reason, as well as others, I stress the need for further research on the sleep patterns in early infancy. On the other hand, the observations made by Moore and Ucko (1957) indicate that during the first weeks of life noise and other forms of disturbances (presumably within certain limits that the War Nurseries may have exceeded) do not tend to interfere with the sleep of the baby. Furthermore, Kleitman and Engelmann (1953) concluded that although there are wide individual variations, the infant sleeps more and for longer periods during the night than during the day even in the earliest weeks. They also noted that these observable differences between day and night increase rapidly during the first three months and only much more slowly thereafter. These data seem to be in line with the observations made at the Hampstead War Nurseries.[2]

More recent studies have demonstrated that the sleep schedule is closely linked to many other physiological regulatory mechanisms which in the human organism follow a twenty-four-hour period that seems to be geared to the rhythmic changes of nature. These mechanisms regulate rise and fall of temperature, heart rate, blood pressure, metabolism, adrenocortical activity, etc., all of which follow a twenty-four-hour cycle of peaks and lows which coincides with the waking and sleeping states. These rhythms can be reversed but only through a prolonged period of adaptation (Luce and Segal 1966). Nevertheless, some of the physiological and endocrinological mechanisms and functions involved are apparently not completely developed at birth and their degree of integration requires further investigation. However, the data already available speak against the completely random and disorganized pattern of the sleep-wakefulness rhythm that Gifford suggests. Other authors, e.g., Moore and Ucko (1957), concluded that babies do not have to "learn" to sleep through the night but "that there is a natural tendency for infants to lengthen their period of continuous night sleep while curtailing that taken by day" (p. 341). Yet their own observations seem to point in the direction that certain

2. Parmelee et al. (1964) studied the sleep patterns of forty-six infants from birth through the sixteenth week. The infants slept an average of 16.32 hours daily during the first week and 14.87 hours by the sixteenth week. The average longest period of sleep per day was 4.08 hours during the first week and 7.67 hours in the twelfth week. The average longest period of wakefulness per day was 2.39 hours in the first week and 3.11 hours in the twelfth week.

specific factors in the infant's relationship to the mother may facilitate or hinder the establishment of an appropriate sleeping rhythm during the evening. Moore and Ucko also found that a number of the factors generally assumed to influence or interfere with the sleep rhythm of babies do not seem to be operative before the third month of life.

From the third to the twelfth or fourteenth week. In the second phase described by Gifford (1960), that of "precursors of ego functioning," there is a sharp decrease in the hours of sleep during daytime and in the frequency of night feedings and a proportional increase in the hours of night sleep. Thus the number of total hours of sleep remains similar, while at the same time a more organized sleep-wakefulness rhythm develops. To Gifford, "This configuration suggests an integrated process of adaptation to the 24-hour cycle, more complex and organized than reflex responses to crude external stimuli can account for. The 'physiological' basis for this process is the maturation of the perceptual apparatus, perhaps constitutionally determined, and its psychological or 'learned' basis is the result of a developing emotional interrelationship between the infant and his mother. An alternative explanation, that the evolution of the sleep rhythm is entirely the result of neurophysiological maturation, fails to account for sleep disturbances before the third month when the mother-child relationship is disturbed, as in Rank and Mcnaughton's atypical child [1950], or in the frequent lesser disturbances that occur in normal and neurotic families. If a disturbed maternal relationship can interfere with the development of the sleep-wakefulness pattern, it may be assumed that a relatively normal relationship can exert a favorable influence" (p. 25).

On this point there still exists some controversy. Moore and Ucko (1957) concluded that babies do not have to "learn" to sleep through the night. They state: "What we have called the 'settling' process, a form of learning at the level of biological adaptation, requires no consciously directed training by the parents" (p. 347). Luce and Segal (1966) concluded that "the mounting evidence suggests that the twenty-four hour rhythm is a reality, ticked off by the central nervous system, and that a baby begins to sleep through the night, not because his parents train him but because his brain has sufficiently matured" (p. 55). Parmelee et al. (1964) assert that the development of the sleep pattern "is a normal phenomenon of neurological maturation and rather independent of training and feeding efforts" (p. 582). On the other hand, Oswald (1966) assumes that the "recurrence of inactivity every twenty-four hours constitutes a rhythm which the body has 'learned' through experience" (p. 10). He believes, as does Kleitman, that babies acquire or learn (through the pressures of social life, etc.) the twenty-four-hour rhythm.

Whereas Gifford assumes that an important modification of the previously random and disorganized pattern of the first three weeks takes place, our observations do not support this early disorganized pattern. On the other hand, our charts indicate a reduction of the sleeping time during daytime and a more continuous sleeping period in the evening.

I also question Gifford's use of atypical children to draw conclusions concerning normal development. His argument, that his view can explain the frequent minor sleeping disturbances observed in babies of normal and neurotic parents, is sharply contradicted by the findings reported by Moore and Ucko. Their study of 200 babies from birth onward shows that there are grounds to question many of the generally accepted assumptions about the influence of parental handling (under reasonable conditions, that is, excluding instances of extreme mishandling) on the so-called sleep disturbances in babies *before the third month of life*. These authors established empirically that the age of thirteen weeks is a turning point in the process of adjustment to sleeping through the night.[3] They designate the point at which this change takes place as the "age of settling" and refer to the developments that lead to the change observed by the thirteenth week as the "settling" process.

Several other findings of the Moore and Ucko study are of

3. Moore and Ucko define sleeping through the night as undisturbed sleep between 12 A.M. and 5 A.M. in the morning. Although this interval may be considered to be arbitrary, the substantial body of their observations and conclusions is nevertheless of interest.

special interest. The sexes show no significant differences in the age of the first settling (at the thirteenth week). However, if the whole year is considered, it is apparent that boys wake significantly more often than girls and that these tendencies are already present, though not statistically significant, in the waking scores for the first three months. This finding is also in agreement with Kleitman's observations although Moore and Ucko cover slightly different spans of time in the life of the children observed.

Moore and Ucko also studied the effect of illness on sleep during the first three months of life, that is, before the age of settling; they concluded that illnesses seem to have no lasting effect on the night sleep during this period, although ill health may cause a few broken nights. The sleep pattern was resumed as soon as the acute phase of the illness was over.[4]

Analysts have postulated a connection between sucking and sleep. Moore and Ucko's findings also suggest such an interrelationship which deserves further study.[5]

Their observations also indicate that before the age of three months, i.e., before the age of settling, seasonal changes in light and temperature show no relationship to the age of settling.[6]

Sharing a room and noise had no demonstrable effect on the

4. This finding was in sharp contrast to their findings with regard to the effect of illness on the sleep rhythm during the later part of the first year of life. At that time illness can induce sleep disturbances that may last several months.

5. One of my patients has a baby, aged seven and a half weeks, who at five weeks already slept through the night. This baby is allowed as much sucking time as he desires. His last feeding, consisting of the breast first and then a bottle, is usually taken between 9 and 10 P.M., whereupon he falls asleep until 5 A.M. in the morning. Then again he has the breast and a bottle. This baby is fed on demand and the mother allows him to suck at the breast for any length of time, even when her milk is finished.

6. In the adult sleep-rhythm disturbances have been observed when the 24-hour periodicity of day and night disappears, e.g., in northern Scandinavia and among Arctic explorers (see Gifford 1960).

My own children moved from a country in which there are no significant seasonal changes between day and night to England where at the peak of the summer it is still daylight until 10 P.M. When we moved the children, three and four years old, objected for some time to going to sleep at their usual hour (between 7 and 7:30 P.M.) on the basis that it was still daylight. The opposite was never observed; that is, in winter when it was dark by 3:30 P.M., they were never ready for bed before their usual time.

Anna Freud observed at the Hampstead War Nurseries that when double summertime was introduced, there were great difficulties in getting the children to sleep in daylight.

settling age; the authors in fact thought that it was remarkable "how easily those babies that sleep in the living room would go to sleep with the whole family present making no special effort to be quiet" (p. 338). They refer to Irwin and Weiss (1934) whose studies have shown that continuous fairly strong stimuli—visual, auditory or cutaneous—have an inhibitory effect, at least on the newborn infant.

Further, Moore and Ucko found that a change of cot or sleeping room did not produce any noticeable effect on a large number of infants under three months, whereas *from the third month* on such changes frequently produced temporary disturbances.

On the other hand, they noticed that minimal changes in routine, such as shifting the bath time from morning to evening, proved helpful in settling some of the babies, while in other cases a temporary change such as a holiday upset a previously good sleeper. Generally, however, they found that this type of upset tends to pass easily when it occurs before the third month of life, while at a later age it can be the starting point of prolonged difficulties.

The child's position in the family was significant in terms of the age of settling, but the significance started only with the third child and not with the first two. Moore and Ucko concluded that the mother's experience of having had *two* children is more important than her age or education, which were not significant. The third child usually settles better.

The age of weaning from the breast showed no relationship either to the settling age or to the tendency to wake during the first three months. Breast- and bottle-fed babies behaved similarly. Moore and Ucko state that "actual weaning had a settling effect on sleeping in at least a dozen cases. In no case did weaning from the breast before three months, however sudden, lead to increased waking (we are not here considering other effects of weaning)" (p. 339). Flexibility or lack of it in respect to feeding times (demand versus clock feeding) showed no special relationship to the age of settling; the three groups classed as "demand fed," "clock fed," and "latitude allowed," contained approximately the same number of settlers and nonsettlers and children with high and low waking scores. Certain children, however, benefited (in terms of settling) from a more reasonable adaptation of the timing of feeding in contrast to an early one that had proved too rigid.

Moore and Ucko found that *for most children an adequate amount of interplay with the mother is an important factor conducive to the establishment of an appropriate sleep rhythm.* They referred to this form of contact as "excess nursing time," that is, a measure of the time given by the mother to the baby for contact and play over and above what he may need for feeding. The babies who received the least excess nursing time had the greatest tendency to wake, and those who received and excessive amount were the next most wakeful group, while those who had ten to twenty minutes in addition to the feeding time settled best. The mothers in the third group, it seems to me, had the best functional adaptation to their children. In *Early Childhood Disturbances, the Infantile Neurosis, and the Adulthood Disturbances* (1966), I emphasized that the mother's role in furthering the development of the child consists not only in satisfying his more fundamental needs and protecting him from unnecessary or harmful stimulation but in providing diverse types of stimulation which facilitates the development of specific ego functions.

I am inclined to think that before the third month of life the mother's stimulation, or lack of it, affects the infant's ego development in toto and that the result of this can be observed in the delayed appearance of the smiling response, the age of settling, motor skills and coordination, etc. I do not mean to imply that certain specific forms of stimulation preferred or neglected by mothers may not further or hinder the maturational processes of certain ego apparatuses and functions in preference to others, but I mean to say that a minimum general form of stimulation is necessary for harmonious development. There is sufficient evidence from studies of neglected and institutionalized children to warrant the assumption that extremely disturbed mothers, who cannot provide this basic minimum of overall stimulation and comfort to their babies, or who overexcite them, affect far more of the child's ego progress than just the age of settling. This will be just one of several areas affected.

Finally, Moore and Ucko found an important relationship between night waking and the circumstances of birth. For example, asphyxia at birth was encountered in forty infants (according to the obstetric records), nineteen of whom (47 percent) failed to settle by three months, compared with only 28 percent of non-asphyxiated infants. The asphyxiated group continued to display a greater tendency to wake throughout the year. (The authors point out that the diagnosis of neonatal asphyxia is a somewhat subjective matter and that these records have to be considered with caution.) They quote Preston who also found that children who have suffered a mild degree of anoxia during (child) birth show a permanent tendency to hyperactivity and overresponsiveness, with much crying and disturbed feeding and sleep in infancy, while those with a greater depth of anoxia show serious apathy.

Birth weight, weight at three months, and weight increment over this period were not related either to age of settling or to waking scores for this period.

Discussing the age of settling and sleep disturbances during the first three months of life Moore and Ucko were surprised by the large number of babies who adhered to the norm, especially in view of the fact that more than one adverse factor was present in children who slept throughout the night. In their final assessment Moore and Ucko list the factors associated with continued waking during the first three months and the failure to settle: (1) *lack of wisdom in the parents:* insufficient nursing by the mother due to lack of time or inclination; excess of anxious oversolicitous mothering; erratic behavior due to fecklessness or ambivalence to the child; rigid controlling attitudes leading to the imposition of unsuitable regimes; (2) *some cause within the child:* asphyxia or other birth trauma, constitutional sensitiveness, etc. The interaction of these numerous factors is so complex that, in the opinion of these authors, it is seldom possible to say definitely that the failure to sleep is due to any one particular cause.

Some hypothetical correlations between EEG findings and psychoanalytic observations. Many of the surprising findings of Moore and Ucko are perhaps more easily understood if we keep in mind that the electroencephalographic pattern characteristic for most of the first three months of life—the delta waves—corresponds to a state of somnolence in the adult. In view of this fact it is possible that during this early stage of development the impact of some maternal attitudes on the child has been overestimated, while that of other environmental factors has been neglected. This statement is in no way intended to minimize the significance of the mother-child interaction from the very beginning of the infant's life. However, this statement is intended to specify the nature of this interaction. At first the mother acts as an organizer and stimulator of maturational processes (of a physical and psychological nature) which steer development into appropriate channels and at the same time open the way to later different types of interactions.

Furthermore, as has been pointed out, the functional condition of the infant's brain with its delta waves resembles that of the somnolent states in the adult. The delta waves disappear only at moments when the child is attentive in a special way by the second or third month, at which point the functional capacity is heightened and the alpha waves appear. The stimuli that cause the infant to emerge from the somnolent state can be assumed to be increased internal needs or discomfort, at which point the mother will come to him. The communication between mother and child thus takes place during a stage of heightened alertness and functional capacity. It is plausible that the baby's experiences under these functional conditions are more significant and that the contacts of baby and mother at such points (when the alpha waves displace the delta pattern) facilitate not only ego development but also a beginning awareness of the object.[7]

7. Oswald (1966) remarked that "the alpha rhythm is an indication that the brain is functioning at one particular level of efficiency, alertness or 'vigilance'.... When the alpha rhythm is lost in drowsiness, the brain is functioning at a lower level of effectiveness" (p. 21). He also refers to the experiments of two American psychologists, Emmons and Simon, who tested the commercial "sleep-learning" claims. They played taperecorded answers to questions while the subjects were asleep and also took EEG records. They conclude that we do not learn while asleep (slow waves and spindles). However, the authors found that in the morning answers played while alpha rhythm was present (the subjects were not sleeping at this point) were recalled easily, whereas those played while the alpha rhythm was waning often were not recallable.

It is perhaps not without significance that the institutionalized baby will miss this opportunity of contact with another human being at the times when he is in a state of functional alertness. These occasional states of alertness during the first few weeks of life usually charm mothers who respond intensely and in kind to the child, as all those who have had the opportunity to observe babies and their mothers will confirm. I believe that this interaction has a chain effect: such states of alertness tend to arise more frequently when the child is responded to; the mother's response leads to increased alertness and to the wish for more contact. Conversely the lack of response to these early occasional states of alertness in the institutionalized child may well contribute to, and perhaps determine, his later withdrawn attitude, lack of alertness and interest, and even fear of contact which Spitz and others have described so well.

On the other hand, many ministrations of the mother take place when the functional condition of the baby's brain is of the somnolent type (delta waves pattern); therefore, their impact on the infant must be of a different quality. At such points things happen to him when he is not as alloplastically orientated as in the previous state. Nevertheless, the ministrations of the mother under such conditions still provide him with a wide range of new sensory stimulation, contributing to the functional awakening and development of different ego apparatuses and, at the beginning, more especially the perceptual one. Through these ministrations the mother also provides a good deal of the necessary and basic conditions of minimum comfort and well-being, without which ego development cannot proceed normally.

It seems too that by the second and third month, specific aspects of the mother's behavior, certain types of stimulation and play will have an arousing capacity similar to that of internal needs. The careful study and interpretation of electroencephalographic findings in neonates and their correlation with psychoanalytic observations may help to clarify both the essential needs of the child and the role of the mother as a stimulating agent for further development. As mentioned, the observations on neglected and institutionalized children have demonstrated the damage done to the child resulting from the lack of the necessary stimulation;

significantly, this damage becomes more evident from the third month on. Other observations seem to point to the fact that there is an "ideal" amount of stimulation which has the most beneficial effects. Not only lack of stimulation but also excessive amounts of it interfere with the child's well-being, as has been pointed out earlier with regard to sleep. Provence and Lipton (1962) state that the infants in the institution they studied slept longer hours and with fewer interruptions than babies reared in families. They received similar reports from the foster mothers of children coming from institutional settings. The foster mothers felt that for several weeks the children slept for excessive periods of time. Furthermore, a reduction in the total hours of sleep accompanied the general improvement in the child's development as a response to the improvement in the nurturing care.

At the very early stages of development the infant's response to the mother and to the environmental handling should be understood in the above context and not as a specific symptomatic emotional and psychological response of a complexity that is possible only at a somewhat later stage when the child's ego development and object relations have reached the appropriate levels. Anthropomorphic and homuncular interpretations are thus avoided.

From the Third Month Onward

Kleitman described the important changes in the sleep-wakefulness rhythm of the baby that take place around the twelfth week. These changes correspond to the age of settling as defined by Moore and Ucko in the thirteenth week. Thereafter the development of the child's ego proceeds at a faster rate. As shown above, many of the factors that did not significantly influence the age of settling and the sleep patterns before the third month trigger more or less serious sleep disturbances after the third month. All authors agree that from this time on, many such factors are increasingly capable of having this effect.

From the twelfth or fourteenth week to the twenty-sixth week. Gifford describes the "third phase" of development in terms of the beginning of object relations. The early stages of this phase are in a continuum of development with the last stages of the previous one (Gifford's second phase of early ego development) since many of the achievements begin to appear at the very end of it and will proceed further during this third phase. Some of the landmarks of development appear at this point for the first time, e.g., the hand-mouth coordination.

With regard to the development of the sleep-wakefulness pattern Gifford quotes Kleitman, who emphasized the importance of perceptual maturation in the adaptation of the waking state to the activities of the daytime. This maturation and development of the perceptual apparatuses and processes provide the infant with new sensory experiences and objects of interest in his immediate surroundings. Gifford and others consider the period between the twelfth to the twenty-sixth week as one when rapid advances in perceptual integration take place. The infant becomes increasingly aware of his surroundings and begins to communicate visually with his mother. Among other advances in ego development, Gifford refers to the smiling response (which appears around the tenth to twelfth week) and the development of the hand-mouth coordination, which, according to Hoffer (1949), usually does not take place intentionally before the twelfth week and is well established between the twelfth and sixteenth week. As Gifford points out, the exact chronological relationship between the smiling response, the hand-mouth coordination, and the change in the child's sleep pattern around the twelfth week has never been systematically studied and the possible interaction between these factors has not been established. In any event, as Gifford states, "the infant's capacity for purposeful self-gratification by bringing the hand to the mouth, according to Hoffer [1949], contributes to the organization of the ego, by defining its surfaces, parts, and functions. This capacity for self-gratification increases his independence from his mother's feedings and enables him to sleep through the night . . . [there is] a reduction in the number of night feedings, from over three to about one at the twelfth week" (pp. 31-32).

Rochlin also expressed the view that there seems to be a correlation between structural maturation and sleep-wakefulness behavior. He thought that as the child grows, his needs become more insistent and the periods of wakefulness increase (see Friend 1956).

Gifford quotes Gesell who described "the period between the sixteenth and twenty-fourth week as one of rapid organization within the central nervous system, with the loss of the tonic-neck reflex, the development of occular fixation and the 'recognition' of familiar faces and sounds" (p. 32).

The sleeping time during the day continues to decrease, while the frequency of night feedings and hours of night sleep remain unchanged, thus reducing total sleep by slightly more than one hour. There are well-defined morning and afternoon naps, with the longer period of unbroken sleep between 8 P.M. and 8 A.M.[8] Thereafter a mean ten hours of sleep during the night remains more or less constant during childhood since any reduction in the total sleeping time is due to the disappearance of daytime naps.

Moore and Ucko (1957) point out that during this period about half of the infants who settled at the appropriate time revert to night waking. They quote Shepherd who emphasized the large number of new causes for night waking in the period between six and nine months.

Our own observations at the Hampstead Clinic confirm these findings. Among the many factors capable of triggering disturbances of sleep, particularly after the third month of life, are: changes of environment; the mother's tension, depression or ambivalence to the child; seriously disturbed marital relationship; a new pregnancy; separations, etc. As we have mentioned earlier, their effect on the very young child is not necessarily a direct one, but may be due to the impact of such events on the mother in whom they elicit anxiety, tension, anger, depressive reactions, guilt, shame, etc., that interfere with the previously more satisfactory relationship to and care of her baby.

Perhaps even more striking is the fact that some of the distur-

8. Our own charts from the Hampstead War Nurseries confirm Kleitman's observations, in spite of the fact that our children, unlike those observed by Kleitman, were living in a communal environment.

bances initiated in this way remain with the child for many years, as the following example will illustrate.[9] This example further shows how some of the factors referred to above trigger off a disturbance of sleep or make it worse. It should also be noted that the form in which the disturbance manifests itself can change at different points according to the new dimensions introduced by the new stages of the child's development and the nature of the underlying conflicts of which the original disturbance has become the vehicle.

I.F.was first seen at the Well Baby Clinic *at 9 months.* The mother's general tenseness and her ambivalence to the baby girl were observed; tension was also seen in the baby who trembled and wriggled. The relationship between mother and child was obviously disturbed and battles took place in several areas.

At 10½ months: Difficulties in falling alseep were noted; the child cried unless Mrs. F sat with I until she fell asleep; this had started when the family stayed with the maternal grandmother but continued after they returned home.

At 15½ months: I still needed her mother to stay in the room until she fell asleep.

At 20 months: I tended to awake after one or two hours of sleep demanding company.

At 25 months: The child must have mother sit with her for as long as two hours before falling asleep. The father no longer can settle her, whereas previously I had been more responsive to him than to the mother. She tends to wake frequently during the night and takes a long time to settle. She cries desperately when she is left alone.

From the twenty-sixth week onward. During this period development generally proceeds as rapidly as during the previous phase. More and more factors of increasing complexity can operate as possible sources of interference with sleep or development in general.

Hirschberg (1957) described some of the parental anxieties that frequently accompany the sleep disturbances of children. He

9. I am grateful to Dr. Stross and the staff of the Well Baby Clinic for making available their observations.

found that sleep disturbances in the very young infant (up to one year) frequently affect the mother's narcissism. As a result she will be fearful, make excessive efforts to change, or feel utterly helpless, hopeless, and defeated. Mothers frequently associate their care and acceptance of the infant with his sleep patterns, feeling that if they truly accepted the baby, he would sleep well; or that if they really enjoyed feeding and gratifying the child, he would sleep well. When the infant does not sleep properly, some mothers tend to feel unworthy, doubt their capacity as mothers, and become more ambivalent to the child and to motherhood in general. Hirschberg occasionally found mothers who wanted their infants to sleep uninterruptedly and who reacted with anger and annoyance when the children were awake and demanded food, warmth, and care. These mothers tried to avoid any relationship with the child by having him sleep.

Other mothers regarded the young infant as a part of their own bodies, worried about the effect of the sleep problem on the health of the child, and at a preconscious level feared for his bodily integrity, which unconsciously implied his death; or they experienced strong oral-sadistic impulses as unconscious threats of disintegration and death of their own selves. Still other mothers equated the child's sleep disturbance with oral deprivation, some of them having at the same time unconscious fears of "being swallowed" by the babies.

It is inevitable that these fantasies influence the mother's response to her child.

SLEEP DISTURBANCES IN THE SECOND
YEAR OF LIFE

A detailed consideration of the relevant literature and reports on sleep disturbances in this age group impresses the reader with a certain imbalance in approach: while several writers describe gross disturbances of sleep such as nightmares, pavor nocturnus, somnambulism, and extreme anxiety dreams, the well-established fact that virtually every parent anticipates some form of sleep

interference after the first year of life is often given scant acknowl-
edgment in the literature. While it is obviously important to
survey the etiology and course of the more severe disturbances, I
shall consider difficulties and disturbances around sleep in this
age group principally from the viewpoint that such malfunction-
ing is only one of many possible expressions of infantile anxiety.
This "infantile anxiety" may arise from conflicts of a neurotic
nature, but it may also be an expression of developmental imbalances in the personality. For this latter group I reserve the term
developmental disturbances[10] which can manifest themselves in
many ways, one of them being "sleep disturbances."

Gesell and Ilg (1943), on the basis of their behavioral studies,
consider the reluctance to go to sleep as well as night waking
developmental features of the age group fifteen to thirty months.
Anna Freud's references (1965) may be understood as an extension
of this viewpoint to encompass the psychoanalytic approach to
child development:

> However carefully and successfully an infant's sleeping habits and
> arrangements have been handled in the first year of life, difficulties
> with sleep, or with the ease of falling asleep, intervene almost
> without exception in the second year. . . . falling asleep is no longer a
> purely physical affair as the almost automatic response to a body
> need in an undifferentiated individual, in whom ego and id, self and
> object world are not yet separated off from each other. With the
> strengthening of the child's object ties and of his involvement in the
> happenings of the external world, withdrawal of libido and of ego
> interests to the self becomes a prerequisite for sleep. This is not
> always accomplished without difficulty, and the anxiety aroused by
> the process makes the toddler cling all the more tenaciously to his
> wakefulness. . . . These [symptomatic manifestations of the state of
> wakefulness] again disappear spontaneously when the child's ob-
> ject relationships become more secure and less ambivalent, and
> when his ego becomes stabilized sufficiently to permit regression to
> the undifferentiated, narcissistic state necessary for sleep. [pp.
> 157-158]

10. For a detailed exposition of the early developmental disturbances, developmental
conflicts, etc., see Nagera (1966).

During the second year of life the physical maturation of the central nervous system continues and will be fairly complete toward the end of this period. Only then does the child reach that level and degree of maturation of the organic structures of his central nervous system which most other mammals possess at birth. Only at this point do the *physical structures underlying* the mental apparatus reach the level of completeness and maturity which is necessary for the normal functioning of the mental apparatus in the human. This completeness, however, refers only to the basic organic structures; in functional terms there are great differences between the child and the adult. To fill the functional gap between the two requires a long and arduous process of experiencing, learning, exposure to the most diverse sources of physical and psychological stimulation, opening new functional pathways of an ever-increasing complexity (for which the structures are now getting ready). We have sufficient evidence to postulate that the mother and her stimulation are necessary for the normal maturation of the central nervous system of the child, side by side with the natural and innate physical forces tending toward the physical maturational completeness of this system. Similarly we know that the mother is essential for the awakening of the functional capacities of this structure. This is an extremely complex process which we do not yet understand. Suffice it to say that the mother exerts an influence, directly and indirectly, on the development of the child's ego apparatuses and drives, both of which run parallel and interact with each other (see chapter 1.)

Sleep disturbances (as well as other disturbances) cannot be properly understood without paying due regard to the peculiarities of the developmental stage. In this way we learn what factors in the child's personality favor or contribute to the sleeping difficulties which are so characteristic for this period and which have to be considered a developmental disturbance. Anna Maenchen suggested this appraoch in 1955.[11]

Among the different factors that need to be considered is the

11. I am grateful to Dr. Maenchen for allowing me to examine the unpublished paper "Sleep Disturbances and Ego Developments." For an abstract of this paper, see Friend (1956).

degree of ego development reached, i.e., the child's capacity to understand the happenings in the world around him, the level of his thought processes, the existence of an early capacity for internalization, the capacity to bind and deal with anxiety, etc. In addition, we must assess the child's drive development and its influence on his ego processes and object relations. Similarly, we have to consider the fact that in the second year of life there normally exists a relative imbalance between these three lines of development and that this imbalance is bound to provoke certain types of responses in the child when he is confronted with certain experiences.

With regard to object relations, there has been a gradual development from the stage of need satisfaction to that of object constancy. Because of this development (itself the result of complicated maturational advances) it is no longer the child's "needs" and the object's need-fulfilling functions that are all important. The object, independently of its need-fulfilling aspects, has become the child's primary concern. Obviously, the transition from the phase of need satisfaction to object constancy is a very slow and gradual process which starts in the third or fourth month, gains further impetus during the second half of the first year, and reaches its full development during the second year of life. In most cases it is already well established toward the end of the first half of the second year.

At this point most of the child's interest is concentrated in the mother, a situation of the greatest significance for the evaluation of the child's reactions. On the other hand and in spite of this unique tie to his mother, the child takes notice of and relates to other persons in the family, especially when these persons make efforts to earn the toddler's sympathy. In this way, father, grandparents, older siblings, and others become part of the toddler's enlarged world. It has perhaps not been sufficiently realized that these other relations take place only under the shadow of the relationship with the mother. The two-year-old child will spend much time playing with the grandparents away from the mother (if they take the trouble to come down to his level and appeal to his interest), secure in his knowledge that the mother is around the house though not necessarily in sight. This behavior may suggest the child's independence from his mother. However, if she were to leave the house, the child would demand to go with her and refuse to play with the grandparents; and if he is left behind he will break down in tears and anxiety.

Similarly there are certain times and activities that belong exclusively in the context of the relationship to the mother. At these points the toddler demands his mother and will not accept a substitute—not even those persons to whom he has a good relationship at other times. It is due to this special type and quality of the cathexis attached to the mother that the toddler finds it difficult to settle down to sleep. He is very reluctant to relinquish contact with this precious object. This explains his constant demands for the mother to lie down with him, hold his hand, sit beside his bed, read him yet another story, etc. The presence of the mother is required not only at bedtime but also when the child wakes from his sleep, when he is unwell, has hurt himself, or is frightened, etc. On all these occasions the child demands his mother. In fact, fathers, grandparents, and other relatives are shocked by his rejection, by his extreme distress and despair if the mother is not available, and by their complete inability to soothe and comfort him. This reaction is a direct consequence of the developmental stage the child has reached in his object relations. His reaction is further clarified if we examine it against the background of ego development in order to see what the latter can do to cope with the experience.

From our observations we have to conclude that especially during the first half of the second year there is little the ego can offer. When the child is distressed and anxious, the ego is still easily put out of action and cannot make use of the scarce resources available. Earlier during this period the ego still lacks the capacity to distinguish between absence and complete disappearance or to link absence with the subsequent return of the object. A child at this age has no concept of time. From his egocentric position he cannot understand that the mother is not there when he requires her presence (a feeling justified by his previous experience since normally the mother has been available to him); he has not developed the capacity to delay his affective response, to pause and consider the meaning of, and the reasons for the mother's absence. Because of his limited capacity to comprehend and draw inferences, the child's ego, especially when under the stress of anxiety, can do little to master the experience and the automatic affective response that follows it.

Yet, only a few months later when the ego has developed further, the child's response is of a very different nature. The link between the mother going out and her return has established itself, his experiences have been broadened, and his thought processes have further matured. His ego is then in a much better position to deal with the problem. Thus we have observed children who in the first part of the second year of life were overwhelmed by the mother's absence, but in the second part of the same year were able to cope with it by ego means.

In one of the cases I have in mind, the child woke up during the evening and went searching for the mother. His grandmother told him that mummy had gone out but had left the message for him that she was going to be back soon. The little boy turned around and walked to his bed, repeating to himself two or three times, "Mummy will be back soon," adding, "Mummy went to cinema." He fell asleep again without any difficulty or distress. He could now master the meaning of her absence as his own explanatory addition to the mother's message "went to the cinema" shows. It is of interest not only that he could, by means of meaningful thought processes, bind the anxiety which otherwise might have arisen, but also that at this stage "cinema" was for him a place where mother went occasionally and from which she returned soon. He did not really know the concrete meaning of "cinema." As is well known, the ego's capacity to tolerate anxiety and to bind it by means of thought processes increases markedly during the second year because language, though still limited, makes important contributions (A. Katan 1961).

Another child started to say "mummy holidays" whenever the mother was absent. This simple mental link greatly helped the child to cope with the mother's absence because this link had a concrete meaning to him—mummy was not gone or lost forever but away for a short period and would come back. With the help of this associative link, his ego was able to bind the anxiety.

In view of the fact that the toddler's ego becomes increasingly able to cope with the anxiety engendered by the mother's absence, it is necessary to emphasize this especially vulnerable and critical period in the early part of the second year of life. This period, usually of short duration, is characterized by the high cathexis of the object at a time when ego development is still limited. Special efforts must be made not to expose the child to negative experiences during it. The child has for developmental reasons no tolerance for the absence of the object. This is feared per se. But added to this is the fact that when the child is confronted with the mother's absence, his automatic response is an anxiety state which may reach overwhelming proportions. Repeated traumas of this type cannot fail to have serious consequences for his later development, quite apart from the fact that they may lay the basis for later sleep disturbances as in a case reported by Anna Freud (1966). This child developed a sleeping disturbance at two and a half years. The parents led a very secluded life and had never left the infant until that age. They arranged to go out expecting that the child would not even wake up, but she did wake, found a stranger, and reacted with a screaming attack. From that moment on the child clung to her mother and had many difficulties in settling at sleep time. Anna Freud once suggested to the parents that they play games of hide and seek with the child, but this proved impossible because the child went into a panic each time a parent disappeared. The following years were very painful for the child and the parents. At latency the picture changed and the child reacted with excessive independence and a great deal of hostility to the parents.

These considerations apply to all "separations" during the day or at night. They are of particular significance at nightime when the ego is in a regressed state.

Similarly, other types of sleep disturbances at this period are largely dependent on the developmental stage reached by the ego. Children in this group are occasionally overexcited and stimulated by the parents. This creates states of inner tension to a degree that the primitive ego cannot cope with or bind. Something similar may happen if the child has been exposed to overexciting or frightening experiences during the day. Furthermore, such experiences may lead to disturbing dreams. At this early stage the child's ego is frequently not yet able to distinguish between dreams and reality and may therefore express fears about going to bed and sleep. Luce and Segal (1966) quote the sympathetic comment of a child psychiatrist concerning this problem: "If you went to sleep one night and found a tiger in your bed, would you want to go back? True, the tiger is not in the bed before sleep, yet the child knows that when he closes his eyes it may return to pounce upon him" (p. 23). Even exciting positive experiences during the day may lead to broken sleep. This happened in one of my children who was then eighteen months old. He woke up from a dream in the middle of the night looking for a horse he had seen in the living room of the house. He was most upset when he did not find the horse. The overexcitement about the horse was a residue of his actual experiences during the day preceding the dream. Naturally with the increase in ego development and the establishment of a clear-cut distinction between dreams and reality this type of developmental disturbance will disappear.

This view is at some variance with that of Mack (1965) who assigns a symbolic and highly conflictive content to the child's "nightmare" in the first half of the second year; such content implies a degree of structuralization and a use of dream work which are more commensurate with a somewhat later stage of development (beginning at approximately eighteen months). As Freud (1901) has shown, a common element in children's dreams is that they are "simple and undisguised wish-fulfilments" (p. 644). Another characteristic of such dreams is "their connection with daytime life. The wishes which are fulfilled in them are carried over from daytime and as a rule from the day before, and in waking life they have been accompanied by intense emotion. Nothing unimportant or indifferent, or nothing which would strike a child as such, finds its way into the content of their dreams" p. 645). These comments suggest a more appropriate explanation of dreams occurring from approximately twelve to eighteen months: that they contain either a direct wish fulfillment or an expression of more archaic fears and anxieties which were evoked by relatively commonplace daytime events and which were not adequately assimilated into the child's experience at the time they occurred.

The type of interference with the ease of falling asleep due to increasing ego development, which nevertheless is not yet sufficient to master many of the situations confronting it, is already apparent in some children from the thirteenth month on and increases during the second year. The sleep pattern charts of children at the Hampstead War Nurseries show this clearly. Anna Freud (1966) referred to similar experience in her experimental nursery in Vienna. She noted that before the thirteenth month many children fell asleep spontaneously almost any place they were and needed to be carried to their cots, while afterward the pattern changed and the children tossed and turned in their cots for a long time before going off to sleep. She thought that this change in sleep pattern had to do with ego development.

As Margaret Mahler appositely put it: "precisely the most cherished and relatively farthest advanced partial function of the individual ego may be the one which is most vulnerable and therefore the troublemaker. To guard the integrity of functions in the organs which execute them, the child is reluctant to go to sleep, or awakens" (see Friend 1956, p. 519).

Some children in this age group (second year) resort to obsessionallike arrangements before going to sleep. These "rituals" are the result of specific interactions between ego and drives and are especially pronounced when the move into the anal-sadistic stage coincides with advanced ego development and a tendency to internalize early toilet-training demands. These obsessionallike arrangements are an expression of the anal-sadistic conflicts and the defense activity directed against them, as well as the child's strong ambivalent feelings toward the objects that interfere with his anal pleasures. Some of these children fight falling asleep or wake up from sleep because of the fear of not having control over their sphincters. As Selma Fraiberg (1950) stated, "The conflicts of the anal period play an important role in symptoms of sleep disturbances. . . . When pleasure in soiling must be relinquished for fear of loss of the mother's love, the conflicting tendencies may produce another type of anxiety dream which results in interruption of sleep. Here the fear of soiling in sleep breaks through. In two such cases [described in the paper] it was seen that the wish to soil was manifest in the dream . . . but fear of loss of the mother exerted a more potent influence at the critical moment, so that the wish-fulfilling function of the dream failed and anxiety broke through, resulting in the interruption of sleep" (p. 308).

Anxiety over loss of sphincter control and the fear of gratifying forbidden instinctual wishes need not be expressed through dreams. For example, the following account of a child, C A, who attended our Mother-Toddler Group and Nursery School contains material which encompasses both the child's fear of loss of control (early superego concern) and her anxiety over separation from mother and loss of mother's love (which was expressed in attempts to keep mother up during the night).

When C was fourteen months old, her mother returned to work and C was looked after during the day by an au pair girl. "C's toilet training entailed tremendous struggles. When she was two years old and completely untrained, the grandmother and the helper tried to train her, expressing their disgust at C's inability to conform. C described motions as 'gusting' but resisted the pot for seven months. During the latter part of this period she would withhold her stools for several days. At two and a half years C attempted bladder and bowel control during the day. Three months later she demanded to be put to bed without her nappies. When this was granted, she developed a sleep disturbance and demanded her mother's attention for hours. When C was left alone she busied herself with washing the floor in the bathroom and the bedroom, running back and forth to the bathroom to get the pot and empty it. She became very preoccupied with scissors and cut her doll's hair, her pretty hair ribbons, and her clothes, and expressed her usual wish to be a boy while fighting with her elder brother. When she gave up withholding her motions, she started spitting fights with her brother instead." C thus appeared to react aggressively to her mother's absence and the imposed toilet training. As she relinquished the symptom of withholding her motions, she expressed sequentially the conflict over her penis envy and over her competitive relationship with her brother.

Another relevant case was described by Berta Bornstein (1931).

This child's extreme fear of lying down was understood as fear of falling asleep and dreaming, which was determined by fear of loss of sphincter control and of soiling the bed while asleep. Similarly, in a mother guidance case seen over several months at the Hampstead Clinic, a three-year-old boy would call out for his mother several times during the night saying he wished to urinate. When his mother came to him, he appeared tense and anxious, but usually passed only a few drops of urine. When the mother was encouraged to take a more lenient attitude to the occasional wet bed, the boy became less anxious, the calling out diminished, and his sleep improved.

It should be noted that such obsessionallike reactions as described above can also be observed in a different group of children, who are characterized by slow ego development. In spite of the external similarities, the obsessionallike reactions of these children are the result of primitive ego anxieties which lead to a need for uniformity, for exact repetition of every step in the sleep arrangements. These rituals are related to the ego's primitive fear of change and of the unknown. In a minority of cases they are the first signs of what will later prove to be an atypical ego. In still others they indicate a special type of imbalance between the levels of ego development and object relations, and more specifically a different quality of the object relationships. At the beginning of the toddler stage normal children can and do take on trust a great deal from their objects. On the basis of this relation most of the normal ego fears of this phase are automatically alleviated and controlled by the mere presence or reassurance of the object. The primitive ego fears of the other children, however, are not reduced by such reassurances because this automatic trust is lacking and as a result they have a very disturbed presleep period.

In the sleep disturbances described so far I have stressed their developmental background. That is to say, most of them are manifestations of developmental interference rather than the result of conflicts of a neurotic nature. An exception are those disturbances which are due to early internalization of parental demands, for example, with regard to toiler training.

In still another group of cases, the so-called disturbed sleep of children between the first and the second year of life started, for example, when the family returned from a holiday during which the child was allowed to sleep with his mother or parents. On his return the child, naturally enough, refuses to sleep in his own bed. Here again there are no neurotic reasons for the difficulty, the child is only trying to cling to the gratification afforded by sleeping with the parents in terms of skin erotism, warmth, security, etc., gratifications which are in no way conflictive to him at this point in his development. A significant number of so-called sleep disturbances of this period belong in this group.

According to Hirschberg (1957), the parental anxieties about the one- to three-year-old "are concerned with the separation and loss meanings involved in the sleep disturbance, and the aggressive attack implied, and are associated with problems in the parent-child relationships" (p. 138). The records of the Hampstead Clinic show that many factors which precipitated sleep disturbances during the first year of life—the mother's tension, depression, ambivalence; unsatisfactory marital relationships—continue to be a significant influence during the second year, while many others now become operative, e.g., the birth of siblings, hospitalizations of mother or child, the father's absence, etc.

These considerations indicate that the normal physiological process of sleep begins to be interfered with as the development of the mind gains momentum and is increasingly influenced by mental activities and conflicts. Sleep, furthermore, now takes on a diversity of psychological meanings. All these psychological factors can interfere with the physiological process as effectively as— at times more effectively than—the purely physical disturbances of the body.

Analyses of children under five at the Hampstead Clinic have clearly demonstrated that sleep, at first merely vulnerable in infancy, assumes the specific coloring of each successive libidinal phase and can gradually become a major area of neurotic conflict. In many of the children who began analysis at ages of two and a half to three years, the sleep disturbances began either in the first or early in the second year of life, continued into the anal and phallic phases. They were overdetermined and were an expression of the phase-specific libidinal and aggressive impulses and anxieties.

SLEEP DISTURBANCES IN THE THREE-
TO FIVE-YEAR-OLD

Children in this age group are confronted with the phallic-oedipal conflicts and have to deal with the resultant infantile neurosis. Melitta Sperling (1955) remarked that "The occurrence of mild and transient sleep disturbances during the oedipal phase can be considered a typical feature of childhood in our culture. The severer disturbances of this phase, however, especially the acute exacerbations leading to persisting sleeplessness, are pathologic phenomena indicative of serious emotional disorder" (p. 359). This statement has been amply borne out by the children who have been referred to the Hampstead Clinic: it is quite rare to find a child in this age group who is not experiencing some difficulty over sleep, whether it be tardiness in falling asleep, night waking, anxiety dreams, projective fears of ghosts and wild animals, inability to sleep alone, desire to share the parental bed, sleep phobia, ritual behavior at bedtime, etc. In our experience, however, such sleep difficulties frequently do not represent the central core of the neurotic conflict and are offshoots of the symptom formation proper.

Anna Maenchen (see Friend 1956) expressed the opinion that the sleep disturbances in the oedipal and postoedipal stages of development are essentially the same as those of adults, a point of view with which I agree.

In the majority of children aged one to three years, and particularly in those under two and a half years, a disturbance of sleep can most usefully be viewed as a developmental disturbance which either will show spontaneous remission or will improve with more appropriate environmental handling. To some extent this statement is still true with regard to children aged three to five. Perusal of our clinic treatment records discloses, however, that a *consistent* disturbance of sleep is to be understood as a symptom (frequently one of several) resulting from internalized neurotic conflicts and that this symptom cannot be dealt with solely by manipulation of the environment. A more fundamental change in the child's functioning will be effected only by analytic treatment.

Even in this age group, however, there are some "disturbances" which still appear to be based largely on the maternal handling of the child. For example, I have at present a girl, J H, in analytic treatment who was referred at the age of two and a half because of stammering and a lavatory phobia. Mrs. H, in her interviews with me, continued to express concern about the child's wakefulness at bedtime and about her screaming and insistent demands to join her parents downstairs. Whenever we discuss this situation, it becomes quite apparent, both to mother and therapist, that the child's difficulty in remaining in her bed is intimately connected with the mother's inability to be firm with J as well as with the mother's underlying wish to have J present downstairs with her husband and herself. It should not, of course, be overlooked that the mother's handling in this regard coincides with the girl's own desire to participate in the parents' activities and with J's oedipal wishes to separate the parents.

I have previously referred to children who showed an early vulnerability of sleep which assumed neurotic proportions when they moved into the anal and phallic phases of libidinal development. The analytic material of all these children was indexed (Sandler 1962), and the statements listed on some of the index cards are particularly relevant to this study. The following example clearly demonstrates that a sleeping disturbance can be an admixture of the child's own anxiety and neurotic conflict and be determined by inadequate parental handling.

A Z began treatment at the age of two and a half. I quote from material indexed eight months later. "The referral letter described A's symptom simply as difficulty in sleeping. This was amplified by the mother as meaning that he would not go to sleep at the proper time and would waken most nights several times. He was usually taken into the parents' bed, where he thrashed about and kept his parents awake. At the beginning of treatment he slept in the same bedroom as the parents. This problem was dealt with in two ways, first, by interpretation of Tony's fear that the mother might go away while he slept, his wish to separate the parents, and his wish to join their exciting intercourse; secondly, by encouraging the mother to provide another bedroom for him and relieving her anxiety about him. He moved into a bedroom of his own and after a few nights of broken sleep, he slept the whole night through from 6:30 P.M. to 6 A.M.—the first time since he was an infant. Thereafter the pattern varied from time to time. Sometimes he slept all night through, sometimes he awoke during the night. When he awoke, however, the sound of either parent's voice was sufficient to allow him to go back to sleep. During the last month or two prior to indexing his sleep has been sound and there appears to be no difficulty now."

Hirschberg (1957) makes the point that "with the three to five year old, the parents are less consciously aware of their attitudes which are involved in the sleep disturbance since these attitudes are related to [their own] Oedipal anxieties, parent-child competitiveness, and aggressive-castrative wishes on the parents' part" (p. 138). Based on his investigation of forty cases of sleep disturbances studied over a two-year period, Hirschberg maintains that parents tend to view their children's difficulties in terms of specific reality fears rather than as disturbances in drive development and in the children's object relationships to the parents. Our clinical data (both diagnostic and analytic) certainly indicate that parents become increasingly unable to cope with symptoms connected with sleep as the child moves into the phallic phase of libidinal development. Among the factors that may determine the difficulties and induce the parents to seek external psychiatric help are, as Hirschberg postulates: the parents' own unresolved oedipal conflicts and ambivalence to the child; impairment of important areas of ego functioning, particularly cognitive processes which normally show acceleration at this time (in this area one must consider not only the physiological effects of consistent lack of sleep, such as apathy, listlessness, irritability, but also the contamination by neurotic conflict); impairment (frequently sadomasochistic involvement) of the child's relations to his parents and, as a consequence, impairment of his ability to move into the wider world of social relationships.

I have previously stressed that a vulnerability of sleep in infancy can grow into a neurotic conflict and assume the coloring of each phase of libidinal development. While Melitta Sperling (1949) puts the onset of oedipal wishes somewhat earlier than we would be inclined to do, her statement is relevant to our own findings: "Even if toilet training is conducted in an understanding manner, in our culture it represents a frustrating experience to the child who has to give up satisfaction of anal-sadistic impulses and also repress the aggressive impulses which may arise as a reaction to toilet training if it is carried out in a forceful manner. From the ages of two to five, these repressed aggressive impulses are intensified greatly by the addition of repressed sexual impulses of the oedipal phase. Even in the most favorable setting, every child at this age lives through a period of emotional frustration which leads to repression of sexual and aggressive (sadistic) impulses. Under normal circumstances, that is, if repression comes about gradually and not too abruptly, the child is able to pass through this phase without obvious manifestations. If, however, in addition to this, other traumatic experiences are added, particularly sexual overexposure and overstimulation, arrival of a sibling (who is favored by the mother), operation, severe masturbation threats, and similar frustrations, the increased aggressive impulses will be reflected, mostly in disturbed sleep" (p. 33).

This adhesiveness of the sleep disturbance symptom is nicely illustrated in the following example of a girl, G H, who was taken into analytic treatment at the age of two years eight months. The index was prepared two years later. In her case we see clearly the evolution of a sleep disturbance beginning at eleven months which by the time she was three years old contains a complex symptom formation.

On referral, G H could never sleep alone, even with sedation, but awoke crying and got into the parents' bed.

This continued into the second year of treatment, with symptom-free intervals from three to four months, and was seen to express her conflicts on various libidinal levels:

1. The wish to possess mother and displace father. This was a bid for mother's protection from father's physically exciting activity.

2. The desire to possess the mother in the negative oedipal phase and to be mother's sexual partner. She played going to sleep, then awakening and jumping onto the therapist's (mother's) lap, while the father was somewhere nearby. For the most part these instances occurred in regression from the positive oedipal wish.
3. The wish to keep the mother safe, after having observed the primal scene in which she conceived the mother as hurt.
4. The wish to separate the parents to prevent their having another baby. This was connected with the fear of being replaced by another baby; and the oedipal wish to be the one to make the baby: "She wants to be the one to make babies."

Interpretations of fears and conflicts gradually led to diminution of the symptom, and by the eighth month was sleeping alone. Exacerbations arose after G witnessed sexual intercourse and the anxiety caused by the above conflict continued.

However, the persistence of the symptom was due mainly to the parents' use of the symptom; they acted out their own sexual inadequacies via the child. As soon as they were firm in their demand that the child sleep in her own bed, G complied and the symptom disappeared.

Another determinant of G's difficulty in falling asleep was fear of retaliation for her aggressive impulses. These were expressed on several libidinal levels: against the brother's penis; against either mother or father both in the positive and negative oedipal position. The aggressive impulses dramatically broke through in relation to the therapist as well. G bit the therapist as a phallic attack expressed in oral terms. She felt ill. After an interpretation of her outside aggressive impulses, she appeared sleepy. She repeatedly forced her eyes open to see whether the therapist was near before she fell asleep.

This symptom completely cleared after an interpretation of the aggressive impulses arising from the oedipal strivings. Another requirement was that mother not collude with this symptom, i.e., that she not invite it in the service of maintaining her masochistic defense. The mother would berate the child because she was so tired and had so much work to do, but she assumed that she would not go to sleep alone. When the mother insisted, the child immediately complied. The parents' contribution to G's sleep disturbance will be discussed later.

In another child, D B, we see the cumulative and encompassing effect of a sleep disturbance. D attended the Hampstead Well Baby Clinic from the age of ten weeks. Although the pediatrician recorded that sleep began to be a problem toward the end of his first year, Mrs. B dates the onset of the real problem just before D's second birthday when Mrs. B was depressed, unhappy in her marriage, and formed an extramarital attachment. By the time he started treatment at the age of three, he refused to sleep alone and involved the whole family in shifts from bed to bed; he was also unable to separate from his mother during the day even for a short period. When he was two and three quarter years old, a sister was born and her birth added to D's problems (cf. Melitta Sperling's remarks above) in that she became another rival for mother's attention; the therapist who treated D considered it likely that the mother's pregnancy, together with her depression and consequent withdrawal at the time, contributed to the consolidation of the boy's sleep disturbance. What follows is a summary of the various meanings of D's sleeping disturbance as they were understood in treatment (the index was prepared one year and ten months after therapy began.)

D was referred because of his refusal to go to sleep at night without his mother's presence, which started in his second year. It sometimes took up to three hours to get him to sleep. If she tried to leave him before he was asleep, he got up and followed her around. He woke again during the night, and could not sleep again unless he was taken into the parents' bed, or one of them came to sleep in his room. Often having got one parent sleeping in his room, he would again get up and go and wake the other, from fear of the consequences of separating the parents. He was anxious and frightened when left alone, but would become overexcited when his father or mother was with him.

This disturbance was found in treatment ot be overdetermined. It arose originally as a part of his reaction to his mother's emotional and physical absences, which aroused intense hostile and aggressive fantasies, so that D then needed her presence as a reassurance that she was unharmed. It was intensified when D began to move into the phallic-oedipal phase, and then represented also an acting out of his wish to separate the parents and control their sexual activities. It was enhanced and prolonged by the seductive atmosphere of the home, where the parents made little attempt to conceal their turbulent marital relationship and their extramarital affairs. Finally, the disturbance was one manifestation of D's need to use his parents as external ego supports in controlling his own instinctual impulses.

After two years of intensive treatment D's sleep disturbance was resolved.

At the oedipal stage the fear of going to bed or the difficulty in falling asleep may be due to masturbation conflicts. The following extract from an index card of a girl, H J, who began treatment at the age of five, illustrates this. Toward the end of the first year of her analysis she refused to go to bed because "sleep was dirty." When the therapist linked this with H's guilt over masturbation, she replied: "It is even right" and followed this by expressing a wish to see how father goes to sleep and to sleep with him, corrected to: "with mummy and daddy."

At the time of referral the mother reported that H occasionally woke up screaming. Often H was able to recall the terrifying dream from which she woke, e.g., that a thief wanted to take something. Her dreams during the course of her analysis mostly reflected her penis envy and her oedipal strivings, libidinal and aggressive.

Disturbing dreams with an oedipal content are of course frequently noted in children of this age group in treatment at the Hampstead Clinic.

Melitta Sperling (1949) thinks that sleep disturbances at this stage may be more frequent among boys than girls because of its relation to castration fear. Our impression is that there are no great differences between boys and girls in this respect.

SLEEP DISTURBANCES OF THE LATENCY PERIOD

At around five years of age and with the resolution of the phallic-oedipal conflict children begin to move into the latency period. The sleeping disturbances of latency resemble those of the adult, as was the case with the sleep disturbances in the oedipal period. They can be the expression of all sorts of underlying psychopathology and cover the whole range of conflicts to which human nature is exposed.

In the latency period sleep difficulties may manifest themselves for the first time or a previously existing sleep disturbance may disappear or be expressed in a different form. Very frequently at this stage the conflicts around masturbation move into the foreground. They are sometimes associated with unresolved phallic-oedipal conflicts and phallic-oedipal fantasies of the most diverse nature; they are thus frequently found at the basis of a large number of symptoms, rituals, and behavioral manifestations which usually occur during the period immediately preceding sleep. Their performance becomes a necessary and unavoidable precondition of falling asleep. Although other forms of disturbances such as nightmares, somnambulism, and even pavor nocturnus can occur during latency, there is in general a shift of emphasis to the presleep arrangements with a marked diminution of the tendency to go into the parental bedroom and to ask for the company of one of the parents, so typical of the three to five year period. On the other hand, earlier sleep disturbances frequently disappear in the latency period. This is usually due to a combination of several factors, some of which are the result of developmental advances while others are based on cultural patterns and attitudes.

Naturally, many of the sleep disturbances in the preceding phase resulted from the intensity of the phallic-oedipal phase-specific conflicts. And where the sleep disturbance has existed earlier, the phallic-oedipal conflicts usually made a distinct contribution to this disturbance. With the onset of latency and the satisfactory resolution of the phallic-oedipal conflicts, a number of sleep disturbances (as well as other disturbances) tend to disappear. During a normal latency period there is a marked reduction in the activity and intensity of the drives, a situation that frequently changes the internal balance of the personality and the forces involved in conflicts in ways that permit their resolution or at least favor better adaptations. Apart from the fact that there is less pressure from the drives, further ego development takes place. The ego is now in a better position than before to cope more satisfactorily with the drives and with reality. In addition, the ego is now capable of using new and more efficient defense mechanisms.

Similarly, these changes in the drive and ego organization contribute to the important advances in the child's object relationships. Previously the child was almost completely involved with and dependent on the parents. Now he can take a number of steps away from this intense and exclusive tie. He gains some independence, and much of the cathexes previously invested in the parents are now redirected toward the community of peers.

When the child leaves behind the normal and unavoidable stage of his infantile neurosis, we can expect him to leave behind all the symptomatic manifestations that were the direct expression of the conflicts of that phase, including those concerning sleep. In favorable cases, minor disturbances of earlier phases are brought under more satisfactory control. Obviously, qualitative and quantitative factors play an important role in the final outcome of these developmental processes.

Unfortunately in a large number of cases, these qualitative and quantitative factors are such that a satisfactory outcome of the infantile neurosis and a reasonably normal latency period are not possible. When this is the case, the sleep disturbances (as well as others) will find their way into latency, adolescence, and adulthood. Naturally, each period makes a specific contribution to the personality and the nature of the conflicts as well as to the variations in the form in which symptoms are expressed.

Another favorable contribution to the possible solution of the sleep disturbances comes from the side of the environment in the form of a cultural attitude. As the child enters the latency period, the parents begin to show some flexibility in their handling of the child's sleeping arrangements. He is usually no longer "put to bed" but is given a certain leeway. This implies that to some degree the child increasingly assumes responsibility about his going to bed. This allows him to establish his own adaptive ceremonials during the presleep period (what Fenichel [1945] calls the "secondary measures"). Anna Freud once remarked that the young child has fewer coping mechanisms allowed to him, not more sleeping disturbances.

The following case taken from the files at the clinic illustrates the multiplicity of conflicts that can find expression in an extremely disturbed presleep period as well as in the innumerable obsessional rituals and arrangements that were required by this seriously disturbed girl. Because of the severity of the disturbance the behavior observed is a caricature of what in lesser degrees is quite generally present.

J M, twelve and a half years old when treatment began, had among other symptoms numerous rituals and compulsive actions that she was forced to perform at bedtime before she was able to settle down to sleep. Thus, for example, the window curtains had to be arranged to have a fold in the middle. She had to make sure that the arm of the chair did not touch the table and was separated from it by a space of one inch; the tablecloth had to be placed exactly on the middle of the table; the pillow had to be placed exactly in the middle of the bed; the books had to be arranged in a certain manner; other objects had to be placed in such a way that they would not fall to the floor during the evening making noises that would frighten and waken her. Similarly, two clocks in her room had to be kept at a certain distance from each other so that they would not make too much noise during the night and wake her, a preoccupation that was accompanied by an intense fear that one of the clocks might stop altogether, in which case she felt it would be impossible for her to sleep for weeks.

All these manifestations were the condensed expression at anal and phallic-oedipal levels of her libidinal and aggressive conflicts and were due to the contamination of anal fantasies, intercourse fantasies, primal scene fantasies, agressive impulses, conflicts around masturbation, penis envy, and castration fantasies.

When J was a baby she constantly fell asleep in the middle of her feedings and had to be tickled or slapped to wake her to continue feeding. The mother stated that J had no special sleeping disturbance in early infancy. If she woke at that time she would talk to herself for some time without disturbing the parents. At around three years anything new upset her and the special ceremonials began to appear. The routines always had to be followed in exactly the same way. By latency at sleeptime she demanded that the curtains be drawn exactly the same amount, and the parents noticed that she was afraid of new shadows.

During latency many children develop the habit of reading before falling asleep as a defense against engaging in various fantasies (very frequently of an erotic nature) and in order to avoid the impulse to masturbate.

I treated an extreme case of this type where the disturbance grew more severe and continued into adulthood. During the latency period this boy began to read compulsively in bed to avoid engaging in fantasies which usually led to his playing with his penis. In later life he developed the severe obsessional neurosis that brought him to treatment. At this time a large number of obsessional rituals had to be performed before he was ready to go to bed. Once in bed he had to read compulsively the daily newspaper from the first page to the last one, including advertisements and everything else. Usually he fell asleep at some point during the process of reading the newspaper and before he was able to finish reading every bit of it. Consequently the following night he was forced to start reading the newspaper (of the previous day) where he had interrupted it before he could proceed to the paper of the day. There were times when he was several days behind in his reading. This incongruous behavior served the useful purpose of having several old newspapers to read through on those days when the wish to masturbate and the concomitant anxiety were stronger and kept him awake for a longer period of time than was usual. On such occasions he caught up with reading the old newspapers, managed to get exhausted, and fell asleep. The specific aim of this compulsive behavior was made patently clear by the fact that on the rare occasions when he succumbed to the temptation to masturbate in bed he had no need to read the newspapers that evening but went straight off to sleep.

The following case of a latency girl, P C, six and a half years old at the beginning of treatment, shows how a sleeping disturbance that started at one and a half years was used for the expression of phallic-oedipal conflicts during that phase. It further shows how an unsatisfactory resolution of the infantile neurosis perpetuated the symptom into the latency period. P C started to wake three to four times every night at the age of eighteen months. She then shouted for her parents to come and rub ointment on her itching skin or went into the parents' bedroom to wake them. In treatment the analyst could interpret the oedipal fantasies behind this behavior; that is, her curiosity about what the parents were doing together in bed as well as her wish to interfere with it; and the sexual gratification she derived from having the parents, especially the father, rub the ointment on her body. The symptom cleared up; P now had undisturbed nights for the first time in her life.

It should be noted that in this case the interpretation of the oedipal content was sufficient to clear up the symptom, although the sleeping disturbance had been present long before it could have had any phallic-oedipal significance. As we have seen, sleeping disturbances that begin early in life and persist serve different purposes and have different contents and meanings at different times. I believe that in this case and many similar ones the interpretation of the later and more significant layers of content was sufficient (in therapeutic terms) because earlier the "symptom" had no specific psychological content, in terms of a "neurotic conflict" situation, and acquired significant content only during the phallic-oedipal phase. At first the "symptom" appeared in conjunction with the skin complaints and was retained because the child's skin erotism was gratified, a gratification that at that particular stage of her development was not necessarily conflictive (as it became later when the phallic-oedipal fantasies were attached to it).

This observation and similar ones make it clear that some of the earlier "sleeping disturbances" are not always due to compromise formations arising from specific neurotic conflict situations but are attributable to factors of a completely different nature. Although in their outward manifestations there are no apparent differences between the earlier and later disturbances, there are very significant metapsychological differences which account for the later vicissitudes of these different "symptoms."[12] We further believe that many of the nonconflictive determinants of the early disturbances disappear as development progresses. If the symptom is nevertheless retained, it is due to the psychological conflicts that may have attached themselves to it in the meantime. For this reason the interpretation of the current psychological conflict rather than the genesis of the symptom is sufficient in therapeutic terms. This is in sharp contrast to those cases in which the disturbance of sleep likewise appears at an early age but is the result of specific "neurotic conflict" situations, for example, the fear of wetting or soiling during sleep when the child has already internalized the wish to be clean and dry. In this type of case, interpretation of the phallic-oedipal content alone will usually not suffice to clear the symptom, although it may bring a measure of relief and generally improve the sleep disturbance. Since the

12. It is clear that to refer to all these different types of phenomena as "symptoms" is not quite appropriate and has only descriptive meaning.

phallic-oedipal significance was superimposed on a symptom resulting from conflicts at an earlier level, the symptom cannot be resolved without interpretation of the anal-sadistic impulses and the wish to set and soil.

Finally, some of the conflicts that appear during the phallic-oedipal stage may find an even more forceful expression during a disturbed latency period. This happens, for example, with regard to conflicts around aggression which at this stage are frequently seen in children who have not resolved their infantile neuroses. These aggressive conflicts lead to massive fear of separation from the mother and can create a particularly difficult situation when the mother has to go out during the evenings, but they are operative even if the mother stays at home. The following example illustrates this situation.

J R had suffered from a disturbed sleep since the age of three and a half years. By the time she was nine years of age these difficulties had greatly increased. Her behavior at that time clearly indicated the nature of the underlying conflicts. After she went to bed she felt compelled to come downstairs to kiss her mother and reassure her that she loved her. When the mother had to go out at night, whether alone or with the father, J showed a great deal of anxiety, asking compulsively, "Will you be all right?" She insisted that her mother wake her up on her return in order to reassure herself that the mother was safely back.

A similar situation exists in those cases in which the child has a sadistic conception of the sexual relationships between the parents that has been reinforced by early primal scene observations and by an unsatisfactory hostile relationship between the parents. In several latency children seen at the Clinic the unconscious fear that the father will harm or kill the mother was the prime motive of their need to sleep in the parents' bed or to separate them during the evening.

GENERAL CONSIDERATIONS

As we have seen, from the second year of life on sleep becomes an increasingly more vulnerable area. When we examined a large number of the files from our diagnostic department, we were surprised by the high frequency of references to difficulties around sleep. In some cases the sleep disturbances were present at the time of referral and were one of the reasons for referral; more frequently they had been present in the past or were considered a minor complaint among the more important ones. It is self-evident that "sleeping disturbance" is no more than a descriptive term covering many different types of underlying psychopathology the specific nature of which must be determined in each case.

A no less striking situation exists in the adult if we consider the amount of ritualized behavior that most human beings go through before settling down for sleep. Luce and Segal (1966) state that "however inconspicuous, almost everybody performs some rituals embodying unspoken and perhaps unrecognized feelings, and without these rituals it is hard to sleep. It may be the ceremony of bedtime ablutions, washing, bathing, brushing teeth. It may be the dog's walk, locking the house, turning on night lights—or something more bizarre" (p. 29). They refer to Charles Dickens's habit or rearranging the furniture of hotel bedrooms in which he stayed; he would push the bed around until its head pointed north according to his compass; the rationale behind this peculiar behavior was that he wanted to benefit from certain magnetic currents. Similarly, Winston Churchill during a Big Three conference in 1953 insisted on having twin beds in his room, sleeping part of the night in one bed and the rest in the other. Fenichel (1945) considers impairment of the function of sleep one of the most frequent neurotic manifestations, to be found in almost every neurosis.

There is no doubt that in the process of socialization and civilization we have sacrificed much of what in earlier times may have been the patterns of sleep, assuming that these patterns were then determined largely by the needs of human nature and not as nowadays by social conventions, fashions, and the progress of civilization. Luce and Segal (1966) point out that the neat bed-clothing and nightdress of today are recent innovations, while previously the sleeper wound himself into a shroud of linen. They also state that beds came into general use throughout Europe only in the ninth century, while the private bedroom was an innovation of the fifteenth century and is not yet the norm of mankind in general. As they say: "A child who is reluctant to be left alone for sleep, who insists on leaving his door open and having a light, may be showing an impulse for protection and comfort that was more readily satisfied during past eras, and today among the less privileged" (p. 25).

Anna Freud (1966) pointed to the difficulties of studying "need patterns" with regard to sleep because social conventions interfere with them from the beginning of life. On the one hand, the infant is "put to sleep" and in this way patterns are imposed. On the other hand, it is not "natural" for the infant to sleep under the conditions imposed—alone and between cold sheets. The human baby is perhaps the only creature (among mammals) who sleeps alone without any skin contact and natural warmth. Present cultural conditions may disregard important aspects of sleep which more closely approximate "natural" conditions. Anna Freud recalled a patient who, in describing how he went to sleep as a child surrounded by his toy animals, said that he was probably trying to re-create a litter. She further remarked on Aichhorn's description of the sleeping patterns in his home for dissocial boys. The first thing many of these boys did was to rip the sheets off the beds in order to sleep in contact with the rough blankets, which may be an indication of the importance of skin contact.

Anna Freud considered it of special importance to assess the degree to which the disturbances of sleep are due to the handling of the child and how much comes from within the child as the symptomatic expression of specific conflict situations. At one point in life every child wants to stay up but is put to sleep. Conversely, there are many occasions in life when a person may want to sleep but is forced to stay up. The same is true with regard to the time of waking. The young child wakes up early; then the child begins to attend school and with it begin the difficulties in waking. She pointed out that while we have feeding on demand for children, we do not have sleeping on demand.

One cannot help being reminded here of the role played by "transitional objects" (Winnicott 1953). Our attention has been attracted by a limited number of observations in which the mother lies with the child for a short while as part of the process of putting him to sleep. These children have never shown any interest in or need for a transitional object, but we cannot say whether this is true in all cases or is just a chance observation.

Some of the cases studied at Hampstead have shown that the sleep problem of the child is sometimes the expression of the psychopathology of one or both parents. In such cases the child's symptom belongs in the context of the family disturbance. I have earlier described the case of a little girl, G H, whose sleep disturbance was multiply determined by inner factors at different developmental stages. Here I want to describe how her "family milieu" helped to create and maintain her symptoms.

Mrs. H was seen weekly in mother guidance. Shortly thereafter the father was taken into psychoanalytic treatment (under the Hampstead Clinic program of simultaneous analysis). We soon discovered that the older brother, P, who was studied by our diagnostic department, also suffered, among other things, from some disturbances of sleep; he frequently woke up during the night and would then roam around the house for long periods of time.

From the analysis of the father we learned that although the marriage was not completely unsatisfactory, he experienced no sexual satisfaction for which he blamed his wife. He described his wife as a very compulsive woman who had to finish a multitude of house cleaning chores before she was able to go to bed. These severe compulsive needs of the wife oscillated, being worse at some times and slightly better at others. As a result she was never in bed before midnight by which time Mr. H had been overcome by sleep. He asserted that this situation ruined his sexual life. He would argue with his wife to persuade her to come to bed early and leave some of the completely unnecessary chores for the next day, but she could not do this. Mr. H's complaints about the difficulties introduced into their sexual life by his wife's disturbances were certainly true, but these complaints simultaneously served the function of a useful rationalization by means of which he could hide his own inner difficulties. As his analysis progressed, it was found that he was riddled with fantasies of being damaged and of having a small damaged penis. Earlier in his life he had had occasional difficulties with his potency which further strengthened his fears. He felt he was an unsatisfactory sexual partner and that he was incapable of satisfying a woman sexually. Unconsciously, this was the real reason for his wife's avoidance of sexual intercourse with him. Mrs. H was seen in weekly interviews throughout the period of the child's treatment. From her material it was clear that there was a great deal of reality in Mr. H's complaints. Her compulsive behavior had as one of its aims the avoidance of sexual intercourse. She too unconsciously very much welcomed the sleeping disturbances of the children because they made it nearly impossible to have a regular sexual life with her husband. As far as the father was concerned, the sleep disturbances of both children and especially that of the little girl, although a conscious motive of complaint (as another source of interference with his marital sexual life), were a most welcome and unconsciously encouraged symptom that helped him to avoid being exposed to what he feared most—his lack of virility. Because of these fears much of his sexuality found an outlet in a number of unconscious fantasies in which he was very potent sexually with women who were small in size (his wife was in fact a very small woman) and with little girls. The discovery of these fantasies in analysis terrified and depressed Mr. H who had been in the habit of getting into bed with his little girl when, because of her disturbed sleep, she called one or the other parent. At the time of the diagnostic evaluation of G H it had already been noted that her father was in the habit of overexciting her at bedtime and that his behavior acted as a seduction and greatly contributed to her inability to fall asleep and to sleep through the night. Furthermore, partly as a result of his homosexual conflicts and partly as a defense against the incestuous wishes for his daughter, Mr. H was in the habit of getting into bed with his slightly older son completely naked, behavior that must have contributed to the boy's sleeping difficulties as well. A further determinant of the child's sleep disturbances, especially that of the little girl, was the fact that the father had an unconscious need to expose the children to primal scene observations as he himself had been exposed in childhood, events of which he retained a vivid recollection. I have earlier pointed out the repercussions which witnessing the primal scene had in the inner life and fantasies of the little girl. At the beginning of his treatment Mr. H expressed surprise at the frequency with which the little girl woke up and walked into the parents' room while they were having intercourse. He was for some time completely unaware that this was usually not accidental. He often managed to wake her up by making excessive noise, etc. It was striking that P frequently roamed about the house while the parents had intercourse, but he never came into the parents' bedroom.

It can be seen that different unconscious needs, fantasies, and conflicts in each of the parents and the conflicts in their relationship to each other have all contributed to the onset and the establishment of the disturbances of sleep in these children. Each parent's psychopathology as well as that existing in their marital relationship required the maintainance of the children's symptoms as significant elements and safety valves for the parents' equilibrium.

It seems probable that disturbances of sleep in children are particularly suitable vehicles for the expression of parental difficulties of a most diverse nature. They add themselves to whatever contributions come from the conflicts of the child himself at the different developmental stages.

In a number of our cases the sleep disturbances of the child have become the battleground on which the parents express the aggression and tension that really belong in the context of their unhappy marital relationship. The child's sleeping difficulties often exacerbate weaknesses that exist in the marital relationship, e.g., when the mother, who is usually the most affected by it, finds herself faced with a chronic shortness of sleep or when the husband resents having his sleep disturbed or refuses to take his share in coping with the situation. In one case the mother unconsciously favored the maintenance of the symptom in the child because it gave her an opportunity to express hostile feelings to her husband. The hostility had its roots in an unhappy marital situation about which she did not feel able to complain. She could use her husband's refusal to share the burden of coping with the child during the night to express much of her bottled-up resentment. On a conscious level she strongly wished that the child's sleep return to normal both for her own sake and because of her awareness of the increasing deterioration of the relationship with her husband. In this respect it must be taken into consideration that fathers usually escape the unpleasantness of their children's disturbances by being away at work; however, having their sleep interfered with is something they can hardly ignore or escape from.

Since the disturbance in these cases must be considered a "family disturbance," the child therapist is forced to ask himself whether individual treatment can substantially influence the disturbance. If he suspects intense parental involvement in the child's symptom, the only answer to the problem probably is simultaneous analysis. It is feasible, on the other hand, that as the child develops further and gains some independence from the parents, he may find means of disengaging himself from this interaction. The child described by Jenny Waelder-Hall (1935) seems to indicate that this may be possible, at least in those cases where the parental contribution has not been too excessive. Longitudinal and follow-up studies of this type of problem will clarify some of these issues—the dependence on parental psychopathology, the possibility of detachment as the personality grows, etc.—but the fact that most adults require special (though mostly unconscious) arrangements and preparations before going to sleep points in the direction that inevitably significant contributions to the later personality come from multiple areas. This fact also leads back to a point made earlier: by now we may have departed from what at one time were more "natural" conditions of sleep in early infancy to such an extent that hardly anyone really escapes unharmed.

In a number of our cases the child's disturbed sleep (which served an essential function in the parent's psychopathology) disappeared when the mother was able to be firm and to correct her attitudes and expectations of the child with regard to sleep, with the help of the child's therapist, her own treatment, or mother guidance. These observations seem to point to the fact that some sleep disturbances are "service symptoms"—that is, they serve a function in the child's external relations; in spite of their apparent severity, these symptoms are essentially not compromise formations resulting from conflicts in the child. Once the child accepts the imposition of the service symptoms, however, they are utilized for the expression of the different developmental and neurotic conflicts that the child may be dealing with at any given time. It must be noted that there are important metapsychological and prognostic differences between sleep disturbances having a service function and those resulting from a compromise formation of internal and internalized conflicts in the child. In the cases in which the symptom has not been suggested, provoked, or somehow superimposed on the child's personality, nothing short of analytic treatment of the child will do away with the disturbance. Anna Freud (1965) pointed to another reason why parents contribute to the maintenance of the child's sleep disturbance: "Parents may also play a part in maintaining a child's disturbance. Some of the . . . sleeping rituals are kept up by the child only in collusion with the mother. Owing to her dreading the child's anxiety attacks as much as the child does himself, the other participates actively in keeping up defenses, precautions, etc., and thereby camouflages the extent ot the child's illness" (pp. 47-48).

It is evident that the tolerance of different parents to having their sleep disturbed by the child's difficulties varies greatly, and what constitutes an intolerable upset for some is not even mentioned by others as a problem. This reaction is significant not only for the child's sleep disturbance itself, but also for how it will affect the mother-child relationship in general. An unsettled mother-child relationship may in turn affect other developmental conflicts and other areas of the child's personality. The therapist must therefore abandon whatever concept of "norm" he himself may have with regard to sleeping patterns and assess each problem on its own merits: How much physical and psychic stress is experienced by the child, the mother, and other members of the family; and what is the threshold of tolerance for disturbed sleep in each family unit.

In this chapter, I have traced the vicissitudes and different forms of expression that the sleeping disturbances acquire according to the degree of ego development, the level of object relationships, and the different developmental stages and conflicts that the child must go through. I noted that during the latency period, partly because of the increasing liberty given to the child to make his own sleeping arrangements, many of the earlier symptoms disappear or are replaced by special arrangements specific to and characteristic of each individual. This process of adaptation sometimes continues in adolescence and adulthood resulting in a further reduction of the earlier symptomatic manifestations. However, not all persons find these happy solutions; in many instances, early disturbances persist and are still manifest in adulthood. In these cases the nature and intensity of the conflicts do not permit of such adaptive solutions referred to above.

One of my adult patients is a good example of this type of case. The patient began analytic treatment at the age of thirty. He complained of anxiety states, faulty potency, and a large number of conversion and psychosomatic symptoms, for which no physical causes had been found in repeated medical checkups. Although he did not complain of sleep difficulties it soon was apparent that sleep was a disturbed area as well. The patient was a bachelor who lived alone. At bedtime he was haunted by fantasies that somebody was hiding in the dark of his flat ready to attack him. He frequently searched the place to reassure himself that there was nobody in the room, but in spite of the search he remained uneasy and anxious and was in no way reassured. Whenever his anxiety became too intense, he took a sleeping pill. In the treatment there soon appeared other fantasies and behavioral manifestations relating to his sleep difficulties. The nature of his work required him to travel a great deal and to sleep in hotels and quite often to stay at the homes of friends or business associates. On all these occasions, and especially when he was a guest in a family, he had to make a number of elaborate arrangements before settling to sleep. He locked his door and placed chairs and other objects behind it and blocked the different approaches from the door to his bed. This behavior was based on a fantasy that the host had every intention of attacking him during the night. His elaborate arrangements would ensure his waking up (through the noise of falling objects) if anybody entered his room or approached his bed. Curiously enough, in spite of his fear (which he consciously recognized as irrational), once he had finished the arrangements described he would take some sleeping pills. During treatment it became clear that the precautions and symptoms reached a peak when his host had an attractive wife who aroused him sexually.

Two different sets of impulses determined this behavior. The first one was his wish to kill the husband and take possession of the wife. This wish was defended against by means of projection: his host had murderous designs on him. The second group of fantasies concerned his fear of sexually assaulting his host's wife in an extremely sadistic way. To protect both himself and them in case he should do this while asleep, he made certain that if he were to take a step out of bed he would wake up. He had to make sure that he could not possibly leave the room. He believed he had had one or two episodes of somnambulism in his early childhood which further increased his fear of his actions during sleep.

These disturbances of sleep had started in his early infancy and had never completely disappeared. A necessary precondition of his falling asleep as a very small child had been his chewing a special piece of cloth which his mother attached to his blanket and which was renewed every two weeks when the previous one was destroyed. After the birth of his sister when he was four years old he became afraid of the dark, a fear which was intensified when he was ten or eleven. He feared that somebody was about to attack him. He traced this fear of the dark to a memory of the age of five: he woke up once and saw an old woman beside his bed sitting in the dark. He was terrified but turned his back on this figure pretending he was asleep. He believed the old woman might have been his grandmother who was living in the house at the time and with whom he had a special relationship. He always liked her and used to play with her breasts a great deal, which apparently he was allowed to do. The anxiety he experienced then turned out to be the result of a displaced oedipal fantasy (from the parents to the grandparents). His grandmother had come to him in the evening "abandoning" the grandfather, and he feared that the latter would come and attack him for the seduction of his wife (that the wife of his host might come to him during the evening was an ever-present fantasy of his.) Furthermore, while he was in treatment he visited his parents for a short holiday after he had been away from home for several years. To his surprise he had to take the same precautions and had the same irrational fear that his father would come to kill him during the night.

The intensity of the unresolved oedipal conflicts which were reinforced by massive conflicts with his strong aggressive and sadistic impulses, made it impossible for this patient to deal with his early difficulties by simple ritualized arrangements (the "secondary measures" of Fenichel). It is of interest that this patient regularly fell asleep during the sessions whenever his aggressive feelings toward the analyst went beyond a certain point.[13] By falling asleep he protected the analyst from his conscious death wishes and possible aggressive attacks; on the other hand, if he were to attack the analyst in his sleep, he could not be held responsible for it.[14]

13. Simmel (1942) also referred to the sleep disturbances arising from important conflicts around aggression.

14. Davison (1945) remarks, "the anxiety which produces insomnia in one individual [and we may add even in the same individual at different times] may be responsible for somnolence in another because he fears that if awakened he will be incapable of resisting the temptation to carry out his powerful incestuous masturbatory or aggressive wishes in reality" (p. 485).

Similarly, whenever a girl friend spent an evening in his flat he felt greatly distressed and suffered from insomnia motivated by the fear of what he could do to her in his sleep. To ensure that nothing could happen he always took some sleeping tablets.

According to our observations, there are many persons who, because of their fear of aggressive impulses, take pills to ensure that they will be immobilized during the night. In this way they assure themselves that they can control the feared impulses during sleep.

Turning to the classification and definition of sleep disturbances, we encounter some difficulties. The developmental approach followed in this paper has a number of advantages, but in some respects it is not sufficient, especially for the study of older children and adults. It should be complemented by a consideration of the specific phase of the sleep process that is affected:

1. Disturbances in the presleep stage, of which many instances were given, the severe obsessional rituals being an extreme example. Sleep phobias should also be considered and the nature of the specific fear must be determined. Is it the state of sleep itself, the room, the bed, nightmares, etc.?

2. Disturbances in the falling asleep period (see Varendock 1921).

3. Disturbances of the sleeping period, including:
    (a) certain types of dreams;
    (b) talking during sleep, general restlessness, etc.;
    (c) night waking, which might imply simple waking during the night with quick return to sleep or hours of delay, anxiety, and agitation;
    (d) nightmares;
    (e) night terrors (pavor nocturnus);
    (f) sleep walking;
    (g) some fuguelike states, in which even crimes have been committed.

4. Disturbances of the waking-up period, including early waking, incapacity to wake, and perhaps hypersomnia that may well require a category of its own.

In this respect it is necessary to mention that the generally assumed relationship between dreaming and sleep talking, sleep-walking, enuresis, teeth grinding, etc., has been disproved by recent and conclusive research. As Fisher (1965) points out, these phenomena do not take place during the REM periods (characteristic of the dreaming periods) but they occur mostly during the NREM periods of sleep. Furthermore, it has been demonstrated that mental activity during sleep is not restricted to the dreaming period. A discussion of these aspects and of the effects of sleep deprivation and dream deprivation, as demonstrated by Fisher and Dement (1963) and West et al. (1962), is unfortunately beyond the scope of this paper. For an excellent summary of the research on sleep deprivation and many other aspects of sleep and dreams in general, see Luce, Segal, and McGinty (1965). The relationship between dream research and psychoanalytic theory has been studied by Trosman (1963) and Fisher (1965).)

Finally, I briefly want to note the similarities between some actual neuroses in adults and those sleep disturbances in very young children which are due to overstimulation or seduction of the child. In the actual neurosis of adults a sleep disturbance may be a prominent symptom, which has arisen from a state of inner tension built up as the result of insufficient drive discharge (not infrequently of libidinal impulses). In the first case, the inner tension is due to the lack of satisfactory outlets either because of unfavorable environmental circumstances or because of other reasons. In the second case, the seduction or overstimulation arouses a degree of excitation for which the child lacks the appropriate channels of discharge due to his limited physical and psychological maturity. Furthermore, he still lacks the ego functions necessary to bind this amount of excitation.

References

Bornstein, B. (1931). Phobia in a two-and-a-half-year-old child. *Psychoanalytic Quarterly* 4:93-119.

Davidson, C. (1945). Psychological and Psychodynamic aspects of disturbances in the sleep mechanism. *Psychoanalytic Quarterly* 14:478-497.

Fenichel, O. (1945). *The Psychoanalytic Theory of Neurosis.* New York: Norton.

Fisher, C. (1965). Psychoanalytic implications of recent research on sleep and dreaming. *Journal of the American Psychoanalytic Association* 13:179-303.

Fisher, C., and Dement, W. (1963). Studies on the psychopathology of sleep and dreams. *American Journal of Psychiatry* 119:1160.

Fraiberg, S. (1950). On the sleep disturbances of childhood. *Psychoanalytic Study of the Child* 5:285-309.

Freud, A. (1965). *Normality and Pathology in Childhood.* New York: International Universities Press.

――― (1966). Personal communication.

Freud, S. (1901). On dreams. *Standard Edition* 5:629-686.

Friend, M.R., reporter (1956). Panel on sleep disturbances in children. *Journal of the American Psychoanalytic Association* 4:514-525.

Gesell, A., and Ilg, F.L. (1943). *Infant and Child in the Culture of Today.* New York: Harper.

Gifford, S. (1960). Sleep, time and the early ego. *Journal of the American Psychoanalytic Association* 8:5-42.

Hirschberg, J.C. (1957). Parental anxieties accompanying sleep disturbance in young children. *Bulletin of the Menninger Clinic* 21:129-139.

Hoffer, W. (1949). Mouth, hand and ego-integration. *Psychoanalytic Study of the Child* 3/4:49-56.

Irwin, O.C., and Weiss, LaB. A. (1934). The effect of darkness on the activity of newborn infants. *Studies in Infant Behavior, vol. l* University of Iowa Studies 9:163-175.

Katan, A. (1961) Some thoughts about the role of verbalization in early childhood. *Psychoanalytic Study of the Child* 16:184-188.

Kleitman, N. (1939). *Sleep and Wakefulness.* Chicago: University of Chicago Press, 1963.

Kleitman, N., and Englemann, T.G. (1953). Sleep characteristics of infants. *Journal of Applied Physiology* 6:269-282.

Luce, G.G., and Segal, J. (1966). *Sleep.* New York: Coward-McCann.

Luce, G.G., Segal, J., and McGinty, D. (1965). *Current Research on Sleep and Dreams.* Public Health Service Publication No. 1389. Washington, D.C.: U.S. Government Printing Office.

Mack, J. (1965). Children's nightmares. *International Journal of Psychoanalysis* 46:403-428.

Moore, T., and Ucko, L.E. (1957). Night waking in early infancy. *Arch. Dis. Childhd.* 32:333-342.

Nagera, H. (1966). *Early Childhood Disturbances, the Infantile Neurosis, and the Adulthood Disturbances* New York: International Universities Press.

Oswald, I. (1966) *Sleep.* London: Penguin Books.

Parmelee, A.H., Wenner, W.H., and Schulz, H.R. (1964). Infant sleep patterns from birth to 16 weeks of age. *Journal of Pediatrics* 65:576-582.

Provence, S., and Lipton, R.C. (1962). *Infants in Institutions.* New York: International Universities Press.

Rank, B., and Macnaughton, D. (1950). A clinical contribution to early ego development. *Psychoanalytic Study of the Child* 5:53-65.

Ribble, M.A. (1943). *The Rights of Infants.* New York: Columbia University Press.

Sandler, J. (1962). The Hampstead index as an instrument of psychoanalytic research. *International Journal of Psycho-Analysis* 43:287-291.

Simmel, E. (1942). In: Symposium on neurotic disturbances of sleep. *Yearbook of Psychoanalysis* 1:194-201.

Sperling, M. (1949). Neurotic sleep disturbances in children. *Nervous Child* 8:28-46.

——— (1955). Etiology and treatment of sleep disturbances in children. *Psychoanalytic Quarterly* 24:358-368.

Trosman, H. (1963). Dream research and the psychoanalytic theory of dreams. *Archives of General Psychiatry.* 9:9-18.

Varendock, J. (1921). *The Psychology of Day-Dreams.* London: Allen and Unwin.

Waelder-Hall, J. (1935). The analysis of a case of night terror. *Psychoanalytic Study of the Child* 2:189-228.

Walter, W.G. (1953). Electroencephalographic development of children. In: *Discussions on Child Development,* vol.1, ed. J.M. Tanner, and B. Inhelder, pp. 132-160. New York: International Universities Press.

West, L.J., Janszen, H.H., Lester, B.K., and Cornelisoon, F.S., Jr. (1962). The psychosis of sleep deprivation. *Annuals of the New York Academy of Science* 96:66-70.

Winnicott, D.W. (1953). Transitional objects and transitional phenomena. *International Journal of Psycho-Analysis.* 34:89-97.

Chapter Fourteen

THE IMAGINARY COMPANION

During the last few years at the Hampstead Clinic we have studied a small number of children who had, at the time of their diagnostic assessment or previously, an imaginary companion. In no case was the imaginary companion the cause for referral. Usually, its existence was elicited more or less accidentally during the course of the diagnostic investigation.

When we explored this fantasy further, we were surprised to learn that only rarely did the imaginary companion play a significant role in the analysis of these children. In fact, we know of only two children who directly and frequently referred to their imaginary companions during the analytic sessions. One such case was described in the literature (Sperling 1954). Since our clinical material is limited, we can only state what our experience was, without drawing any inferences or conclusions as to the meaning of this observation or its general validity.[1]

1. Bender and Vogel (1941) have described a large number of children mostly in latency and late latency who talked quite freely of their imaginary companions in a therapeutic situation. But these children were not in analysis (with its special setting and conditions); they were studied in hospitals where they seem to have been very actively questioned.

In collaboration with Alice Colonna and the Clinical Concept Research Group, whose members are: H. Nagera (Chairman), A. Freud (Consultant), S. Baker, A. Colonna, R. Edgcumbe, M. Foote, W. E. Freud, A. Gavshon, A. Hayman, S. Ini, R. Putzel, and I. Rosen. A number of colleagues helped with the review of the literature and gave permission for the use of their clinical examples. I wish to thank Eva Bry, Lottie Kearney, Elizabeth Model, Dr. Josephine Stross, and T. de Vries.

One possible explanation for the absence of references to the imaginary companion, at least in the treatment of the younger child, is that the imaginary companion frequently plays a specific positive role in the development of the child, and once that role is fulfilled, it tends to disappear and is finally covered by the usual infantile amnesia. Although this assumption is probably correct, several puzzling elements remain.

First, in a successful therapeutic analysis of adults, much of the infantile amnesia is lifted. In fact, the success of the analysis usually depends in part on achieving this to a sufficient degree. Nevertheless, in our experience and in that of a considerable number of colleagues whom I have consulted, memories of an imaginary companion are recovered only rarely. Yet we know that the phenomenon of the imaginary companion is not a rare occurrence in children. According to Harriman (1937), for example, one third of the children he studied had an imaginary companion. Why then is it so rarely recovered?[2]

Second, in a large number of individuals the imaginary companion makes its first appearance in later developmental stages, e.g., in latency, a period that usually is not covered by the infantile amnesia. What has become of these imaginary companions?

There is a third point related to the above. We have come to know of a few adults who clearly and consciously recollected having had an imaginary companion in their childhood and who nevertheless managed to go through what they considered a satisfactory analysis of several years' duration without ever referring in the analysis to their memories of their imaginary companions.

While we have no definite answers to many of the questions raised, we believe that further inquiry into this phenomenon has long been overdue.

2. Perhaps the answer lies (in the case of the very young child) in the fact that what is important is not the content of the fantasy associated with the imaginary companion but the developmental purpose it is designed to fulfill. In this sense it has to be considered part of a developmental process and that is not the type of thing that is recovered by the lifting of the infantile amnesia. Furthermore, what cannot be recovered has to be reconstructed, and there are obvious difficulties in reconstructing the early existence of an imaginary companion. Another possible reason is that in the analyses of adults we do not pay as much attention to this phenomenon as we should.

A review of the psychoanalytic literature discloses only one paper devoted entirely to imaginary companions (Sperling 1954). In addition, several analysts have occasionally referred to this phenomenon (Anna Freud 1936, Selma Fraiberg 1959, Murphy et al. 1962, Harrison et al. 1963). The situation is quite different outside the psychoanalytic literature where one finds a variety of publications by sociologists, psychologists, and educators. "A Study of Imaginary Companions" was published by Vostrovsky as early as 1895. Several authors devoted special chapters or even an entire book to this topic (e.g., Harvey 1918, Hall 1907, Green 1922).

In our experience, the phenomenon of the imaginary companion is observed most frequently in children between the ages of two and a half to three years and nine and a half to ten years, the majority being found in the earlier range. Some authors, e.g., Vostrovsky (1895), claim that the first appearance of the imaginary companion varied from the first to the thirteenth year of life, but her conclusions are not based on direct observations of children.

Hurlock and Burstein (1932) placed the first appearance of the imaginary companion much later. They concluded, "Among the girls, the age at which the imaginary companion is most likely to appear is between five and seven years of age. Boys experienced this phenomenon at a considerably later age than did girls. One third of the group of people studied fixed the age of first appearance of the imaginary playmate at the stage between seven and nine years of age" (p. 385). The discrepancy between our findings and those of Hurlock and Burstein is, I believe, a result of the procedure followed by these authors. Their study is based on questionnaires given to 701 high school and college students whose ages varied from fifteen and forty years, with the median being eighteen to nineteen years. Hurlock and Burstein were not aware of the fact that infantile amnesia usually covers the earlier years; if a person nevertheless remembers the imaginary companion (possibly because he was told about it by his parents), he will tend to place it outside the period covered by the infantile amnesia. Our experiences and that of others whose data were obtained through direct observation of children demonstrate that the imaginary companion appears from two and a half years onward.

Bender and Vogel (1941) described fourteen cases of imaginary companions. At the time of admission to the Children's Ward of Bellevue Psychiatric Hospital the children were five to ten years of age, but in some cases the imaginary companions had been active for several years prior to admission. Harvey (1918) thought that the imaginary companions tend to disappear at two points, either at the ages of seven to eight, or between eleven and twelve. Svendsen (1934) stated that "anything approximating accurate information in regard to the time at which imaginary companions disappear is difficult to obtain, owing to the gradual character of the process" (p. 996).

The imaginary companion phenomenon is not restricted to the age groups so far described. Harriman (1937), for example, reported the experiences of a number of college students in psychology who kept their imaginary companions longer than is usually observed. In one case, the imaginary companion made its appearance when the student was twelve to thirteen years of age and remained active for several years thereafter. In another case, the fantasy of an imaginary companion remained active until the student, a male, was eighteen years of age. In some of the cases described by Harriman the fantasy of the imaginary companion was as vivid and clear at this later age as it had been at the beginning; while in others the fantasy, though still present, had lost much of its former distinctness.

We should add that only two analysts among the many we consulted remembered adult patients who referred to a childhood imaginary companion during their analyses. The special interest of one of these cases is that the patient not only referred to the imaginary companion in his analysis but in fact retained his imaginary companion throughout adulthood. It was the analyst's impression that although this patient's imaginary companion had lost much of its distinctness, it nevertheless continued to play an active role in the patient's psychological life.

Some authors, e.g., Svendsen (1934), believe that the imaginary companion is accompanied by strong visual imagery. Harvey (1918) believes that the imaginary playmate is a visual or auditory idea that becomes as vivid and real as a visual or auditory percept, but that the child nevertheless always recognizes its unreality.

Bender and Vogel (1941) state that they never observed the imaginary companion phenomenon in psychotic children and that they found no instance in which they had any reason to believe that it represented a feature in a prepsychotic state.

Different authors cite different figures with regard to the frequency of the imaginary companion. Svendsen (1934) thinks that about 13 percent of all children show this phenomenon. She arrived at this percentage on the basis of the following definition: "the term imaginary companion, as it is used in this study, implies an invisible character, named and referred to in conversation with other persons or played with directly for a period of time, at least several months, having an air of reality for the child but no apparent objective basis. This excludes that type of imaginative play in which an object is personified, or in which the child himself assumes the role of some person in his environment" (p. 988). Hurlock and Burstein (1932) maintain that as many as 20 percent of all children have imaginary companions, while Harriman (1937) believes that this phenomenon can be observed in about one third of all children between the ages of three and nine. Kirkpatrick (1929) was of the opinion that practically all children have imaginary companions in one form or other.

The discrepancies in these figures, it seems to me, are largely dependent upon the criteria used to define an imaginary companion. A review of the literature makes it clear that there are no uniform criteria and that a variety of fantasy manifestations in children are included by some authors and excluded by others. In what follows I shall use some familiar imaginative activities of children to highlight the difficulties in deciding what constitutes an imaginary companion.

All child therapists with experience in the treatment of children between the ages of two and seven know how frequently they find an ally among their toys or in a lion, a tiger, a crocodile, Superman, etc. These different animals and persons blindly obey their commands and are ready to attack anyone by whom the child feels threatened. Such dangerous beasts frequently appear at those points in the treatment when the child displaces onto the therapist a fear that belongs in the child's relationship to his father, for example, especially when he has managed to project onto the father and therapist his own hostile and aggressive designs.

One of my patients, a four-year-old boy, used a crocodile and a tiger whenever he felt particularly aggressive toward me. I could observe the following sequence: at first he either verbalized his hostile intentions or tried to attack me physically by kicking or hitting. Shortly afterward he would become frightened by his actions and fearful of retaliation by me. He then looked in his cupboard for his crocodile and tiger, warning me that these two powerful allies were ready to defend him and would destroy me if I meant any harm.

Such behavior is common and frequent enough during therapy; although it seems as if this child had provided himself with an imaginary companion, it was at first confined to the analytic hour and, within the analytic hours, to those occasions when his aggression was aroused and he feared my retaliation. This type of imaginary companion is an ad hoc construction designed to deal with a specific situation such as that described and may not even have arisen were it not for the special conditions of the analytic treatment. It is doubtful whether this type of phenomenon in this limited form really deserves to be considered a true imaginary companion. (Furthermore, my patient used concrete objects, a toy tiger and a toy crocodile, while in most cases the real imaginary companion does not require concrete representation.) If one does so consider it, then one must agree with Kirkpatrick (1929) that all children at one age or another have the fantasy of an imaginary companion with greater or lesser intensity.

My little patient's use of the animals, however, did not remain confined to the analytic session. Somewhat later in treatment when his fear of being smacked by the father increased—a fear that had a reality basis—he began to protect himself further by taking the two powerful allies home. If this was not allowed, he took them home in his imagination by pretending that he had put them into his pocket. In the following session he would comment spontaneously or in response to my questions how these animals had frightened his father, who then did not dare smack him. With these developments, the defensive ad hoc fantasy had obviously assumed a more integral part of the child's fantasy life; for a while these two animals were his constant and reassuring companions at school, at home, and, when necessary, during the analytic sessions. Even though this type of behavior is closer to the imaginary companion phenomenon than the former, we very much hesitate to consider it a typical example of imaginary companion.

The literature also contains some figures relating to the incidence and nature of the imaginary companion in boys and girls. In Svendsen's (1934) sample of forty cases with clearly defined imaginary companions, the ratio between girls and boys was three to one. In the fourteen cases that Bender and Vogel (1941) described as a heterogenous and unselected group, there were seven girls and seven boys. Bender and Vogel also quote Jersild et al. (1933) who in their study of 143 children with imaginary companions found that girls gave more definite descriptions of their imaginary companions than boys. Further, the imaginary companions of girls were more frequently of the opposite sex than was the case with boys. However, the majority of both boys and girls had companions of the same sex.

Jersild et al. (1933) found that seventy-nine percent of the 143 children had imaginary companions that were human beings, characters from stories, and, in a few cases, elves and fairies.[3] In twenty-one percent the imaginary companions were anthropomorphized animals, dolls, and other special objects. In a large majority of cases, the imaginary companions went through a variety of metamorphoses and changes in accordance with the child's wishes. Only a few children experienced a strong feeling of a "real presence" in association with the imaginary companion. Burlingham (1945) referred to the fantasy of having a twin, which is occasionally "built up in the latency period as the result of disappointment by the parents in the oedipus situation, in the child's search for a partner who will give him all the attention, love and companionship he desires and who will provide an escape from loneliness and solitude" (p. 205). Although the wish to have a twin usually appears as a conscious daydream (similar to the family romance described by Freud) rather than as an imaginary companion fantasy, we know of a prelatency girl whose imaginary companion was a twin.

We also know that some children have only one imaginary companion, while others have a great number of them simultaneously. Harriman (1937) reports the case of a young woman

3. The theme of an imaginary companion has frequently been used in literature. For a good survey see, for example, Bender and Vogel (1941).

who as a student still had imaginary companions, though they had lost some of their distinctness. At the age of nine she created three imaginary companions, three beautiful girls who in her fantasy lived next door to her own house. These three imaginary girls would visit her in the evening, engage in long conversations, and, among other things, introduce their "friends" to her. According to this student's account, she soon had about twenty-five imaginary companions including a few male ones. She had filled several diaries with a large number of stories about them.

SOME CHARACTERISTICS OF
THE IMAGINARY COMPANION

The imaginary companions of some children play a most active role in the household, tending to interfere a great deal with many of the everyday routines. Some children demand a place at the table or in the car for their imaginary companions and make other elaborate preparations in order to satisfy the "needs" of their companions. All this may greatly interfere with such activities as going out, eating, and sleeping—much to the annoyance of the parents— even if we leave to one side those imaginary companions who are deliberately mischievous and provocative.

One of our cases, Roberta, a girl of two years eleven months, has created her own imaginary family which consisted mostly of TV characters appearing on such programs as *Merlin and Goofy, Donald Duck,* and *Pluto*. They were living in the bathroom cupboard or just under a cot. Once, when the mother had just steered Roberta and the pram across a busy road, Roberta started to howl because "Merlin" had been forgotten on the other side. The mother said that she simply had to go back and get "him."

Katherine, age three, also had many fantasy animals and people who accompanied her even on the street. The mother described to us how after crossing a street they had to wait until Katherine was satisfied that all her imaginary companions had crossed the street as well.

In other cases, the imaginary companions remain unobstrusive and do not much interfere with the daily routines of mother and child. The clinical manifestations of this phenomenon are enormously rich and varied. Naturally, the experienced clinician finds in all the individual details a useful source of information about the inner difficulties, struggles, developmental stresses, and conflicts of the child.

INTELLIGENCE AND IMAGINARY COMPANIONS

Several authors agree that there exists a relationship between the level of intelligence and the production of imaginary companions. It is generally assumed that the better-endowed children produce the most distinct and vivid imaginary companions as well as the most complex and better-elaborated stories around them. Thus, Jersild et al. (1933) found that the children capable of describing well-defined imaginary companions had higher IQs than the others. Svendsen (1934) believes that the phenomenon of the imaginary companion is not limited to highly intelligent children but that it is more prevalent among them. Bender and Vogel's findings on the intelligence level of their group of children would tend to support Svendsen's opinion. Most of the cases we have examined belong in the group of high-average or superior intelligence, but our sample of cases is not a representative cross section of the population.

Harriman (1937) expressed the opinion that "the phenomenon of imaginary companions may well have a genuine relationship" to creative writing (p. 370). We have already referred to one of his cases, the young woman who developed a series of twenty-five imaginary companions. She explained that her elaborate fantasy life was in part motivated by her desire to write novels and her hope to utilize this material for plots later on. According to Harriman, she did in fact keep her records up to date as these imaginary friends progressed through college and became established in life. This case illustrates a shift in the use of this phenomenon: at nine years of age it was used to cope with specific personality problems; later it was in the service of more neutralized aims. One also suspects that, in this case, the earlier phenomenon of the imaginary companions was transferred into what is more properly called a continuous daydream.

AGE OF THE IMAGINARY COMPANION

The imaginary companion usually is of the same age as the child, or slightly younger. In a few instances, they were somewhat older than the child, but we have not come across a single case in which a child's imaginary companion was an adult. On the other hand, the imaginary companions may possess some adult characteristics (strength, power, knowledge, authority, etc.) or be referred to as growing up fast.

PRE-LATENCY IMAGINARY COMPANIONS

Although the significance of the imaginary companion is usually determined by a variety of factors, it seems to play a special role in the development of the child at the age of two and a half to five years. For this reason we have singled out this group from the latency group in which this phenomenon serves different functions.

Selma Fraiberg (1959) described the imaginary companion called "Laughing Tiger," of Jannie, aged two years eight months. He was the last in a long series of imaginary companions. In tracing his origin Fraiberg correctly states that he was "the direct descendant of the savage and ferocious beasts who disturb the sleep of small children" (p. 17). Laughing Tiger had in fact appeared at a time when Jannie had been very frightened by animals who could bite, including some neighborhood dogs. Confronted with the "ferocious" animals (which embodied the projection of her own hostile and cannibalistic fantasies), the little girl chose an active way of dealing with her fears. Aided by her capacity to use imagination and fantasy, she was finally able to master her conflicts and anxiety—at least, it gave her the necessary respite for a sufficient length of time, until her development in other areas allowed for a better control of the impulses and fears that, to start with, she had been unable to manage in any other way. Fraiberg remarks that Jannie could have used a variety of other mechanisms, as children frequently do, in order to deal with the problem. For example, she could have avoided animals in general, she could have avoided leaving her home and the safety of her parents, or going to sleep (i.e., developed a sleep phobia) in order not to meet the feared animals even in her dreams.

By means of fantasy Jannie transformed the ferocious beast into a friendly animal, who showed his teeth not in anger but in laughing. This laughing tiger was afraid of children and he particularly feared his mistress and obeyed her every command. All this naturally allowed Jannie's ego to operate freely, without having to resort to the restrictions imposed by avoidance and phobic symptoms. Fraiberg further states: "Laughing Tiger was a very important factor in the eventual dissolution of Jan's animal fears. When he first made his appearance there was a noticeable improvement in this area. When he finally disappeared (and he was not replaced by any other animal), the fears of animals had largely subsided and it was evident that Jan no longer needed him. If we watch closely, we will see how the imaginary companions and enemies fade away at about the same time that the fear dissolves, which means that the child who has overcome his tigers in his play has learned to master his fear" (p. 19f.).

Anna Freud (1936) described an older child (seven years) who used very similar mechanisms. This boy's imaginary companion, a tame lion, terrified everybody else, but loved and obeyed him. She says:

> From the little boy's analysis it was easy to see that the lion was a substitute for the father, whom he, like Little Hans, hated and feared as a real rival in relation to his mother. In both children aggressiveness was transformed into anxiety and the affect was displaced from the father onto an animal.[4] But their subsequent methods of dealing with their affects differed. Hans used his fears of horses as the basis of his neurosis, i.e., he imposed upon himself the renunciation of

4. Freud (1909) pointed out that this step has great economic value for the whole personality. Little Hans had to see his father constantly, while by displacing his fears onto horses he felt anxiety only when confronted with them; and even this could be escaped by avoiding going out, as he in fact did for some time.

his instinctual desires, internalized the whole conflict, and, in accordance with the mechanism of phobia, avoided situations of temptation. My patient managed things more comfortably for himself. Like Hans in the fantasy about the plumber, he simply denied a painful fact and in his lion fantasy turned it into its pleasurable opposite. He called the anxiety animal his friend, and its strength, instead of being a source of terror, was now at his service. The only indication that in the past the lion had been an anxiety object was the anxiety of the other people, as depicted in the imaginary episodes. [p. 74f].

FUNCTIONS OF THE IMAGINARY COMPANION

1. *As Superego Auxiliaries*

The imaginary companion serves a variety of functions depending upon the special needs of the child who creates it. Not infrequently imaginary companions are used as superego auxiliaries. It is well known that the younger child needs external controls before his superego is fully established; therefore, many young children use the imaginary companion as an intermediate step between the external controls (in the form of the parents) and their own fully developed superego structure. Such children "consult" their imaginary companions, who in turn instruct them to control their behavior in general or certain impulses in particular. Katherine, one of our patients, consulted Susan (the imaginary companion) about whatever she planned to do.

Hammerman (1965) described this phenomenon clearly in his paper on "Conceptions of Superego Development":

Obedience and self-control, however, are not yet the same as self-criticism derived from moral judgment, which is the hallmark of a discrete intrapsychic structure. It seems reasonable that initially the developing superego organization works only under the actual supervision of external objects. *In the well-known imaginary companions of children, we note the projection of prestages of the superego. Even though imaginary, the need for an actual external object is still great.* [p. 327; italics mine]

He also referred to the regressed agoraphobics who frequently need the companion as an external, actual authority.

The use of the imaginary companion as a superego prop or auxiliary is by no means limited to the younger child. Many older children with reasonably well established superegos use such companions in their attempts to cope with particular impulses that seem to escape control because of special situations of frustration, stress or conflicts. Thus Bender and Vogel (1941) describe a ten-and-a-half-year-old boy who had a history of rejection and neglect by his parents. His imaginary companion would ask him why he had been bad all the time and simultaneously threaten him by saying that if he continued to be bad, his parents would never come again.

The differences between younger and older children's uses of this mechanism deserve attention. In both cases the imaginary companion fulfills the purpose of controlling their behavior, but in the young child the imaginary companion is at times an integral part of the developmental steps taken in the direction of internalization and introjection of external commands, and thus contributes to the building up the superego structure. In the older child the imaginary companion acts as a necessary (though temporary) "prop" or "superego auxiliary" to assist an already established superego. In the first case, the phenomenon of the imaginary companion highlights the role of *fantasying* as well as that of the resultant fantasies in furthering the development of both ego and superego structures. This particular role of fantasying, to my knowledge, has not yet received sufficient attention.

2. For Impulse Discharge

Some children use the imaginary companion for purposes that can be considered the opposite of those described above. In their case, the imaginary companion is a vehicle for the discharge of impulses that are no longer acceptable to the child either because he has internalized the parental prohibitions or because he fears the parental attitude to such impulses (before internalization has taken place). By this means the child justifies his "naughty" behavior to himself or the parents, or at least tries to do so when he is accused, for example, of his dirty, messy, destructive behavior. He may excuse himself by saying that "Sam" or "Peter" (the imaginary companions) ordered him to do so. It was not his fault, naturally. This type of response is more frequent in the younger child, but even older children will occasionally try to justify some of their actions in this way.

The following case of Maritza is another example illustrating not only the use of the imaginary companion for drive discharge but also its origin and the sequence that led to its establishment.

Maritza was the youngest child in her family. She had two brothers, Paul, six years older, and Peter, eight years older than she. When she was just over two years old, her brothers taught her to say some dirty words, among them "pupu" (feces). At their suggestion she would repeat this word with a great deal of pleasure. Shortly thereafter Maritza began to tell stories about "Pupu," an imaginary boyfriend with whom she enjoyed doing forbidden things and who could do all the naughty things she did not dare do. Pupu frequently made his appearance at moments of frustration in Maritza's life. For example, on one occasion when her brothers were to go away for the weekend while she had to stay home, she said: "I am going with Pupu to a cottage where there is no lawn mower" (on a previous occasion she had stayed with her family in a cottage and had been frightened by the noise of the lawn mower). From the time Maritza was two and a half years old, Pupu was an active member of the family. The mother felt that Pupu was in many ways a personification of Paul with whom Maritza had an ambivalent relationship. They played a great deal together, tending to tease each other. Maritza admired this older brother and was very jealous and envious of him. On one occasion Paul's shoes had been left in the middle of the room and the brother was about to pick them up when Maritza objected: "No, they have to stay there; Pupu wears those shoes."

On another occasion Maritza was building a village with her wooden blocks. Suddenly she turned to her mother, indignant and crying, "Now Pupu destroyed my village" (the structure she had been building had collapsed). The mother answered: "Well, if he disrupts your buildings, he has to go to his own mother so that you can play in peace." Thereupon Maritza opened the door, pretended to pick up Pupu, and threw him outside. That day she did not refer to the imaginary companion again, but on the following day he was back.

During the next few months Pupu's identity began to change. "Pupu has a new suit," she said, just after her father had bought a new suit. Thus, Pupu represented aspects of her father. She now demanded that Pupu sleep by her bedside, and every evening a cupboard had to be moved close to her bed because "That is Pupu's bed."

Some time later her brother Paul had to go to the hospital for treatment—an event that reactivated in Maritza an early hospitalization experience when her mother had not been able to stay with her. The mother sympathized with Maritza's renewed anxiety and explained that Paul would not have to stay in the hospital. It was very unfortunate, the mother added, that Maritza had had to go to the hospital and that she had not been able to accompany her. Maritza answered immediately: "Pupu's mother did stay with him."

More recently Maritza became ill on a day when she expected to visit her grandfather. She asked her mother to let Pupu know that she could not go. The mother promised to do so, but Maritza insisted, "But he is standing outdoors, you have to tell him now, you see he is waiting for me." Maritza was content only when the mother opened the door and delivered Maritza's message to Pupu.

It should be noted that to start with Maritza uttered the anal word with great delight. Shortly afterward, when she was told this was not nice, the word Pupu was used to refer to her newly created companion who could do all the naughty things she did not dare do any longer, thus allowing her some vicarious gratification of forbidden impulses. Still later Pupu acquired additional roles that in part represented wishes she had in relation to her brother and father.

3. *As a Tool Toward Mastery*

The case of Jimmy is included here by way of contrast. It illustrates how a very gifted child used a different type of fantasy activity to master a variety of situations in which other children might have created an imaginary companion.

Jimmy was an extremely gifted four-year-old child. He had great verbal facility: at the age of eighteen months he already was in command of sixty words, and at two years he was quite capable of carrying on a real conversation.

Jimmy had shown no interest in teddy bears or dolls until his second birthday, when his mother was about six months pregnant. When his first baby sister Julia was born, he became very attached to such toys and always wanted one as a companion. He showed no particular preference for anyone of his many dollies, tigers, and teddies. All he wanted was to keep one of them with him for most of the day.

At bedtime Jimmy would say, "Teddy go sleep." He may in fact have placed several dollies and teddies in his cot, but he usually threw all of them out when he wanted to go to sleep. He was intensely jealous of his sister and frequently tried to interfere when his mother was nursing Julia. He had learned from experience that noises made Julia break off feeding and sometimes cry. Armed with this knowledge, he would come bouncing into the room where his mother was trying to feed the baby, shouting, "Let's make a noise, Teddy," while he and teddy proceeded to bounce up and down the bed, pretending to be "lions." It should be noted that he always use one of his real teddies or dollies for this purpose and never resorted to an imaginary companion.

Some time later Jimmy was trying to sort out whom he could marry. He also wondered whether his grandfather (a widower) could marry a student lodger living in their house. He finally produced his two dollies and asked that one be dressed as a boy and the other as a girl. He had them married and demanded that they make some dolly babies. When he was three he met Jennie, a three-and-a-half-year-old girl. He saw her altogether on three or four occasions and they got on very well together. At first he asked, for example, where Jennie was when she was not in the block of flats where he lived (she came there only to visit her grandparents). Where did she live? Could he go there? He wanted to see her very badly. Finally, he stated that he was Jennie. This represented an identification with the lost object, a mechanism that he frequently used in dealing with losses.

A similar situation developed with another little girl, Katie, whom he saw only very rarely. For months, two or three times a day he demanded to be told a story that had to include Jennie and Katie. During this period he often said that he and his sister were Jennie and Katie, "two sisters living with their parents."

Still later a cousin, about the same age as Jimmy, visited for a few days. After Alexander's departure Jimmy was for two days several times close to tears. By the third day he brightened up after he told his mother that he now was Alexander and should be called by that name.

Jimmy had always liked books, and at about two and a half began to be interested in the contents of the stories rather than the pictures illustrating them. He enjoyed acting the stories over and over again. He became

Tom the Kitten and assigned different roles and names to his mother, father, sister, and various visitors. He became extremely annoyed if he was not always addressed as Tom the Kitten or by the name of the character he was impersonating at the moment. Similarly, the father, mother, sister, etc., had to be addressed by their role names. In turn, he became Percy (the small engine), James (the red engine), and a variety of other characters.

Jimmy's attempt to master through play and fantasy those situations that he found difficult to handle could also be seen in his personification of Pepito, Pepito was "a bad hat" because he did not know how to make friends with girls and went about it in all the wrong ways. At this time Jimmy was most anxious to relate to other children, but found it nearly impossible to do so. Jimmy then asked his mother to invite some girls so that he could learn how to make friends with them. He frequently pretended to have friends around to play. When his mother mentioned in the morning that she had invited two children to come to tea, he would immediately pretend, "The doorbell is ringing! Come and see who it is. Come on in! Mother, we are having a tea party for all our friends." He would then bounce around the room, playing games with these "friends." Yet, as soon as the real ones came, he began to scream because they touched his toys or even because their mothers started to talk to his mother. Yet, after practicing this fantasy game for some time, he did overcome his difficulties in relating to other children.

4. For Externalization and as Scapegoats

Imaginary companions are very frequently used as scapegoats, the recipients of all the badness and negative impulses of the child. This mechanism of externalization is seen more frequently in the young child than in older ones. To externalize, five- to six-year-old children generally select a "real" child or an ad hoc imaginary one, but usually not an *imaginary companion*. In the young child, the imaginary companion seems to represent a prestage or precursor of externalizing onto a real object. This process is probably favored by the very young child's belief in magic, omnipotence, and his animistic conception of the world.

Selma Fraiberg (1959) described this use of the imaginary companion very vividly. She says that the child "acquires a number of companions, imaginary ones, who personify his Vices like characters in a morality play. (The Virtues he keeps to himself. Charity, Good Works, Truth, Altruism, all dwell in harmony within him.) Hate, Selfishness, Uncleanliness, Envy and a host of other evils are cast out like devils and forced to obtain other hosts. . . . When Daddy's pipes are broken, no one is more indignant than the two-year-old son who is under suspicion. 'Gerald, did you break daddy's pipes?' he demands to know" (p. 141).

As Fraiberg points out, although the child knows that Gerald is an invention of his, he achieves a number of gains in this way. First, he tries to avoid criticism from the parents for his misdeeds and unacceptable impulses. Second, he can maintain his self-love. Third, though he cannot yet control his impulses, he addresses the imaginary companion as a naughty boy is addressed by his parents. He shows in this roundabout way the emergence of a self-critical attitude, which eventually will enable him to control his impulses.

One can hardly avoid the impression that in such cases the imaginary companion acts as a "developmental buffer," that is, as something that mitigates for the child's primitive ego what is at times an impossible situation. The young child acts on impulses whose strength can override his primitive and precariously defended ego at a time when he is already aware of the parental displeasure occasioned by some of his actions. Thus, by means of the imaginary companion, he strikes a compromise that makes the situation more tolerable for his helpless ego and temporarily restores some balance. Perhaps we will be less inclined to underestimate the value of the imaginary companion if we take into account that many of the controls that we demand of the very young child are often beyond his limited capacities. In this respect we can again observe definite similarities with the role played by fantasying and fantasies in later life. Both are used in the attempt to solve conflicts and to restore at least a transitory inner equilibrium, before excessive stress forces a path into symptom formation, regression, or other disturbances.

5. *To Prolong Feelings of Omnipotence and Control*

Other examples suggest that a few children use the imaginary companion as part of an attempt to prolong their own feelings of omnipotence and control. For a few, the imaginary companion is a necessary, intermediate step before they can transfer, at least in certain areas, control to their parents while simultaneously accepting limitations to their own previously omnipotent feelings (which now have to be ascribed to the parents). This move from the child's belief in his own omnipotence to a belief in the parent's omnipotence is, as we know, a slow, gradual, and difficult process, the intimate nature of which still escapes us. I suspect that in this achievement fantasying and the world of fantasies play a more significant role than is generally ascribed to them.

6. *Impersonation of Ego Ideals*

Not infrequently the imaginary companion is an impersonation of the child's primitive ego ideals, ideals that may be beyond his reach. The companion is good, clever, strong, clean, unaggressive, lovable, etc. This function of the imaginary companion can occasionally be observed in children who for a variety of reasons feel rejected. By endowing the companion with all the attributes the child lacks, he can vicariously participate in the companion's loving relationship with parents. Occasionally too, the imaginary companion is used as a weapon for defiance and provocation, as a vehicle of the negative aspects of the young child's ambivalence, etc.

7. *To Deal with Loneliness, Neglect and Rejection*

Feelings of loneliness, neglect, and rejection frequently motivate the child to create imaginary companions. In his sample of forty children, Svendsen (1934) found that 55 percent of the children were "only" children at the time they created the companion. Many of the examples given by Bender and Vogel (1941) show a clear relationship between the imaginary companion and loneliness, neglect or rejection. Thus, ten-and-a-half-year-old Charles said: "They [the imaginary companions in the form of a brother and sister] come when I am very lonely, not when I am playing with the boys. . . . They are a great comfort to me when I am all alone" (p. 59).

Several of our own examples also illustrate this point. The obvious importance of loneliness for the creation of imaginary companions may have induced several authors to note the frequency with which they disappear when the child finds suitable real companions. Green (1922) found that this fantasy usually vanishes when the child goes to school. He explained the imaginary companion phenomenon as part of an unsatisfied instinct of gregariousness that is fulfilled by the friendships established at school. Nevertheless, as we have seen, the imaginary companion owes its existence to a great variety of factors; therefore, it can be expected to disappear at entry into school only in those cases where it arose as the result of "loneliness" and for no other reason. Furthermore, the imaginary companion can frequently be observed in children who are by no means lonely, as I hope to show below.

8. *To Deal with the Birth of a Sibling*

In several of our cases the child developed imaginary companions immediately after the birth of a sibling. Tony, ten years old, was referred to the Hampstead Clinic because his teacher complained that he was "terribly dreamy and not with it." As a result his schoolwork was not up to standard. At that time he was suffering from sleep difficulties. The history of Tony's imaginary companion was as follows:

Tony was about three years old when his first sibling, a boy, was born. He was totally unprepared for this event. When Tony saw the baby for the first time, he looked away and from then on continued to ignore the baby. Immediately after the brother's birth Tony pretended to have an imaginary friend by the name of "Dackie," with whom he played and talked for hours at a time. Dackie was around most of the day, getting up in the morning with Tony and going to bed when Tony did. Dackie remained with Tony until he was five years old. Yet, at the age of ten, Tony still remembered Dackie, and when he was reminded of his imaginary companion, he laughed in a shy way.

Caroline was about three years eight months, when her brother Barry was born. Shortly thereafter Caroline invented an imaginary playmate called "Dooley." At first the mother paid little attention to this, but she became increasingly concerned when this playmate took up more and more of Caroline's time and thought. The mother felt that this preoccupation was "beyond the realm of make-believe." Caroline attributed many of her actions to Dooley's suggestions and during the day would spend hours talking to "her." Dooley also was a girl, a fact in which the mother recognized a compensatory factor, for Caroline had wanted a sister, not a brother.

Dooley would tell Caroline "to eat dinner with a spoon and fork because it is quicker." In the beginning Dooley was a little girl, presumably like Caroline, but later Caroline said that Dooley was growing up "like her mother."

Later on, Caroline had other imaginary companions such as "Feeler," who was a big girl, and "Jane" whose characteristics were not known to us. These three, Dooley, Feeler, and Jane, were permanent members of the household, while several additional characters visited each day.

When Caroline was tested at the Clinic, she told the psychologist that "Dooley does not want to do any more." Furthermore, she asked the psychologist what *her* Dooley's name was, taking it for granted that the psychologist also had an imaginary companion.

Graham was about two years eleven months when his brother Peter was born. Shortly afterward, within a period of two months, Graham created an imaginary companion who was also called Peter. Graham, who had expected a playmate, was very disappointed by the size of the baby. He had resented his mother's absence during the delivery, and had clearly shown his dislike of the newcomer by telling his mother: "Put it back in your tummy." When Peter was born, Graham was given a doll called Becky. Becky soon was involved in the accounts Graham gave of his doings with his imaginary playmate "Peter." They were shortly joined by another imaginary companion, a "baby Peter," and thereafter Graham spoke of "my two boys" as he had heard his mother do. He included his companions in all preparations that were made for outings and in all plans for spending the day at home. While Graham openly talked about his companions with members of the family, he did not refer to them in the presence of other people.

On the basis of such examples it is tempting to assume that some

sensitive children find the mother's limited withdrawal of attention following the birth of another child more than they can bear
and that they react to it by creating a more faithful and reliable
figure in the form of the imaginary companion. These children
may well feel lonely because after the arrival of the newcomer the
previously undivided attention of the mother must be shared.

Where the memory of an imaginary companion is revived in the
analysis of an adult patient, it is instructive to see it in all its
complexities, fulfilling more than one need experienced by the
child. For example, in the following material we can see that it
simultaneously serves the purpose of correcting painful reality,
denying and relieving loneliness, and assuaging guilt.

The patient, a man in his fifties, was the fifth of seven children. He had
one older sister, three older brothers, and two younger ones. In the fourth
year of his psychoanalytic treatment he became much concerned with the
fact that, whenever he thought he had found a friend, it did not take long
for him to experience a deep disappointment, as the friend about whom
he had been so happy at first turned against him. The relationship soon
deteriorated, he was enraged about being "let down," no longer wanted,
and he found himself as friendless as before.

At this point he mentioned that as a child he had had a fantasy brother.
He had been smaller and younger than himself, and totally blind. He
thought that he had kept this fantasy going for about two years, between
the ages of eight and ten. Work on this imaginary brother brought to
light the following main aspects. The patient had been severely disturbed
about the arrival of a brother when he was eighteen months old. This
experience had been revived and more clearly remembered again two
years later when another baby brother was born.

The mother had given each of the seven children all her attention and
love as long as they were small. She adored babies and would never hand
over their care to anyone else; but as soon as the next child came this
happy state was suddenly brought to an end and she turned all her
interest and care to the newcomer. It seems that by the time the sixth and
seventh child arrived she no longer felt able to give the older ones enough
interest until much later when she had stopped having babies.

After a phase of great unhappiness and jealousy, in his second to
fourth years, the patient developed a reaction formation against his
jealousy of the younger brothers: he became a fatherly older brother,

trying to make them into his friends, hoping that they would follow him, love him, and be with him constantly. This seems to have been a very successful and happy time at first, when the younger brothers were delighted about his attention and willing to conform to his wishes. However, as they grew up, they refused to be ordered around as before. They freed themselves from their dependence on him and turned against him aggressively. He suffered intensely from "losing" them and tried more and more aggressively to regain control over them.

It is during these years that his "blind rages" occurred. Among his memories there was one in which he violently punched one of his brothers and was accused by the nurse of "nearly blinding him." It appears that the development of the fantasy about having an imaginary blind brother began soon thereafter. Its main features were:

The brother is younger, like his own brothers, but his blindness makes him totally dependent on him; he cannot go anywhere without him and never wants to leave him. Being with his older brother, walking with him, feeling his arm over his shoulders, or sitting close to him, is the happiest experience for the blind brother. There is no one else he wishes to be with, nor anyone else who understands him as well. As they walk together they arouse everyone's attention. At first people say, "Look at the blind boy," but immediately afterward they say: "How fortunate he is to have this wonderful big brother, what an unusual child he is to be so good and helpful to his blind brother!" This part of the fantasy gave the patient the greatest satisfaction each time he thought of it, as it contained both the gratification of his exhibitionistic wishes—everyone looked— and the relief about his guilt for his destructive wishes, when he was praised for his kindness toward the younger brother.

A large part was played by the imaginary brother's constant presence, as the patient had felt extremely lonely among the crowd of children in the house. He had felt so hostile against them that he could hardly bear their company at times. To be alone had been especially threatening during and after the phase when he experienced the turning away of the younger brothers.

The "blind brother" also stood for the incapacitated aspect of himself. The defensive function of this fantasy became clear when the patient accepted his own regressive longing for dependence and saw that the wish to be wanted as a "blind child" by his father had been an important factor in retreating from his dangerous hostility against him.

In the role of the blind brother he also felt relief from his guilt about the fantasies of blinding the favorite brother whose "loss" had caused him intense pain.

9. *To Deal with Changes Generally*

The next example shows some aspects of the coping mechanisms that a little girl evolved as a reaction to a sudden change in her living conditions that also involved losses. She engaged in a continuous daydream involving the participation of a variety of subjects (animals and people), many of which acquired the status of imaginary companions.

Zeeta was one of the children at the Hampstead War Nurseries,[5] where she had been for eighteen months, from the age of seventeen months to three years. She was a colored baby girl whose cultural background was especially good. Zeeta was described as a delicate and gifted child whose emotional and intellectual development showed some unusually interesting features.

At the end of World War II Zeeta left the Nursery and went to live with her mother and a new father, a man she had met many times before. The first few weeks at home were difficult. Zeeta missed her nurse intensely and found it difficult to make friends with her new daddy. It was then that she began to play elaborate fantasy games. The mother reported that at three years, two months, Zeeta developed a new animal fantasy. "She has a brood of imaginary animals, cats and chickens which live with her and share all her activities. It is quite uncanny the way she looks at them, just as though she could really see them. Often she tells me off for clumsily kicking one of them or I have to lift them up over the pavement and am told that 'they are too small, they can't manage.'" In her report Dr. Hellman wondered whether this child had replaced the group life at the Hampstead Nursery by the imaginary chickens and cats that accompanied her everywhere and, for example, made her walks very similar to those she had taken with the other toddlers whom she had had to leave at the Nursery.

In the ensuing weeks Zeeta's fantasies developed further, as the mother reported: "The cats have gradually disappeared, but the chickens have remained and a husband and father have been added. The husband's name is Percy and the father's Ninny. They seem to be very feeble characters; she only allows them to call at the back door and, when asked about their occupation, she says: 'They do washing up at the office where

5. The account here given of this case is a condensed version of the Fifth Half-Yearly Report (1949) of the Hampstead Nurseries (After Care) written by Dr. I. Hellman.

my Daddy works.' Sometimes they bring rings and brooches to her, but they usually take them away again. On the whole she treats them more like a burden or even a liability, whereas the birds and cats she liked to care for and was most loving with."

Until her fourth year Zeeta was surrounded by an ever-changing population of small animals and tiny babies. They needed a great deal of care and comfort and accompanied her everywhere. By that time she had overcome her initial difficulties with her new father and was on extremely good terms with him. The mother said: "She absolutely idolizes her Daddy; it amuses me to see how her former hostility has changed." Zeeta then had a husband, George, who stayed with her for many months. During the second half of the fourth year the mother wrote: "You will be interested to hear that we now have a pony living with us. It has red ears, a red nose, and red legs, and sleeps in the corner standing on two legs. Of course, he accompanies us everywhere, buses included, but I can generally persuade him to go into my shopping bag when the bus is too full."

Anna Freud and Dorothy Burlingham concluded the report on Zeeta by stating: "Life in a community, which to many young infants is merely a burden, evidently stimulated Zeeta's fantasy life to an unusual degree. . . . As Dr. Hellman remarked, these daydreams seemed to reflect her early attitude to her small companions; they reveal at the same time that this attitude was a motherly one. In comforting the other infants, in helping them and in looking after their needs, Zeeta seems to have given the others the intimate care and protection which she missed owing to the absence of her own mother."

10. *To Avoid Regression and Symptom-Formation*

The following example is particularly instructive in that it shows how a child at a time of serious stress in her life managed to create an imaginary companion who helped her avoid regression and symptom formation. This was in sharp contrast to the reaction of her two older siblings who responded to the same traumatic situation with regression and symptom formation. In this case the imaginary companion fulfilled the same role as that ascribed by Freud (1908) to many daydreams: they are temporary measures compensating for a frustrating or difficult external reality and prevent the development of a full-blown neurosis. That this child's imaginary companion fulfilled the same function is not as surprising as it may seem if we consider that this phenomenon is a special type of fantasy with specific characteristics that distinguish it from other daydreams. In her case, the imaginary companion served a variety of functions such as superego auxiliary, scapegoat, for externalization, etc.

Miriam was the youngest of three children; her sister Laura was eight years old; her brother, nine and a half years old. The parents were a highly intelligent, young, professional couple.

The imaginary companion, Susan, appeared when Miriam was five years old, shortly after her parents divorced each other and the mother suffered a mental breakdown that required several months of hospitalization. The children were sent to their grandparents. At first they lived in the grandparents' cottage, but they were soon moved to a caravan (with an au pair) just outside the grandparents' cottage. The situation was further aggravated by the fact that at that time in her life Miriam was extremely attached to her father. The latter left soon afterward for America, where he has since remarried. The two older children reacted to the events described with different overt symptoms such as school difficulties, sleeping disturbances, and regression (bedwetting), while Miriam developed no such symptoms but created Susan, her imaginary companion, who stayed with her for almost nine months.

Miriam had been very close to Laura, but with the advent of Susan she withdrew markedly from her sister, much to the latter's distress. Laura would beg Miriam to play with her. Miriam, engaged in lengthy conversations with Susan, would reply: "Leave us alone." In contrast to Laura, the elder brother took no notice of the imaginary companion.

Miriam was described as a competent, well-organized, active, and friendly child. Nevertheless, during the difficult period at home she had to attend a new school where she was unable to make friends. Further, according to the reports, she was very reality-oriented and had a clear knowledge of what is reality and what is fantasy, but she always tended to deal with difficult experiences by temporary withdrawal into intense play with her dolls. She usually emerged from this preoccupation after some time reentered her active life at school. She repeated this behavior after a recent visit with her father in the States, which had been more disturbing to her two older siblings than to her.

Miriam had always been devoted to the maternal grandmother. She used to ask her mother to be allowed to stay "at the hotel with Gran," taking her doll and Susan with her. The grandmother entered into the fantasy of the imaginary playmate and consequently heard a good deal about Susan. For instance, when asked whether she had slept well, Miriam would reply in the affirmative, adding: "Susan slept well too. In the night she was cold and I put an extra blanket on her bed." At meals she might say, "We have to think about Susan [who might be hungry]. . . . Ah, well, never mind. I will make her some dinner later." She and Susan would go off to play together in the woods for the afternoon. At other times she talked for hours with Susan. Miriam made it clear that Susan had no family and belonged exclusively to her.

It was obvious that Miriam mothered Susan, thus restoring in fantasy, at least to some degree, her earlier relationship to her now withdrawn, depressed, and absent mother (who was hospitalized). That Susan was created to cope with the puzzling events and the sudden absence of the mother was further confirmed by the many conversations in which Miriam asked her imaginary playmate what had happened to her mother. She was heard saying, "What happened to Mummy?" and "Mummy wants us to do ——— ." We do not know what factors in Miriam's personality determined her choice of this specific fantasy as a way of coping with the stress situation; nor do we know why, in her case, this was a sufficient and apparently very successful device.

The imaginary companion also embodied some superego aspects and in this sense occasionally took the mother's place. Miriam would frequently say: "I have to consult Susan about doing [whatever it may have been that was on her mind] or "Susan would like me to ——— ."

By means of the mechanism of externalization.[6] Susan also became an outlet for feelings that Miriam could not have expressed otherwise. For example, she said: "I think Susan is very unhappy these days" or "Susan has no family, poor Susan." At other times Miriam stated: "Susan is terribly angry, she hates her teacher. She even hates me. Of course, I am angry with her too, but we will make it up later." I mentioned earlier that Miriam found the change of school when her parents separated especially difficult. At that time she said: "I hear Susan. She doesn't want to go to school," thus expressing her own difficulties by attributing them to Susan. In fact, with the exception of this brief period, Miriam enjoyed and loved school.

Miriam's imaginary companion faded away when she acquired a very close friend at school. Now, nearly four years later, Miriam says of her imaginary companion, "I invented her . . . of course, she was real."

---

6. Sperling (1954) pointed out that the "child finds it easier to project his own fears and hopes onto the imaginary companion and to communicate them in this form instead of confessing that they are his own fears and wishes" (p. 252).

IMAGINARY COMPANIONS AND TRANSITIONAL OBJECTS

The following example shows clearly the simultaneous presence of an imaginary companion and a transitional object.

Mary, a young adult, had no conscious recollection of her imaginary companion. Her knowledge of it came from stories her mother had told her at different times. In contrast, she had clear memories of a rag doll named Whoopee, her transitional object.

The imaginary companion (whose name was forgotten) appeared when Mary was two to three years old. At that time the family consisted of the father, the mother, and three children, Mary, Paula (age ten), and Eva (age eleven). Mary was actually an only child; the two older girls in the family were close relatives of the parents who adopted these two children when they became orphans. When Mary was born, Paula was already a member of the household. Eva joined the family two and a half years later—at about the time when Mary created her imaginary companion. Unfortunately, the exact sequence of events could not be ascertained.

Due to the gap in the ages between Mary and the two older girls, on the one hand, and the closeness in ages of Paula and Eva, on the other, the latter naturally tended to play together and to exclude Mary. As an adult, Mary distinctly remembered playing by herself while Paula and Eva played together.

When the imaginary companion made its appearance Mary's mother was under severe strain and perhaps somewhat depressed following a quick succession of several serious accidents, illnesses, and various deaths in her immediate family. Mary probably felt very lonely at this point because the mother's attention was concentrated on nursing relatives.

The mother remembered that the imaginary companion had been a little girl with whom Mary played in the garden and the house. The imaginary playmate had to have a place at the table and be given meals; however, Mary did not take her along on outings. The mother was not worried about the imaginary playmate and gladly provided food, etc. The imaginary companion began to disappear about a year or so later when Mary acquired two real companions. One was a girl of her own age, and the other a boy about a year older; both lived near her.

What is of special interest in this case is that throughout the period in which the imaginary companion fantasy was active Mary also had a transitional object, the rag doll called "Whoopee" which she had been given when she was a baby and which she remembered very well. Whoopee had acquired her name by virtue of the way in which she had been mistreated. While throwing her up in the air, Mary would yell: "Whoopee." She kept Whoopee until she was six or seven years of age, in contrast to her imaginary companion whom she kept for only one year. It should be noted that the transitional object was important before, during, and after the phase of the imaginary companion.

This example, as others, shows that an imaginary companion appears in situations of special stress or of a traumatic character. Murphy (1962) described the stress situation during which Sam, three years, three months old, created his imaginary companion "Woody."

Sam had had an unfortunate accident in the bathroom. The tip of his finger had come off when the door was shut on it. The day the stitches had to be removed the doctor proceeded forcibly to take the screaming child away from the mother. Murphy says:

As an outgrowth of this separation situation a little elf named "Woody" appeared in Sam's fantasy. On August 22 Sam told me about him—that Woody was with him in the treatment room because I couldn't be there. In the next three weeks Woody turned up in many different situations and served many different purposes— sometimes a companion, sometimes a helper, sometimes a scapegoat:

Playing doctor, Sam said to me, "You take your medicine and you won't have to have penicillin." "You'll have to stay in the hospital all day and all night." When I asked him how I could manage to do that he told me there was a little elf, "Woody," who would stay with me, just like it was at Dr. H's office—Woody was there with him because I couldn't be with him.

At Dr. H's office he cried hard when leaving me and while soaking his finger—this was one of the times when he had gone to sleep on the bus on the way to the office. Before putting a bandage back on today, Dr. H held up Sam's two little fingers next to each other to compare the length. Later Sam asked about this, "Why did Dr. H *measure* my finger?" "Why is it pink at the tip?"

I asked him why he had made a fuss at the doctor's office, and he said "Because Woody wasn't there—he was on vacation."

Later, when we were making brownies he said, "Woody used to make brownies when he was a little boy—he told me that up at Dr. H's office."

The creation of such a satisfying externalized image to stay with him at the time his mother was forced to leave suggests both the importance of the strong support from mother, and the strength in his own struggle to maintain the feeling of support during her absence. Later he said to his mother one day, "You know Mommy, Woody was really you." [p. 124f]

Some time later when he was introduced to nursery school, he showed considerable hesitation and uncertainty and was overwhelmed by the large group of children. Murphy described how "Once in a while his imaginary elf-friend, 'Woody,' showed up; on October 3, 'Woody was at school today—nurse said he didn't have to open his mouth—he's still a little shy,' but he didn't seem to be needed much of the time" (p. 64). "He used his mother as an anchor to familiarity, for help, as a playmate, and as a love-object during the early period of getting acquainted in the new situation. His imaginary companion 'Woody,' an elf, also helped him" (p. 66).

FANTASIES, DAYDREAMS, AND IMAGINARY COMPANIONS

I have earlier stated that the imaginary companion phenomenon is a special type of fantasy (and fantasying) that has all the characteristics of daydreams. Like ordinary daydreams, the imaginary companion fantasy is an attempt at wish fulfillment of one sort or another, is ruled by the pleasure principle, can ignore the reality principle, and need not be reality adapted, yet the fantasying person remains fully aware of the unreality of the fantasies that are being indulged in. In other words, reality testing remains unimpaired.

Nevertheless, there are a few significant features that are typical of the imaginary companion phenomenon and which are not necessarily characteristic of other forms of fantasy. First, although the imaginary companion is an attempt at wish fulfillment, the type and quality of the wishes involved, especially in the case of the younger child, are different from those that give rise to fantasies in older children. In the latter the wishes are concerned with the gratification of instinctual impulses or specific component instincts that have become conflictual. In many young children, the imaginary companion fills the emptiness, neglect, loneliness, or rejection which the child seems to be experiencing. In this there is nothing conflictual in the neurotic sense. The child is claiming what is after all a genuine right of his—attention, love, and companionship. For this reason he probably can talk quite freely about the imaginary companion, a fact that is in sharp contrast with the reluctance of older children to communicate their fantasies, which are so jealously guarded precisely because they involve impulses that are conflictual (in the neurotic sense) and objectionable. Consequently, they must be kept as secrets. This difference in attitude is one of the most significant differences between the imaginary companion fantasy and other fantasies. While other fantasies can be vivid and intense, that of the imaginary companion has a special quality in this respect. This can perhaps be better understood if we take into account the younger child's animistic conception of the world and his strong belief in magic and in the omnipotence of thoughts. This does not imply that even the young child is not aware of the unreality of the companion; rather I wish to emphasize that in spite of this awareness and coexisting with it, these fantasies have a special quality of vividness and reality for him.

A related factor is the frequency with which the imaginary companion seems to occupy a physical space in the actual world of the child, while other fantasies involving objects are better and quite clearly contained within the realm of imagination and do not require a quasi-physical presence.

We should also note that an intense fantasy life frequently implies a withdrawal from the unpleasant real world into a more satisfactory inner world. This use of fantasying usually also involves a certain withdrawal from the world of real objects. In the imaginary companion fantasy, however, the intial withdrawal from the real world of objects is quickly followed by a return to reality and to the object world. Having found a new solution, the child brings his imaginary companion back into his real life and tries to have it integrated with and accepted by his object world.

I shall end by quoting from Selma Fraiberg (1959):

> There is great misunderstanding today about the place of fantasy in the small child's life. Imaginary companions have fallen into ill repute among many educators and parents. Jan's "Laughing Tiger" would be hastily exiled in many households. The notion has got around that imaginary companions are evidence of "insecurity," "withdrawal" and a latent neurosis. The imaginary companion is supposed to be a poor substitute for real companions and it is felt that the unfortunate child who possesses them should be strongly encouraged to abandon them in favor of real friends. Now, of course, if a child of any age abandons the real world and cannot form human ties, if a child is unable to establish meaningful relationships with persons and prefers his imaginary people, we have some cause for concern. But we must not confuse the neurotic uses of imagination with the healthy, and the child who employs his imagination and the people of his imagination to solve his problems is a child who is working for his own mental health. He can maintain his human ties and his good contact with reality while he maintains his imaginary world. Moreover, it can be demonstrated that the child's contact with the real world is *strengthened* by his periodic excursions into fantasy. It becomes easier to tolerate the frustrations of the real world and to accede to the demands of reality if one can restore himself at intervals in a world where the deepest wishes can achieve imaginary gratification. [p. 22f.]

References

Bender, L., and Vogel, F. (1941). Imaginary companions of children. *American Journal of Orthopsychiatry* 11:56-65.

Burlingham, D. (1945). The fantasy of having a twin. *Psychoanalytic Study of the Child* 1:205-210.

Fraiberg, S. (1959). *The Magic Years.* New York: Scribners.

Freud, A. (1936). *The Ego and the Mechanisms of Defense.* rev. ed. New York: International Universities Press, 1966.

Freud, S. (1908). Creative writers and day-dreaming. *Standard Edition* 9:141-156.

——— (1909). Analysis of a phobia in a five-year-old boy. *Standard Edition* 10:3-152.

——— (1910). Five lectures on psycho-analysis. *Standard Edition* 11:3-158.

Green, G. H. (1922). *Psychoanalysis in the Classroom.* New York: Putnam's.

Hall, G. S. (1907). *Aspects of Child Life and Education.* Boston: Green.

Hammerman, S. (1965). Conceptions of superego development. *Journal of the American Psychoanalytic Association* 13:320-355.

Harriman, P. L. (1937). Some imaginary companions of older subjects. *American Journal of Orthopsychiatry* 7:368-370.

Harrison, S. I., Hess, J. H., and Zrull, J. P. (1963). Paranoid reactions in children. *Journal of the American Academy of Child Psychiatry* 2:677-692.

Harvey, N. A. (1918). *Imaginary Playmates and Other Mental Phenomena of Children.* Ypsilanti, Mich.: Michigan State Normal College.

Hurlock, E. B., and Burstein, W. (1932). The imaginary playmate. *Journal of Genetic Psychology* 41:380-392.

Jersild, A. T., Markey, F. V., and Jersild, C. L. (1933). Children's fears, dreams, wishes. *Child Development Monograph 12.* New York: Teachers College, Columbia University.

Kirkpatrick, E. A. (1929). *Fundamentals of Child Study.* New York: Macmillan.

Murphy, L. B., et al. (1962). *The Widening World of Children.* New York: Basic Books.

Nagera, H. (1966). *Early Childhood Disturbances, the Infantile Neurosis, and the Adulthood Disturbances.* New York: International Universities Press.

Sperling, O. E. (1954). An imaginary companion representing a prestage of the ego. *Psychoanalytic Study of the Child* 9:252-258.

Svendson, M. (1934). Children's imaginary companions. *Archives of Neurology and Psychiatry* 2:985-999.

Vostrovsky, C. (1895). A study of imaginary companions. *Education* 15:383-398.

Chapter Fifteen

CHILDREN'S REACTIONS TO THE DEATH OF IMPORTANT OBJECTS

A BRIEF REVIEW OF THE LITERATURE

A review of the literature on children's reactions to the death of close relatives must also include papers dealing with their reactions to transitory losses because these have also been described as mourning. Furthermore, the very young child always reacts strongly to separation from the important object (mother), regardless of whether he understands the causes of the mother's absence or the meaning of the death. Naturally, at certain stages of his development, as Freud (1926) pointed out, the child "cannot as yet distinguish between temporary absence and permanent loss. As soon as it loses sight of its mother it behaves as if it were never going to see her again; and repeated consoling experiences to the contrary are necessary before it learns that her disappearance is usually followed by her re-appearance. . . . In consequence of the infant's misunderstanding of the facts, the situation of missing its mother is not a danger-situation but a traumatic one. Or, to put it more correctly, it is a traumatic situation if the infant happens at the time to be feeling a need which its mother should be the one to satisfy" (p. 169f.).

The reaction of children of different ages to separation from the parents under a variety of conditions has been studied and described by Anna Freud and Dorothy Burlingham (1942, 1943), Spitz (1945, 1946), Spitz and Wolf (1946), James Robertson (1958, 1962), Bowlby (1960, 1961a, 1961b, 1963), Mahler (1961), and others. Bowlby (1960) considers the reaction of infants, when separated from important objects, as identical with the adult reaction of mourning, a point of view that has been questioned by Anna Freud (1960), Schur (1960), Spitz (1960), and Wolfenstein (1966). Other authors, e.g., Shambaugh (1961), in sharp contrast to Bowlby, agree with Helene Deutsch, who believes that the "process of mourning as seen in adults apparently differs from that seen in children" (p. 521). Rochlin (1959) states that the adult type of mourning is not common in children.

Fleming and Altschul (1963), studying the effects on adult personality structure of object loss in childhood, found a wide range of repercussions in terms of arrested development, faulty reality testing, impulse control, etc.

McDonald (1964) described the reaction of nursery school children to the death of the mother of one of the children in the group, while Barnes (1964) described the reaction of that child and her younger sibling to the death of their mother. Cain et al. (1964, 1966) studied children's reactions to the death, natural or through suicide, of sibling and parents. They pointed to the multiplicity of dangers encountered by such children during their psychological development.

There is some disagreement in the literature as to the age at which children are able fully to comprehend the concept of death, grasping as well the idea of its finality. Wolf (1958) believes that something similar to the adult comprehension of death is not observed before the ages of ten or eleven, while Furman (1964a) holds the opinion that a two- to three-year-old is capable of "mastering the meaning of death" and a three-and-a-half- or four-year-old has the capacity to mourn. Wolfenstein (1966) has questioned Furman's timetable with regard to mourning. Wolfenstein (1965) described a child's reaction to the death of a parent as an inhibited emotional response and designated as "mourning at a distance" the apparent contradiction existing between the intensity of the grief shown for someone far away (such as President

Kennedy) as contrasted with that shown in respect to a close relative (p. 80).[1] Wolfenstein (1966) stated that mourning as "described by Freud did not occur" in the cases she studied (p. 96). In fact, "The painful and gradual decathexis of the beloved parents which the adolescent is forced to perform serves as an initiation into how to mourn. . . . Until he has undergone what we may call the trial mourning of adolescence, he is unable to mourn" (pp. 113, 116).

Laufer (1966) observed in analytic treatment the response of an adolescent whose mother died suddenly of a coronary thrombosis. He stated that the "loss of the oedipal object in adolescence may constitute a developmental interference in the sense described by Nagera (1966)" (p. 291). It is from this angle of *developmental interferences* that I shall approach the question of children's reactions to the death of close relatives.

This brief review of the literature allows us to conclude that different authors disagree on the age at which children are capable of mourning. There are those, e.g., Bowlby (1960), who believe that mourning (in the adult sense) is possible and can be observed from the sixth month of life onward, or, like Furman (1964), who think that mourning can be observed only from the third or fourth year of life onward. There are others, e.g., Shambaugh (1961) and Rochlin (1959), who believe that the mourning process differs in children and adults, and Wolfenstein (1965, 1966), who believes that mourning becomes possible only with the resolution of the adolescent phase, after the appropriate detachment from the parental figures has taken place.

My own view is closer to that of Wolfenstein, that is, mourning as defined by Freud (1917) and as observed in the adult is not possible until the detachment from parental figures has taken place in adolescence. This does not imply that some aspects of the mourning process of the adult mourner cannot also be observed in

1. Harrison et al. (1967), studying children's reactions to President Kennedy's death, found it necessary to sound a warning note about the relibility of "the descriptions of children's bereavement reactions given by mourning adults." In their data "it was impossible to distinguish between adult misperceptions and confusions, the children's reaction to the tragedy, and the children's reactions to the changes in the adult" (p. 596).

children as a reaction to the loss of important objects, but I do suggest that there are important differences between the so-called mourning of children and that of adults.

DEATH OF A RELATIVE AS A DEVELOPMENTAL INTERFERENCE

For the adult, the death of a close relative is frequently a traumatic event.[2] For the child, death of a close relative such as father or mother can also be a traumatic event, but even more important, it constitutes what I have described (1966) as a developmental interference and a very serious one indeed.

The mourning that accompanies the loss of an object in adulthood has been rightly described as a process of adaptation (Pollock 1961). For a time, while the adaptation is worked through, everything else is temporarily suspended until the mourning is completed and the adult mourner resumes a normal life. But the child is not a finished product like the adult. He is in the middle of a multipicity of processes of develpment in all sorts of areas and directions—processes that require, for their normal unfolding, the presence of the suddenly absent object. Naturally, in these circumstances it is not sensible to expect that all development will be stopped or a pause produced so that the mourning process, leading to adaptation to the loss, can take place and normal life can be resumed again afterward as in the case of the adult. The pressure of internal developmental forces interferes with the possiblity of a pause for mourning. Thus whatever "mourning" is

2. As we know, the mere act of talking about a recently lost love object fequently leads to a painful breakdown of the ego. This breakdown is in many ways similar to a traumatically overwhelming experience, with crying, sadness, intense pain, inability to think or to react in an orgnaized and normal way. As time goes by and as the work of mourning proceeds further, the same person will be able to talk coherently about the event without the ego breaking down.

Naturally, the reaction to loss differs according to the intensity of the cathexis, the nature of the relationship, the intensity of the ambivalence, the existence of hostile wishes, and other conflicts. Similarly, as Pollock (1961) points out, the sudden, unexpected death of the love object is usually more traumatic than death following prolonged illness.

possible under this multiplicity of developmental pressures must take place simultaneously with, and in subordination to, such developmental needs as are appropriate to the age of the child, a situation that is complicated by the immediate distortions and repercussions of the loss suffered. It is not sufficiently taken into account that if the relevant objects are absent, especially during certain stages, it is in the nature of many of these develpmental processes to re-create the objects anew: to make them come to life in fantasies or to ascribe such roles as the developmental stage requires to any suitable figures available in the environment. It is partly this developmental need that opposes the normal process of mourning and the process of gradual withdrawal of cathexis from the lost object. Thus, relevant objects are brought to life again and again in order to satisfy the requirements of psychological development. Anna Freud and Dorothy Burlingham (1943) described how "Our parentless nursery-children . . . do their utmost to invent their own father-and mother-figures and live in close emotional contact with them in their imagination. But these products of their phantasy, necessary as they are to the child's emotional needs, do not exercise the same parental functions. They are called into life by the infant's longings for the missing love-object, and, as such, satisfy its wishes. They are the personification of inner forces, moving in the child, and as such give evidence of successive stages of development" (p. 126).

This does not mean that children who have lost one or the other parent do not withdraw some cathexis from the memories of such objects and do not try to find alternative or substitute objects to disrupdo so, but this process is frequently interfered with by internal forces that re-create, sometimes in idealized forms, the relationship to the absent object at the slightest disappointment with the world outside or the substitute object.

Parents have to educate their children, impose restrictions on the amount of gratifications allowed (instinctual and otherwise), make demands, etc. This situation leads, at times, to clashes between the child and the parents. It is at these points that there is a readiness (or facilitation) for certain developments to take place that usually complicate and introduce more or less serious disruptions in the emotional growth of these unfortunate children. They may feel, for example, that all these limitations are imposed on them, or that all these demands are made, because "she" or "he" is not their real mother or father, or that all these "unpleasant things" happen because they are not really loved, since they are not their "real" children. Their real mother or father would have been so much nicer, more tolerant and understanding. In short, there is a facilitation in the direction of the idealization of the dead parent and a tendency to split the ambivalence with the positive feelings cathecting the idealized dead parent and the negative ones the substitute parent.

Naturally, this negative cathexis of the substitute parent will have repercussions on the present and future relations between the child and the substitute mother or father. Furthermore, the child's future psychological makeup and future object relations may be similarly harmed by these unwelcomed tendencies.[3]

Another significant factor in children is that the same event, the same developmental interference, will influence development differently. Thus the absence of the father, for example, will acquire new meanings and be reinterpreted in phallic-oedipal terms when that phase is reached, in contrast to the fantasies that accompany the father's absence during the toddler stage.

In this way, developmental interferences, of a detrimental nature, may influence or determine the outcome of subsequent developmental and neurotic conflicts. In the case of the death of a parent, the child is forced to carry on with his psychological development in the absence of one essential figure. This frequently leads to distortions of development and at least tends to complicate the resolution of many of the otherwise normal and typical developmental conflicts of childhood and adolescence. In this way the ground is prepared for a variety of neurotic conflicts

3. A similar situation exists in the case of adoptive parents. Although early adoption by suitable parents is a most desirable event from the point of view of the infant, the adoptive parent should be aware of the developmentally destructive or at least damaging tendencies that fate has imposed on those unfortunate children who have lost their parents through death or abandonment.

that take, as their point of departure, the inappropriate resolution of such developmental conflicts. We have only to consider, for example, that a child who loses his mother or father during or just before the phallic-oedipal phase will find himself handicapped in his attempts to resolve this otherwise typical and normal developmental conflict. Meiss (1952) has described some of these difficulties.

Naturally, the child's need for the parents is quite different from one developmental stage to the next. In the earlier stages the loss of the mother is directly and immediately significant. This is not so in the case of the father except insofar as the mother's mourning and distress will affect her relationship to the baby. Nevertheless, the father's death and consequently the father's absence will become significant in its own right later on, when nature assigns him a variety of roles to play in the development of the child and he is not there to play them.

Finally, in my view, one of the most important differences between the mourning reactions of children and those of adults consists of the fact that the child frequently reacts to the death of a primary object with abnormal manifestations, which in many instances greatly resemble those observed in the case of neurotic conflict or neurosis proper. In other words, they react with anxiety, with multiple forms of regression on the side of the drives, occasionally by giving up certain ego achievements, and by developing abnormal forms of behavior. Though the child is, generally speaking, quite incapable of the prolonged and sustained mourning reaction observed in the adult, he frequently produces instead symptoms of the most diverse nature. They demonstrate the special situation of developmental stress in which he finds himself. Bonnard (1961) has given examples of children who reacted to the parent's death with truancy and stealing. They were seeking punishment out of their sense of guilt for the parent's death. In normal adult mourning such a reaction is not usually observed.

Thus, it seems reasonable to conclude that the death of important objects will, of necessity, produce a serious disruption of the developmental processes per se, quite apart from the special significance that the event may have for the child, according to age, quality of the relationship, intensity of the trauma, special circumstances surrounding the death, the reactions to this event by the remaining important family members, and possible changes for the worse in the child's life circumstances.

THE YOUNG CHILD'S REACTIONS TO LOSS

Many factors contribute to the specific form of "mourning reactions" observed in children following the loss of important objects. They vary, as I pointed out earlier, according to the different levels of development reached in a number of areas of the personality at different ages. It is for these reasons that I question the validity of some comparisons made between the mourning of adults and children. Naturally, such comparisons show many similarities. Unfortunately, there is an occasional tendency to misconstrue them into identities, or to assume that identical metapsychological processes underlie these superficial similarities.

The Development of Object Relations

In order to understand the reactions of children to loss, it is necessary to examine the role that such objects play at different stages in the child's physical, psychological, and emotional development. By specifying the functions of the object and its contribution to the normal functioning of psychological development, we can highlight what can go wrong or actually goes wrong in the child's development when the object is missing.[4]

Many of the reactions observed in the child have to be understood as the result of the absence of one of the elements required for his normal development and not necessarily as a mourning reaction to the loss of the object (as will be the case in the adult

4. For example, Hoffer (1950) has pointed out that an adequate libidinization of the child's body within the mother-infant relationship is important for the development of his body image.

personality). *In short, we must distinguish, in the overt manifestation of the child's reactions to loss, those that are the result of the developmental disturbance introduced by the object loss and the "true mourning reactions to that loss."* At the present time, there seems to be a readiness to lump together these two completely different types of phenomena. Further, as Anna Freud (1960) has clearly pointed out: for a true mourning reaction to the loss of an object to occur, the ego and object relations must have reached a certain degree of development.

Loss during the first few weeks of life. It is easier to ascertain what goes on in the child once he is capable of verbalization. It is more difficult to establish what goes on during the first year of life. Any such attempt has to be tentative and highly speculative. Having this in mind, let us ask what "object" means to the young infant.

Many analysts hold the view that the object has no existence of its own to start with in the psychic life of the child. According to Hoffer (1952), it is included as a part of the self, or rather, as an extension of the "internal narcissistic milieu." If we accept this view, a loss of the object at this particular point in the development of the child can presumably be experienced only as a loss of something pleasurable, as a qualitative change in the "internal narcissistic milieu" since no differentiation exists as yet between self and object. Usually, when such a loss occurs at this early stage, a substitute object takes over the mothering function, and if the substitute object is appropriate, the transitory disequilibrium is restored. When suitable substitute mothering is not available, as, for example, in the case of babies living in institutions, we know that although their physical needs may be well attended to, many of the ingredients of "good mothering" are missing. We also know that the development of such babies is affected in a variety of ways because of the lack of appropriate stimulation.

The mother's presence is thus required for the normal development of a number of ego achievements. Her absence through death or abandonment acts as a developmental interference affecting several areas as well as complicating the development of object relationships beyond the need-satisfying stage. For children growing up in institutions, the distance between the quality of the "ideal mothering" (received by babies growing up with their mothers) and the quality of the "substitute mothering" (offered by the institution) is in direct proportion to the developmental retardation and damage observed. In our culture, somebody in the immediate family frequently takes over the mothering function. When this is the case, the baby may show signs of distress with the change of object, but it seems that, at least in the first few weeks of life, a substitute is more or less readily accepted after a short time (Anna Freud 1952). The distress signs are probably due to his perception of the qualitative differences in handling, general mothering, and the resulting sensory experiences of the "substitute mother figure." The baby's reaction is not based on an awareness of the mother's disappearance as an object but on the perception of a change in the quality of his sensory experiences. It is as if the change had taken place in a part of the child's internal narcissistic milieu—that part or extension of what we later on call his self and which, at this undifferentiated stage (in terms of self-object), is still fused with the mother.

Loss after the second or third month of life. At a later stage, the object *acquires a mental representation of its own in the child's mind as a part object,* according to Melanie Klein, *or as a need-satisfying object,* according to Hartmann (1952) and Anna Freud (1952). The object is now valued on the basis of its role as a need-fulfilling entity. It is these need-fulfilling functions of the object that are important and not the object per se. If during this stage the object is lost or changed, the child will react with more or less marked distress, a response that is probably still due to the marked preference for the familiar and known which are now missing. Although the baby's needs can be satisfied by a substitute object, this is a new, unfamiliar object. The significant difference between the first few weeks of life and this stage is that the object has now acquired a mental representation of its own, even if only as a part object. Nevertheless it has become something independent, identifiable in its own right. It is at this point too that the object starts to be associated with the thing that brings about a particular sensory experience. Thus the baby at the need-satisfying stage notices not only the qualitative changes in the sensory experience of satisfaction (as the younger baby did), but this change is now associated with the change of object. Little by little he becomes more able to discriminate and differentiate such things as differences in the muscular tone, skin warmth, pitch of voice, and breathing rhythms.

Loss in the second half of the first year and onward. With further development the object is valued independently of its need-fulfilling functions. Toward the end of the first or the beginning of the second year the child reaches the stage of object constancy (Anna Freud 1952). If at this point the object is suddenly absent, the child's distress is due to the new type of cathexis, which has a special quality, more permanence, and no longer attaches itself automatically to substitute objects even if the child accepts their ministrations. The example quoted by Bowlby (1960), from Anna Freud and Dorothy Burlingham's book *Infants Without Families,* illustrates this point. It concerns a seventeen-month-old girl who on being separated from her mother, said nothing but "Mum, Mum, Mum," for three days, and who, although she liked to sit on the nurse's knee and have the nurse put her arm around her, insisted throughout on having her back to the nurse so as not to see her.

Strictly speaking, it is only at the point when object constancy has been reached that the nature and quality of the cathexis directed to the object can at least in rudimentary form be compared to the level, nature, and quality of the cathexis directed by the normal adult to his closest objects. It is this special type of attachment cathexis that determines the intense suffering observed when the object is lost. It is this cathexis that must be withdrawn from the innumerable memories of the lost object and made available for the recathexis of some new objects. The quality of the cathexis and the level of the object realtionship are special, and very different from that attached to objects during the early stage of need satisfaction. This is partly explained by the further development of the ego which allows for a better discrimination of the object's qualities and a more clear-cut separation between self and object.

Thus, in my view, it is only from the stage of object constancy onward that the conditions exist, in terms of object relations, which make it possible to observe *some aspects* of mourning in children as the response to the psychologically meaningful loss of an object. In this respect it shows many resemblances to the mourning responses of adults with clear signs of the three phases described by Bowlby (1961b), that is, protest, despair, and denial. Superficially similar responses in the much younger child are based on completely different reasons and mechanisms, as I have tried to show.

Thus, once object constancy has been established, a common denominator has been acquired that persists throughout life. Nevertheless, it would be a mistake to conclude that, from this point onward, children's reactions to death could be expected to be uniform or identical with those of adults. Many other factors, to be examined next, determine the multiplicity of variations in response observed at different ages.

Other Relevant Factors and Considerations

The child's low capacity for the tolerance of acute pain. Human beings generally have a limited capacity for the tolerance of acute pain, and in children this capacity is even lower. Wolfenstein (1966) referred to the "short sadness span, which is usual in children." This short sadness span, which can be considered from another angle as a greater flexibility and mobility of the child's attention and interests based on his intense curiosity and the momentum enforced by the developmental processes, can be observed in a variety of ways. Wolfenstein (1965) described how children in the age range from latency to adolescence cannot tolerate intense distress for long, and quickly bring forward opposite thoughts and feelings. (According to our observations the same applies even more so to prelatency children). As she says, "They do not seem able to sustain the process of protracted mourning that we know in adults" (p. 77).[5] She further refers to children aged nine and ten who cried when they heard the news of Kennedy's assassination and yet could not understand why their parents refused to go to the movies that evening as previously planned or were impatient when they could not find their usual program on television.

I have made similar observations in three children (whose ages ranged from four and a half to thirteen) on the occasion of the death of their grandfather, who had lived at their home for three years. Though there was no question that the three children were upset by the grandfather's death, the youngest tried to listen to some music on the radio early the next morning, as he was in the habit of doing. He accepted the explanation that the other members of the family were still very sad and did not really feel like having the radio on. It was clear that in the following days (until the funeral took place) he was frequently tempted to turn either the radio or the television on. Occasionally he turned it on and off, telling those around that the radio should not be on because his grandfather had died. (This boy's reactions are described in greater detail in the last part of this chapter (see the case of P).)

The other two children, aged twelve and thirteen, showed clear signs of some sadness at different moments as well as a great deal of empathy at the obvious pain of their grandmother. They would undoubtedly have liked to watch their favorite TV programs, but did not do so out of empathy with the adults. The knowledge that they could watch TV again the day after the funeral also helped them to control the wish.

This type of behavior is, in my experience, quite common up to and including adolescence. It cannot be construed to mean that

5. Helene Deutsch in her paper "Absence of Grief" (1937) was one of the first analysts to call our attention "to the phenomenon of indifference which children so frequently display following the death of a loved person." In trying to account for this she did not consider as completely valid either of the two explanations usually given to account "for this so-called heartless behavior," namely, the child's intellectual inability to grasp the reality of death and the still inadequate formation of object relationships. Her own hypothesis is "that the ego of the child is not sufficiently developed to bear the strain of the work of mourning and that it therefore utilizes some mechanism of narcissistic self-protection to circumvent the process" (p. 13).

children do not grieve at all for the lost objects or that some aspect of mourning is not taking place; but it demonstrates Wolfenstein's point that they are hardly able to keep up the process of protracted (and sustained) mourning as we know it in adults. As she points out (1966), "The different ways of reacting to loss according to age often lead to conflict and misunderstandings in the family. The adult . . . cannot understand the seeming lack of feeling on the part of the child. A mother weeping for the father who has died reproaches the child, suffering from an affective inhibition, for remaining dry-eyed" (p. 73). It should not be forgotten that much of the behavior of the adult world under bereavement conditions is a conventional and generally accepted, ritualized type of behavior. This makes little sense to the young child who has not yet come across it and has not introjected it as the appropriate code of behavior under such circumstances. Although many of these rituals are disappearing, in some countries all sorts of rules still exist determining the "official" length of mourning and the severity of the restrictions imposed, according to the closeness of the dead relative, etc.

Object loss plus separation from other familiar objects and surroundings. We know from the observations of Anna Freud, Dorothy Burlingham, J. Robertson, Spitz, Bowlby, and others of many touching examples of intense and more sustained reactions to the loss of the object because of hospitalization of the child or mother or because of absence of the mother for other reasons. But there seems to me to be an essential difference between this group of children and those who have remained in the familiar surroundings of their homes, keeping their rooms and possessions. They have remained as well in the company of other familiar objects even if these objects are, in terms of the mental economics of the child, of less importance than the one lost. The observations of children, by the different authors mentioned, concerned instead children who had suffered not only an important loss in terms of an object but who simultaneously found themselves placed in unfamiliar surroundings with strange people, and who were in some cases faced with the added stress of hospital procedures and medical manipulations.[6] I believe that we tend to underestimate the tremendous importance of perceptual and environmental constancy for the human being and especially for the child. Familiar surroundings and objects, familiar possessions (room, bed, toys, etc.), familiar noises, are important for our well-being.

At Hampstead we have seen many young children who reacted strongly to changes of environment, for example, during holidays. Although they remained with their parents and other relatives, such situations occasionally seemed to trigger a variety of disturbances. Similar distress in the very young child is frequently observed as a response to change of room, cot, or bed. Naturally, children's reactions in this respect tend to vary according to age and specific idiosyncrasies.

I believe that some of the differences observed in the reactions of these two groups of children (i.e., those separated from home and familiar surroundings and those staying at home) to the loss of objects can be accounted for partly by the factors mentioned.

Denial as a reaction to loss. It is natural and normal for the young child to excessively use certain primitive types of defenses such as various forms of denial (in words, actions, and fantasy, or of affect). This factor itself further contributes to making the mourning process of the child somewhat different from that of the adult. As we know, children practically up to the latency period very readily have recourse to denial, especially in traumatic or stressful situations. The low tolerance of the younger child for

6. Anna Freud's and Dorothy Burlingham's observations at the Hampstead War Nurseries concerned children separated from their parents largely as the result of the war conditions. A few children were assigned to a substitute mother and every effort was made for the child to have his "special" person. Robertson's and Bowlby's observations concern mainly children living under hospital conditions, while Spitz's observations concerned, in one case, the reactions to the accidental separation of delinquent mothers and their children who had been living together in a correctional institution. His other observations concerned the development of children in a foundling home in the absence of their mothers and without adequate mother substitutes. Anna Freud (1960) has pointed out that we know in fact little of children's reactions to loss when they remain with the surviving relatives and in their own familiar surroundings.

psychological pain makes this a welcome defense.[7] If denial is the child's primary reaction to loss, its further impact on his development will to a large measure be determined by how the environment deals with this. We know, for example, how frequently adults wish "to spare the child" and withhold important facts from him or, unable to tolerate their own sadness, forbid the child to mention the painful event. (For a further discussion, see footnote 8.)

Another important factor is which element of the experience is denied—e.g., whether it is the affect associated with it or the event itself. If it is the latter, it presupposes some understanding of reality, which of course is a function of the child's age.

Reality testing, reality awareness, reality adaptation, and reaction to loss. Anna Freud (1960) and others have emphasized the importance of relating a child's reaction to loss to his reality awareness. We know, e.g., that at least during the beginning of the second year of life, many children are not yet able to distinguish between dreams and reality. Consequently, events taking place in the dream are treated as pieces of reality, with the result that the child is greatly confused (see chapter 13). We do not know the implications for the further development of the child at this age if, as is bound to happen, the lost mother reappears in his dream life; or in which ways this will affect his understanding of the loss and the process of detaching cathexis from the object. Naturally, this type of problem does not exist for the older child in whom reality testing is well established and who can clearly distinguish between what goes on inside himself and what belongs in the outside world.

But even in older children one can see difficulties that seem related to the child's limited capacity to grasp intellectually and fully the reality, significance, and finality of death. Freud, in a footnote added in 1909 to *The Interpretation of Dreams* (1900),

7. Adults subjected to extreme stress also may resort to denial while the ego gains some time to pull together all its resources in order to cope with more adaptive mechanisms. Frequently the denial lasts only a few instants and takes the form of incredulity, disbelief, the hope that there has been a mistake, or that one is really having a nightmare.

refers to the remark of a highly intelligent boy of ten after the sudden death of his father: "I know father's dead, but what I can't understand is why he doesn't come home to supper" (p. 254). Recently I had the opportunity to observe the reaction of a four-year-old girl to the sudden death of her father. Her mother was naturally extremely distressed and for several days found herself completely unable to tell the children about the father's death. Once she told them, the little girl seemed to understand and to accept the reason for his absence. Nevertheless, several months later, on her birthday she reacted strongly to the fact that her father had not come to her party or sent her any presents. She was angry and cried bitterly, unable to understand why her father had been so neglectful.

In order to understand her reaction at this point, it is relevant to consider the terms in which the father's death was explained to her. The little girl had been going to Sunday school where she had been told that when good people die they go to God in heaven. Thus, she had been told that her father had been very ill, had died, and had gone to heaven. The mother's adviser who recommended this course of action had a number of considerations in mind. First, the children should certainly be told, and it was necessary to overcome the mother's hesitation in this respect. She seemed agreeable to telling the children in this particular way and reluctant to do it in what she referred to as a "cruder way." Second, they should be given the news in the least traumatic fashion possible. Third, they should be told, so far as possible, in words with which they were already familiar so that they could grasp at least some of the meaning and significance of the event.

Nevertheless, it can rightly be said that the information conveyed to this four-year-old girl was itself an elaborated piece of denial. The story told conveys that the father has changed his physical location to heaven, not that he no longer existed. Yet this is a cultural piece of deception having an almost universal character. Religious and spiritual beliefs are based on the existence of an afterlife. This very fact points to the difficult emotions confronting the human mind when coping with the phenomenon of death and to a certain inability or reluctance to comprehend and accept its finality. Perhaps this can be understood on the basis of the narcissistic and omnipotent elements from the early stages of development persisting in the adult where they work against the acceptance of a final and total destruction of the self. It is not difficult to see how much more difficult it must be for the child to come to terms with these facts. Further, at a certain stage, all children believe in the omnipotence of the adult world and especially that of their parents, a belief contrary to the idea of the annihilation of the parents. This explains why Peter (four and a half), a child in the Hampstead War Nurseries, having been told that his father had been killed and that he could not come anymore, said: "I want him to come. My Daddy is big, he can do everything."

It is questionable how much the four-year-old girl, referred to above, would have understood if the straight forward facts had been given to her or what she would have made of them. We know that excessive information in certain areas, for example, in the sexual sphere, or information conveyed in terms that are beyond the ego's ability to grasp, occasionally have a traumatic effect on the child. In other cases when the information is beyond the child's comprehension and realm of experience, he just ignores it and continues to build up fantasies whose content is determined in part by the phase of drive development he happens to be in, and in part by his ego ability to organize the data of the observations and experiences into a set of theories meaningful to him (see Freud 1907).

The child's thought processes and reactions to loss. The capacity for abstract thinking is acquired slowly and very gradually. The younger child's thought processes are concrete. Furthermore, even if the child has reached a satisfactory level of abstract thinking, there may still be pockets where, for a number of reasons (not infrequently of a neurotic character) thinking and judgment remain highly concrete. In stituations of neurotic conflict, stress, or under the impact of anxiety, there is a tendency in young children to revert to concrete forms of thinking. Barnes (1964) described many instances showing a four-year-old girl's concretization of thought processes and their influence on her reaction. Thus, for example, the child objected to wearing a dress which she had previously liked after her little cousins insisted that her dead mother was now an angel in heaven. The dress had been bought by the mother and was of a type known commercially as an "angel costume." According to Barnes, the anxiety aroused by the synonymity of angels and death made the child refuse to wear the dress. Similarly, the girl became reluctant to take naps at nursery school and preferred sitting on the teacher's lap. She finally explained: "You cannot get up when you want to," a limitation that she associated with being dead and more especially with her mother's death.

Another characteristic of the young child's thought processes is open egocentricity so that he tends to evaluate every event in terms of the repercussions it may have on him. Somewhat later, when the typical egocentricity of the toddler stage has to some extent receded, the child's increased psychological awareness of his own helplessness and dependence on the world of objects leads to the same result.

Anna Freud and Dorothy Burlingham (1943) gave many examples of orphaned children in the Hampstead War Nurseries who at the appropriate developmental stage (phallic-oedipal phase) talked "about their dead fathers as if they were alive or, when they have grasped the fact of death, try to deny it in the form of phantasies about re-birth or return from heaven. In some cases this happens under the direct influence of mothers who hide the truth from the child to spare it pain; *in other cases phantasies of an identical nature are the child's spontaneous production*" (p. 107; italics mine). The authors further commented: "Visits from the dead fathers are, if anything, mentioned more often than the visits of ordinary living fathers" (p. 108).

The form in which the children expressed the wish for their fathers' return can be understood as a denial of death, but a number of other significant factors must be taken into account. In the examples cited by Anna Freud and Dorothy Burlingham, some children were unable to grasp the full significance and implications of death. In order to give some meaning to it, they used models based on their previous experience and knowledge. For example, for four-and-a-half-year-old Susan, "deaded" is gone away, "far away to Scotland," which does not exclude the possibility of a subsequent return. The different fantasies (perhaps it would be more correct to say theories) that she verbalized can in part be understood as an attempt to grasp the facts.

Thus, Susan must have heard about the army where daddy-soldiers were and that the army was far away. Hence her hope for his return expressed itself in the fantasy that her daddy (who had been in the navy) was in the army which was too far away for him to come back. When she thought of him as gone with the navy, she logically concluded that he couldn't come back because "there is too much water."

Thus, while the child's thought processes tend to be concrete and egocentric, they are not illogical in terms of his factual knowledge in other respects, as the following illustrations show.

Freud, in a footnote added in 1919 to *The Interpretation of Dreams* (1900), refers to an observation of a highly intelligent four-year-old girl who was able to distinguish, in contrast to Susan, between being "gone" and being "dead." "The little girl had been troublesome at meal-time and noticed that one of the maids at the pension where they were staying was looking at her askance. 'I wish Josefine was dead.' . . . 'Why dead?' enquired her father soothingly; 'wouldn't it do if she went away?' 'No,' replied the child; 'then she'd come back again'" (p. 255).

For Bertie, another child at the Hampstead War Nurseries, death meant that father had been dismembered into bits and pieces. Knowing that broken objects can be mended and believing what he had been told (that God can do anything He wants), he rightly asked what was delaying God in putting father together. Again, on the basis of his factual information concerning the scarcity or complete lack of many things because of the war, he further concluded: "We have to wait until after the war, then God can put people together again."

All these examples show clearly the degree to which the child's age-adequate thought processes influence his understanding of and reaction to death. He obviously makes efforts to understand the painful events on the basis of his previous knowledge. It is not his fault if the adult world feeds him a great deal of distorted and misleading information.[8] His attempts at mastery can only be based on that information. On the other hand, his needs and wishes may at times distort and override factual knowledge (as I have also shown in the section on denial.)

Ambivalence and reaction to loss. Freud (1917) and Helene Deutsch (1937) pointed out that the presence of strong ambivalent feelings leads to a more intense, excessive, or delayed form of mourning in the adult. While we know that in children generally, and especially in the young child, strong ambivalent feelings toward the object world are the rule, we know far too little about how this factor influences the mourning process in the young child,

Having returned to an element of object relations—the theme with which I started my discussion—I will once more proceed with developmental considerations.

THE OLDER CHILD'S REACTIONS TO LOSS

The Latency Period

Many of the factors described as playing a role in the reaction of the younger child in the death of a close relative are still operative,

8. In one of our discussions at Hampstead a colleague described how on a walk he and his two-year-old child had found a mockingbird on the roadside. He tried to shield the child by not referring to the fact that the bird was dead, but the child noticed. The father then decided that they should bury it together. The little boy wanted to know whether the bird was now safe and wished to make sure that no cars could run over it. He also wanted to know whether the bird was a baby, a mummy or a daddy bird, deciding it was a mother bird. More recently he has begun to kill worms and talks freely about this. Anna Freud, commenting on this example, thought that adults frequently try to keep contact with death away from the child at a time when he is interested in and can approach the subject (at his own level). By doing so one surrounds death in mystery, as a dark and secret subject not to be puzzled out and understood. She thought the subject should be treated like the questions about sex. The child should be free to approach it at any age. She further pointed out that the two-year-old frequently approaches injury and death not with horror but with fascination. In the anal-sadistic phase he is most interested in maimed and killed objects. Anna Freud thinks that the adults, by such behavior, are really protecting themselves from the child's sadism.

though in a modified form, during the latency period. These modifications and the relative importance of the different factors involved are highly variable from one child to another.

It is always important, but especially so in latency, to distinguish clearly between two different aspects of the mourning process. The first one concerns the extent to which anybody can experience and express the feeling of loss with the consequent signs of sadness and grief. The second concerns the withdrawal of the cathexis previously attached to the lost object so that the freed energies are available for the cathexis of a new object. The last process, I believe, is easier for the adult than the child. Complete withdrawal of cathexis from the lost object will leave the child in a "developmental vacuum" unless a suitable substitute object is readily found. His emotional development requires the existence of, for example, a mother figure and her physical death does not alter this fact in any way and cannot lead to the type of decathexis that will be observed in the case of the adult. In the latency child, developmental imperatives will tend to keep her alive in spite of the ego knowledge of the reality of the object's death and irretrievable physical disappearance.

How does the latency child normally handle these two components of mourning? Most observations indicate that latency children deal with serious losses, through death, with massive denial, including denial of affect and not infrequently even reversal of affect. This situation seems to be favored or encouraged by our cultural attitudes to death at the present time.

Yet, we will probably agree, on theoretical grounds, that for the further healthy development of the latency child, it will be better if he can, within appropriate limits, express and experience the pain, sadness, anger, and other feelings and conflicts associated with the loss.

Some authors (e.g., Shambaugh 1961, Furman 1964b) believe that children in this age group can, with profit, experience, and express feelings accompanying the loss of the object if helped to do so in analysis. At the same time, many of the unresolved conflicts concerning the lost object can be dealt with, and possible obstacles to further normal development can thus be removed. But the evidence in this respect is still limited, and only further research and controlled observations can clarify the issue.

As to the second and more important aspect of mourning in adults, that is, the slow decathexis of the lost object, the evidence seems to point to the fact that the latency child strongly cathects a fantasy life where the lost object may be seen as alive and at times as ideal. (Not infrequently this fantasy relationship to the lost object is kept secret by the latency child. In one case treated at Hampstead, the therapist, A. Bene, discovered only after many months of treatment that the patient had kept secret an intimate fantasy relationship to a dead sibling for several years of her life.)

Naturally, a fantasy object is not a suitable substitute for an absent parent, but it may well be an unavoidable alternative, especially if suitable substitutes are not readily available to the child. There is also evidence showing how the child makes simultaneous attempts to cathect certain objects in reality and to give them the mother's role (for example, teachers and, in the case of children in analysis, their therapists), especially if their sex favors such a displacement. Unfortunately, neither teachers nor therapists can perform this role appropriately. Furthermore, in cases where a substitute mother is introduced into the life of the child and the father's remarriage restores the family organization, we can observe very quickly a process of disappointment in the new object which is only partly dependent on the object's ability to play a substitute mothering role. This disarray in the object cathexis may have to be considered as one of the unavoidable consequences of object loss, at least when it takes place at certain times in life. Nevertheless, provision must be made for the fact that some children are more able than others to find the most adaptive solutions amidst these difficulties.

Although the overt, superficial behavior of latency children seems to deny more or less completely the importance of the loss suffered, the child's inner life may undergo significant changes that could seriously affect his later development. There is often, in this age group, no apparent grief or sadness shortly after the event, though an immediate and short-lived sadness reaction is occasionally seen. In the foreground one frequently observes not only denial but a reversal of affects as well. Shambaugh's description (1961) of his patient Henry is typical: "I was struck by his affect. He did not look like a boy who had suffered a loss. Instead, he came to his first interviews as if he were full of energy. He was hyperactive and gay, sometimes even to the point of euphoria" (p. 512). Henry did not talk during the sessions about his home or the mother's death. If this imposed censure was threatened, he reacted with anxiety and anger and on one occasion ran from the office when the analyst alluded to the mother's death.

Nevertheless, as Shambaugh points out, an experienced observer could detect behind this facade many ominous signs. Our experience at Hampstead confirms that latency children frequently respond in this way to the death of an important object. They may not show many overt signs of mourning, but a closer examination shows important evidence of serious disturbances, behavioral disorders, and symptom formation.[9]

ADOLESCENCE

There can be no question that by the time the adolescence phase sets in, all the factors named by different authors as necessary preconditions for mourning in the adult are well established. The adolescent's ego development is such that he can understand the full implications and finality of death. His reality testing is firmly established. His awareness of reality and capacity to adapt to it are sufficiently developed. Nevertheless, adolescents shy away from the type of mourning that we know from adults. Their overt behavior and response to loss are significantly different from that of the adult mourner. Yet, they are greatly affected by the loss and react in strong and specific adaptive ways of their own.

How are we then to explain the difference in the mourning response between them and the adult? The significant difference, to my mind, is that the adolescent, as Wolfenstein points out, is

9. Arthur and Kemme (1964) studied the families of eighty-three disturbed children where death of a parent had occured. They found "a high incidence of both intellectual and emotional problems either directly or indirectly related to the loss" (p. 48).

still tied to his infantile imagos, generally and more especially so to the parents. He has not yet completed his psychological and emotional development. Their presence is required for his development to unfold normally until it is finally completed. As with the younger child, the sudden loss of such an object through death creates the same situation of developmental stress that I described earlier as a developmental interference.

The adolescent also tends to recathect the image of the lost object when experiencing certain needs or developmental pressures as was the case with younger children. According to Wolfenstein (1966), "instead of decathecting a lost love object, which is what happens in mourning, children and adolescents tend to develop a hypercathexis of the lost object." According to her, "fantasies of the parent's return are either more clearly conscious or more readily admitted in adolescence than at earlier ages." As she pointed out in 1965: "the death of a parent would find the young adolescent still far from ready to give him up. At the same time conflicting feelings towards the parent would further interfere with pure regret and sadness."

Wolfenstein (1966) and Laufer (1966) have described vividly the reactions of an adolescent girl and an adolescent boy to the death of their mothers. There are many similarities in the reactions of these two adolescents to the loss. I will select from Wolfenstein's case, for the purposes of illustration, some specific aspects of this girl's reaction.

Typically, according to Wolfenstein, Ruth found herself no longer able to cry shortly after the mother's funeral. "She felt an inner emptiness, and as if a glass wall separated her from what was going on around her. She was distressed by this affectlessness, and was subsequently relieved when, comparing notes with a friend whose father had died some time earlier, she learned that the other girl had had a similar reaction" (p. 100).

Again rather typically, after the event Ruth came to her sessions in an elated mood. "She had written a successful humorous composition in which she congratulated herself. . . . [She] proceeded to detail various embarrassing predicaments she had got into, which she turned to comic effect" (p. 101).

She showed the same tendency as Laufer's patient to isolate her feelings of sadness and despair from thoughts of the mother's death. Any such links established by the therapists, if accepted intellectually, were supplanted by a struggle to capture more pleasurable moods. Similarly, obvious denial of the finality of the loss was overtly or covertly maintained by them.

CLINICAL ILLUSTRATIONS

A Young Child's Reactions to Loss

The first example shows the reaction of a normal boy, four years and eight months to the death of his maternal grandfather. This example is significantly different from all the others, probably because the lost object was not a primary object. The child had a very close relationship to his grandfather as a favorite playmate, but at no time had the grandfather become entangled in the boy's phallic-oedipal development, which was lived out with his real father and mother as the objects of this struggle. Furthermore, the realtionship with the grandfather was free of negative and conflictual elements, as could not easily have been the case with a sibling. The case demonstrates not only the difficulties a child of this age has in comprehending the phenomenom of death, but also its repercussions on his phallic-oedipal struggles with the real parents.

P was a well-developed, likable child whose characterisitic approach to life was to master things intellectually. He usually tried very hard to understand what he was confronted with. This attitude also extended to anxiety-provoking situations or events.

Prior to the grandfather's death, P had had some contacts and experiences with death. The family lived close to a crematorium and P had often watched the funeral processions and listened to his older siblings' discussion of them. These had stimulated P's curiosity at an early age and led him to ask many questions about death.

His more direct experiences with death related to animals, birds or fish. For example, he was greatly impressed by an incident that took place when he was three years of age. His siblings kept cold water fish in an open tank. Once P heard them saying that the tank was dirty and the water smelly, whereupon he proceeded to put soap powder and perfume in the fish tank, with the result (unexpected, as far as he was concerned) that all the fish died. His siblings, who were greatly upset, accused him of having killed the fish. He was puzzled and guilty. His intention had obviously been to make the water tank clean and he had no idea of the implications of his actions.

Similarly, he had occasionally watched cowboy films on TV with his older brother and sister. When he saw people being shot at and falling down dead, he showed some concern and asked many questions. Until his third birthday, he did not tolerate being shot at by his brother. Although he enjoyed other imaginative role play, he became angry and distressed when his brother pretended to shoot at him, asked not to be shot at, and refused to pretend to be dead. He would, nevertheless, shoot at others and enjoy their pretending to be dead. After P had moved into the oedipal phase, he no longer objected to being shot at or to pretending to be killed. At the same time he developed the habit of shooting at his father, saying, "You are dead." It was not thought that the child had at this point an intellectual grasp of the meaning of death beyond the fact that it was something bad, that it implied being still, and that one shot only "baddies," enemies or rivals.

The grandparents came to live in P's household when he was two years of age. A special relationship developed quickly between the child and his grandfather. They spent many hours playing together every day and a strong tie developed between them. When, at the age of three, P started nursery school in the mornings, he would immediately upon his return home again be engaged in a game with his grandfather.

Unfortunately, at the time P was three years of age, the grandfather suffered a stroke which left him handicapped. When they resumed play, P's demands were, at times, a strain on the grandfather's strength. Shortly after the stroke, the grandfather developed a serious heart condition that required several prolonged hospitalizations. This further weakened him and greatly reduced his playing with P, but some joint play activities continued to his end.

The grandfather's several prolonged hospitalizations helped to lessen somewhat the intensity of the tie the child formerly had had with him. P was always concerned about the grandfather's absences and talked about the grandfather a great deal. Since, on more than one occasion, the family had serious misgivings about the grandfather's life, the children had been made aware of the possibility of his death.

On the day of his death, which happened suddenly, the grandfather, feeling very ill, had returned from a short walk with his wife. He sat in the living room to rest for a moment, but grew worse very quickly. P's mother sent P upstairs with his sister, after explaining to him that the grandfather was ill and the doctor had to be called. P was soon put to bed and was asleep when the grandfather died.

The next morning P went to school as usual, still not knowing about the grandfather's death. His mother went to fetch him at the end of the morning, and once they were in the car on the way home, she finally told him.

Mother: P, do you remember that yesterday the doctor came to see grandfather because he was very ill?

P: Yes.

Mother: Well, he became worse and worse and since he was so old too, the medicine he was given did not help him to get better and he finally died.

P's expression became very serious and thoughtful. Then he asked as if to reassure himself he had heard properly: "Did grandfather died? . . . Did he died? . . . Poor grandfather. . . . " Between each phrase there was a pause during which he obviously was thinking hard. Then he asked: "When did he died? Was he at home or had he gone to the hospital?" The mother explained that he had died at home, that it had happened so quickly there was no time to take him to the hospital. After a few moments P asked: "And where was he when he died?" The mother explained that he was in the living room where P had last seen him the previous evening. P was thoughtful again for a few seconds and then asked: "Was he sitting or lying down?" The mother explained that at first he was sitting in the big chair and later was taken to the sofa where he lay down. P then asked whether the grandfather spoke when he died. He was told he spoke a little just before dying. P went on: "Did he close his eyes?" "Yes, he did," the mother answered. He remained silent for a while and then asked again: "Did the Rolls Royce from the crematorium come? Did they take him away in a box?" When these different questions were answered factually, he continued his inquest, asking: "How was he, was he dressed up?" He listened with great interest to his mother's reply, then continued: "If I open his eyes and touch them, will he feel it? . . . Does he remember our street?" The mother gave him factual answers. He then said: "Today is a sad day because he died. . . . " After another silent pause, he proceeded to inquire whether each family member knew and what their reaction had been. He excluded only his father.

At this point they arrived home. P went immediately to the living room and wanted to know exactly in which place the grandfather was sitting before he died. Then he lay down on the sofa where the grandfather died, closed his eyes and said, "Let's pretend that I am grandfather and I am dead." After a moment, he got up and went upstairs to the grandfather's room where he took a close look at everything without saying a word.

During the following days he was slightly excited, after which time he was his usual self again. For two or three days, he talked to the other children in the neighborhood about his grandfather's death. When an uncle arrived from abroad, P commented that he knew why he had come. When asked why, he replied, "Because grandfather died." As mentioned earlier, he made frequent comments as to why it was that they could not listen to the radio or watch TV until after the funeral.

He said to his father, one or two days after the grandfather's death, on one of the occasions when he was more excited than was usual for him, "It would have been better if you had died too, because then I could do all the naughty things I want."

If we consider his reaction up to this point, it could be said that in his immediately following behavior and verbalizations he showed sadness, "Poor grandfather." There was no feeling of secrecy concerning the death (nor did his family attempt to keep anything from him: all questions he posed were answered). He did not use manic or jocular defenses, as young children often do, nor were there any indications of attempts at denial. Further, as was usual for him, there was a strong attempt to master intellectually all the implications of what had happened and, to some extent, the meaning of death, by very actively asking a number of questions. Like many children of his age, he associated death with stillness and lack of movement. He also knew, in some way, that in terms of absence, death had a permanent character in contrast with the grandfather's earlier absences through hospitalization. He vaguely inferred that there was more to it that was unclear to him, hence his questions as to what would happen if opened the grandfather's eyes, or whether the grandfather would feel his touching them, or could the grandfather still think and remember things.

He did not react with the common neurotic responses—usually

due to conflict or guilt in respect to the dead person—such as fear of sleep, fear of closing the eyes, or refusing to enter the room where the lost object had died. On the contrary, he was curious and questioning without showing any overt fears, except for the fact that he was slightly uncomfortable when he pretended to be the dead grandfather lying down on the sofa.

In the following days and weeks, while riding in the car, P would occasionally point out places where he had been with his grandfather or which he knew the grandfather had visited. On the other hand, immediately after the death of the grandfather, P stopped his early morning visits to his grandparents' room which he had previously made daily as soon as he woke up. They had usually chatted and, while P had pretended to play his guitar, sung together. At other times of the day which were less reminiscent of this "special" hour, P continued to go to their room.

Although P's reaction to the grandfather's death was surprisingly normal, it nevertheless strained his relationship to his father in the oedipal context. To start with, he moved closer to him and sought his company more frequently as a substitute playmate for the grandfather, but P's oedipal rivalry showed clearly and at times interfered with his ability to play with his father.

At about this time the father had to be away from home for three weeks. P seemed to associate the father's oncoming absence with the grandfather's earlier absences due to hospitalizations and with the fact that these absences were followed by his grandfather's death. His immediate reaction—and he was now obviously under great internal stress—was to try to convince the father to take him along on that trip. He insistently told his mother and siblings that his father would be taking him, though they had explained to him several times why this was not possible. He seemed to accept these explanations. Unfortunately the elder brother teased him occasionally by saying that P was not going because he was too little but that he, O, and C were going. P's faith was somewhat shattered by his brother's teasing and playful statement. Nevertheless he was able to go to his father whenever this happened, asking, rather pathetically, whether it was true that O and C were going. Once reassured, he regained his usual gay composure. However, at the same time he began to reassure the father about how much he liked and loved him, clinging to him more than was usual.

Shortly before the father's trip, P heard about riots taking place in a city he knew his father would be visiting. He listened very attentively to all comments about these riots and the father's plans for visiting that city. One or two days before the trip, when the father was preparing his luggage, P said: "Daddy, you better be careful when you are in that place. They can kill people there." In this condensed statement he was able to express simultaneously both his concern and love for the father and his death wishes.

The father's absence passed uneventfully. However, since the father's return—and this may have been a temporal coincidence only—P showed strong signs of moving away from the "oedipal" mother to other female objects (such as friends of his older sister or other female visitors). He performed for them the phallic-exhibitionistic feats typical for children of his age and usually ended by stating how much he liked them and that he would marry them when he grew up. One cannot but wonder whether this sudden move may have been forced by his need to protect his father from his oedipal hostility and rivalry after his experience of the loss of the grandfather. Be that as it may, one is left with the impression that P's oedipal conflicts were greatly reinforced by the grandfather's death. Previously P had shot at his father, frequently crying out that he was dead. Now, after the actual experience of having lost his grandfather, a new real dimension had been added to his hostile wishes and his ideas about death and rivals.

P is an example of a reasonably normal child who, though showing signs of strain, coped with the event of death in an adaptive way. Many children are less fortunate. The impact on their personality development and the reinforcement of conflicts (developmental or neurotic) will distort their further psychological growth and lead to serious psychopathology, especially so when the object lost is a primary one.

Older Children's Reactions to Loss

B was five and a half years of age when analytic treatment started.[10] He was six and a half when his mother was operated on for cancer of the breast, resulting in the removal of one breast and

10. I am indebted to Mrs. C. Kearney, B's therapist, for the preparation of the condensed summary of the relevant aspects of the case here presented.

the surrounding tissues. He was seven when the cancer recurred in the form of skin and lung metastases, discoloration of the skin, breathing difficulties, and severe coughing spells. He was seven years eight months when his mother died. I shall focus on his behavior during the period preceding the mother's death and his reaction immediately afterward (for a period of two months).

At the time of referral there was clear evidence of massive oral fixations, disturbances of mood and social-emotional responsiveness with vague fears of being attacked. He was preoccupied with fears and ideas of death, separation, and punishment long before the serious illness became manifest. B's mother was aware of the nature of her illness and her impending death (until a few weeks before she died, when she began to deny it). She usually helped B to deny her impending death when it seemed to her that he needed to do so. Yet, at other times, she was equally sensitive in presenting the truth in a manner designed to alleviate his anxiety and possible guilt. In fact their relationship was, at this point, better than ever before. This seemed due to the fact that she included rather than excluded him from her life—as she had previously tended to do. She was now making a courageous and conscious attempt to help him, wanting to be remembered as a "good mother" after her death.

The analytic material in the months before the mother's death could best be described as seesawing back and forth between denial and awareness of the impending object loss, the latter gaining in momentum the closer the reality of his mother's death drew. For example, B made elaborate plans for what he would do with his mother when he reached the age of ten: or he would figure out what his mother's age would be when he was in college and living away from home, preparing himself, as it were, for the inevitable separation by projecting it into the future.

After the therapist had discussed the possibility that his mother might die even though the doctors were trying everything to make her better, B said calmly, "Even if everybody dies, Mommy and Daddy, my uncles and aunts, even you, it still wouldn't matter because we are very rich and we would have all the money we need . . . and we would still have each other," referring to his older brother.

B suddenly became interested in God and professed his religious beliefs. Previously, neither he nor his family had shown any religious interest. He asked, "Would you like better to be liked by God or have many friends? I would like to be loved by God because God can do anything for you . . . He can even make you alive after you die."

Motivated by his desire to make restitution to others while his mother was still alive, he began to champion good causes. He identified with deprived children, organizing a "helping club" among his friends to collect money to send to the "starving and homeless children of India." He wanted to invite a boy who had just lost his mother to his house because "nobody wants to talk to him about his mother." In this way he was expressing his understanding of the void created by his (and the other children's) apprehension over the death of this boy's mother. B asked his own mother to buy a gift for this child which he then took to his house.

B was particularly impressed with Jesus, who "gave up His life to a bum for stealing a loaf of bread . . . to help him," he added. That he was similarly preoccupied with his mother could be surmised when he told the therapist of the games he was playing with his older brother. They would lie down in the street and, at the last moment, would roll aside to escape approaching cars (counterphobic elements were evident in this behavior). Instead of having to die like the mother he was able to escape death at will. He reassured himself further by stating that boys, having no breasts, cannot die of breast cancer. When his identification with Jesus was discussed, he wanted to know if the therapist would give everything she had, "even your life, to make Mommy well." The therapist said that she could not do that, even if she wanted to, because everybody had to live his own life, including him. He would feel sad, but eventually he would be all right again.

Looking back at the material and the child's behavior, one is struck by the fact that B began looking for another object even before his mother died, and increasingly so as her physical and mental deterioration and withdrawal became worse. This was most noticeable in his relationship to the therapist who became much more of a real person for him. He did not want to leave at the end of his sessions, though he would comment, "Your next customer is here." He implied that the therapist was paid for seeing him and wondered if the therapist would see him "even if my Daddy gets poor all of a sudden." On another occasion he suggested that the therapist could ask a famous baseball player for his autograph, adding, "You could tell him it is for your son . . . he may then give it to you."

B became more active in seeking physical closeness with the therapist. He came over to her side of the table and ended up sitting on her lap, asking personal questions and looking in her drawers. When he was gently discouraged, he said, "You couldn't marry my Daddy anyway because you are much too old." He wanted the therapist to call him by endearing names, provided it was "not 'honey' . . . because this is what my Mommy calls me." He gave the therapist permission to call him "Nectar" instead. The loyalty conflict was intensified by the fact that his mother's condition (when he did not deny it) was discussed with him and he then wanted to protect her from his knowledge of it. When the therapist discussed the various aids (e.g., oxygen) his mother needed and mentioned having spoken with her that day, B cautioned the therapist not to tell his mother about his revulsion when he saw her physical condition. She had develped a deep purplish rash on her neck which he called "a crocodile skin."

B had had very little contact with his mother during the week before she died. Although she was at home, she was under heavy sedation and often out of contact with reality; the nurse who looked after her tried to keep the children away from her bedside.

The day before she died, she was taken to the hospital, at a time when B had his therapy session, and the therapist told him of his mother's hospitalization. B wanted to talk with his mother on the phone and was able to do so just before she left home by ambulance. He asked her whether it was really true that she was going to the hospital. He turned to the therapist in desperation when he could not hear her low voice and then screamed into the receiver in an effort to reach her, "Speak louder, I want to hear your voice. . . . Mommy, when will you come home?" B's face was flushed after this brief last talk with his mother. Holding back the tears, he wanted to play at something: "I don't want to talk about Mommy." With an air of confidence which barely disguised his desperation, he repeated what his mother had just told him, that she would be back within a few days. Following the therapist's comment that this was what his mother would wish most to be able to do—to come back to her family—B started to cry and, as if he were an outsider observing his own reaction, remarked in wonderment that this was the first time he had cried since coming to his sessions. He accepted the therapist's verbalization of his sadness over the realization that perhaps his mother would not be able to come home by shaking his head affirmatively and asking why she could not die at home. The therapist talked about the special care she needed, the attention of doctors and nurses, the relief of pain. He then confided that he had heard his mother's moaning and coughing at night during the last two weeks, adding, "She caught a cold from me . . . but it wasn't my fault, I caught it from X." When the therapist explained the cough as the symptom of the mother's illness, B remembered the course of her illness, the "make-believe breast," which had so frightened him originally. He expressed some concern about having been contaminated in his comment, "Can I get her skin?"

B's mother died early the next morning. When his father told him, on coming home from school, his first reaction was to call all his friends on the phone to tell them about it. When he came for his session that afternoon, his mood was one of excitement during the beginning of the hour. It seemed that he was turning painful affects into the opposite. He was smiling, giggling, hyperactive with rapid speech. All his mother's things were now his and his brother's; he said, "All her money is ours . . . her clothes . . . we are rich now . . . even her bed and pillow." Laughing hysterically he said, "We'll take her bed and Daddy can roll over and fall off his bed . . . what will we do with all her clothes . . . to whom shall we give them? If Daddy gets married, we won't give her Mommy's clothes . . . would Daddy marry someone we like, would he ask us, how would we know we like her?" B asked for candy: "I'll need a whole lot today, three, four, six, I'll eat hers, can she still eat candy? . . . She is dead, she can't eat anymore. What would she say if she saw me now? [Therapist: "She could understand that you are really very sad."] I would give everything to make her better again." Correcting himself, he added that he just could not believe that his mother was dead: "I'll never see her again, never talk to her?" He finally broke down crying following the therapist's remark that he would think and talk about his mother because this was the best way not to miss her too much.

In this hour with B it seemed as if now that the incomprehensible reality had intruded fully, he did not know how to react. A feeling of helplessness rather than sadness seemed to overwhelm him: "Why did R say 'who cares' when I told him my mother died? What's the date? Write it down." He encircled the date on the therapist's desk calendar and wanted her to put the whole page in his file. When the therapist talked about the bewildering fact that he had talked to his mother only yesterday, he said, "She asked me to speak loudly. I screamed. Daddy said she couldn't hear well anymore—how come?" B wanted to know whether the therapist would cancel all her appointments to go to the funeral and why she wanted to go when he didn't.

During this session, B established a pattern of mood swings which he repeated daily for many weeks after his mother's death. He usually began his hour in an excited, maniclike mood, and it often took more than half of his session for him to allow sad feelings to emerge.

It seems to me that B reacted like a traumatized child, who was overwhelmed by a sudden shock in spite of some preparation for it. He was now under the compulsion to recreate it again and again in order to assimilate it. The traumatic effect seemed related to the overwhelming affects he experienced in spite of the fact that he had "known," discussed, and even reacted, to a certain extent, emotionally to the expected loss.

His behavior continued to show denial and reversal of affect. "I don't mind that Mommy is dead—I can look at TV now; Daddy lets me." He laughed and in a mock effeminate way paraded up and down the room. "I have her quilt and backrest. I want her jewels. I'll be very pretty. I slept in her bed last night." Externalizing the vague inner excitement which had replaced the previous denial of affect, B giggled and laughed, and often spoke of how glad he was that his mother had died; yet, he would frequently ask what she would say if she could see him now. This was often the cue that he was ready for interpretations of the sad feelings when they were phrased in terms of what his mother "might" think about him, i.e., that she would understand his wanting her things because he missed her terribly much, or her understanding that it hurt him to be sad.

B described this struggle as follows: "You know, I cried this morning when I woke up . . . because I remembered that Mommy was dead. I read . . . then I remembered again . . . then I went into Daddy's room. [In a sudden panic:] What if my Daddy dies? He could, you know, it's possible. Where will A [his brother] and I live? With aunt? I would love that."

B constantly worried about what would happen to himself and to objects close to him, as part of the expression of his helplessness and loneliness. "Maybe I am going to be kidnapped. When you went out [of the room] just now, I thought somebody could come in the window and steal me, and you wouldn't even know it because you would believe I was hiding to scare you [a favorite game of the past] and the kidnappers would kill me." He was similarly preoccupied with fears of getting stuck in the elevator of the therapist's office building (like in a casket?), that he might be there for hours and nobody would find him—or miss him. B tried to keep a picture of his mother in his mind, but her changed appearance during the last few weeks of her life intruded as too painful a memory. In an effort to block out this more recent and realistic image, he brought the therapist pictures showing his mother before her illness. He did this following a visit to the mausoleum, where he seemed to have been overwhelmed by the incomprehensible fact that she was in the casket but unreachable to him. He had wanted to open the coffin: "Would she look funny? She wouldn't have a pink skin. Can she breathe in there? If Mommy wakes up, how will she be able to get out of the casket? Does Mommy have a blanket and sheets in there? Does her sickness go on even when she is dead? I left a peanut butter sandwich there for her."

B expressed death wishes against the therapist, which the therapist interpreted as a reflection of his sadness and his wish that she had died instead of his mother. He replied, "What if a man came in and tried to murder you? I would run out. If you had magic, you would make Mommy alive again and make her live forever. But everybody would want to do this and there are too many people already.

The therapist had the impression that, although the child was sad and occasionally cried, his mourning process was different from that of the adult. B more often seemed to feel helpless and lost rather than bereaved. The painful affects of sadness could not be tolerated for extended periods. He would either deny them, reverse them, or try to find substitutes for the mother (without having detached his cathexis from her). After the mother's death, he became a "collector" of friends and had little toleration for being on his own because of the fear of having to face his sadness. When left alone, he was hyperactive, on the run, apparently experiencing an intense feeling of emptiness.

The strong identification with the lost object and the wish to take over all her belongings were partly motivated by strong feelings of guilt due to ambivalence conflicts in his relationship to her. Some time after the mother's death, he verbalized the fantasy that he bit his mother's breast when he was a suckling infant, thus causing her illness and death. With the mother's death, earlier fantasies of terrible things happening to him returned. He had fantasies of retaliation for his own aggression and suicidal thoughts, saying, "What will happen if I jump out of your window? I'll commit suicide by locking myself in the car and suffocating" (his mother had much difficulty in breathing). He finally said, "I'll be buried next to her," thus expressing his wish to be reunited with her.

A was sixteen years old when he began his analysis.[11] His mother had died when he was ten years old. His overt mourning response was extremely brief. He immediately developed symp-

---

11. I am indebted to Dr. J. Novick, the therapist of this case, who wrote the condensed summary here presented.

toms and character distortions, which subsequently had an impact on the developmental processes during adolescence.

A was not told anything about his mother's condition and, just prior to her death, he was sent away to friends on "the pretext" that she was ill. He was informed of his mother's death after the funeral. He was told that she had died of pleurisy. Yet he probably knew that she was seriously ill because he recalled many details connected with her illness (e.g., visiting her in the hospital, her needing an oxygen tank, seeing her read the confessional prayer). Nevertheless, he was extremely resentful about not having been told and felt that he had been deceived.

A's immediate reaction to the news of the death was to cry, but he soon got over it. At first he missed her and would resent others having a mother. Later he seldom thought about her, and it often seemed to him that he had never had a mother. He probably had no support during the period immediately following the mother's death. It seemed likely that the father's mourning was also aborted. The lack of real mourning in the family and the lack of support during his own mourning combined with other factors to produce in A a pathogenic reaction to the loss.

Following the loss of his mother A developed symptoms and serious disturbances. To start with, the loss of the mother revived earlier feelings of oral deprivation. The awareness of oral wishes led to sadness and the consequent frustration of these needs pushed him into a defensive, anal-based, pseudoindependence from the object world. Building on earlier identifications with the mother, A massively identified with the lost object and lodged his own and the fantasied hostility of his parents within the superego, thus substituting an internalized for a lost relationship and also reinforcing the negative oedipal relationship to the father. A adopted the mother's rituals, her extreme orthodoxy, her hypochondriasis, her intense fear of death, and her her avoidance of social contact. She was said to be unintelligent and mentally ill. A, despite his extremely high intelligence, felt he was stupid and feared that he would become mentally ill. His continuing psychosomatic ailments had numerous determinants, but a basic one was the identification with the hypochondriacal mother. He had a breathing difficulty which, although in part due to a catarrh, probably related to the mother's breathing difficulty during her last few days. He frequently complained of having trouble with his liver—the locus of his mother's cancer.

Finally, the following interferences, in terms of his later development, seem significant. The mother died when A was in latency. The material suggests that a somewhat brief and fragile phallic-oedipal level of organization had been reached and maintained. The dissolution of the oedipus complex had led to a considerable move into latency with a setting up of the father as the ego ideal, the displacement of cathexis onto oedipal substitutes (aunts, older girls), interest in friends, and the sublimation of drive energy into school, sports, and other activities. However, to a certain extent, phallic-oedipal anxieties resulted in regression to the anal and negative oedipal position. It is probable that A's pathology, prior to the mother's death, was within normal limits and did not constitute a threat to further development. The full pathological impact of the mother's death emerged with the onset of puberty and the revival of oedipal feelings. The identification with the mother reinforced an earlier negative oedipal attitude, and the onset of puberty was accompanied by intense homosexual anxiety. The ambivalence previously split between oedipal objects was now directed at the father. Castration anxiety was reinforced by the fantasy that the father had killed the mother. The castration fear was intensified by A's identification with the dead mother and by reality events (he had two hydrocele operations). The revival of phallic-oedipal feelings at adolescence led to anxieties of such intensity that A retreated permanently to the relative safety of the anal position. The death of the mother thus constituted a severe developmental interference.

SUMMARY

In the first parts of this paper I discussed the various factors that determine children's reactions to object loss. The cases cited in the last part demonstrate some of the characteristic responses: the short sadness span; the incapacity to sustain mourning; the massive use of denial and reversal of affect; the inability to grasp the reality of death; the search for substitutes (before the event, if the child was aware of the oncoming death, and after, if he was not); the simultaneous (overt or insidious) symptom formation and the creeping character distortions; the fear of "contamination" causing their own death, often side by side with fantasies of reunion.

Whatever the immediate response, we can conclude that the loss of an important object represents a developmental interference. In the case of P, a normal child, it complicated the ongoing oedipal relationships and perhaps somewhat prematurely pushed the child into relinquishing them. In the case of the two older children who were studied analytically, it was especially apparent that the personality changes introduced by the loss interfered with their subsequent development.

References

Arthur, B., and Kemme, N. L. (1964). Bereavement in childhood. *Journal of Child Psychology and Psychiatry* 5:37-49.

Barnes, M. J. (1964). Reactions to the death of a mother. *Psychoanalytic Study of the Child* 19:334-357.

Bonnard, A. (1961). Truancy and pilfering associated with bereavement. In *Adolescents*, ed. S. Lorand and H. I. Schneer. New York: Hoeber.

Bowlby. J. (1960). Grief and mourning in infancy and early childhood. *Psychoanalytic Study of the Child* 15:9-52.

——— (1961a). Childhood mourning and its implications for psychiatry. *American Journal of Psychiatry* 118:481-498.

——— (1961b). Processes of mourning. *International Journal of Psycho-Analysis* 42:317-340.

——— (1963). Pathological mourning and childhood mourning. *Journal of the American Psychoanalytic Association* 11:500-541.

Cain, A. C., and Cain, B. S. (1964). On replacing a child. *Journal of the American Academy of Child Psychiatry* 3:443-456.

Cain, A. C., Cain, B. S., and Fast, I. (1966). Children's disturbed reactions to parent suicide. *American Journal of Ortopsychiatry* 36:873-880.

Cain, A. C., Cain, B. S., Fast, I., and Erikson, M. F. (1964). Children's disturbed reactions to the death of a sibling. *American Journal of Orthopsychiatry* 34:741-752.

Deutsch, H. (1937). Absence of grief. *Psychoanalytic Quarterly* 6:12-22.

Fleming, J. et al. (1958). The influence of parent loss in childhood on personality development. Read at the December Annual Meeting of the American Psychoanalytic Association, *New York*.

Fleming, J., and Altschul, S. (1963). Activation of mourning and growth by psycho-analysis. *International Journal of Psycho-analysis* 44:419-431.

Freud, A. (1952). The mutual influences in the development of ego and id: introduction to the discussion. *Psychoanalytic Study of the Child* 7:42-50.

——— (1960). Discussion of Dr. John Bowlby's paper. *Psychoanalytic Study of the Child* 15:53-62.

Freud, A., and Burlingham, D. (1942). *War and Children.* New York: International Universities Press.

——— (1943). *Infants Without Families.* New York: International Universities Press.

Freud, S. (1900). The interpretation of dreams. *Standard Edition* 4/5:1-630.

——— (1907). The sexual enlightenment of children. *Standard Edition* 9:129-140.

——— (1917). Mourning and melancholia. *Standard Edition* 14:237-260.

——— (1926). Inhibitions, symptoms and anxiety. *Standard Edition* 20:77-178.

Furman, R. (1964a). Death and the young child. *Psychoanalytic Study of the Child* 19:321-333.

——— (1964b). Death of a six-year-old's mother during his analysis. *Psychoanalytic Study of the Child* 19:377-397.

Harrison, S. I., Davenport, C. W., and McDermott, J. F. (1967). Children's reactions to bereavement. *Archives of General Psychiatry* 17:593-598.

Hartmann, H. (1952). The mutal influences in the development of the ego and the id. *Psychoanalytic Study of the Child* 7:9-30.

Hoffer, W. (1950). Development of the body ego. *Psychoanalytic Study of the Child* 5:18-24.

——— (1952). The mutual influences in the development of ego and id: earliest stages. *Psychoanalytic Study of the Child* 7:31-41.

Laufer, M. (1966). Object loss and mourning during adolesence. *Psychoanalytic Study of the Child* 21:269-293.

McDonald, M. (1964). A study of the reactions of nursery children to the death of a child's mother. *Psychoanalytic Study of the Child* 19:358-376.

Mahler, M. S. (1961). On sadness and grief in infancy and childhood. *Psychoanalytic Study of the Child.* 16:332-351.

Meiss, M. L. (1952). The oedipal problem of a fatherless child. *Psychoanalytic Study of the Child* 7:216-229.

Nagera, H. (1966). *Early Childhood Disturbances, the Infantile Nuerosis, and the Adulthood Disturbances.* New York: International Universities Press.

——— (1967). *Vincent Van Gogh.* New York: International Universities Press.

Pollock, G. H. (1961). Mourning and adaptation. *International Journal of Psycho-Analysis* 42:341-361.

Robertson, J. (1958). *Young Children in Hospital.* London: Tavistock Publications.

——, ed. (1962). Hospitals and Children. New York: International Universities Press.

Rochlin, G. (1953). Loss and restitution. *Psychoanalytic Study of the Child* 8:288-309.

—— (1959). The loss complex. *Journal of the American Psychoanalytic Association* 7:299-316.

Sandler, J., and Joffe, W. G. (1965). Notes on childhood depression. *International Journal of Psycho-Analysis* 46:88-96.

Schur, M. (1960). Discussion of Dr. John Bowlby's paper. *Psychoanalytic Study of the Child* 25:63-84.

Shambaugh, B. (1961). A study of loss reactions in a seven-year-old. *Psychoanalytic Study of the Child* 16:510-522.

Spitz, R. A. (1945). Hospitalism. *Psychoanalytic Study of the Child* 1:53-74.

—— (1946). Hospitalism: a follow-up report. *Psychoanalytic Study of the Child* 2:113-117.

—— (1960). Discussion of Dr. John Bowlby's paper. *Psychoanalytic Study of the Child* 15:85-94.

Spitz, R. A., and Wolf, K. M. (1946). Anaclitic depression. *Psychoanalytic Study of the Child* 2:313-342.

Wolf, A. W. M. (1958). *Helping Your Child to Understand Death.* New York: Child Study Association.

Wolfenstein, M. Death of a parent and death of a president. In: *Children and the Death of a President,* ed. M. Wolfenstein and G. Kliman, pp. 62-79. New York: Doubleday.

—— (1966). How is mourning possible? *Psychoanalytic Study of the Child* 21:93-123.

Chapter Sixteen

CHILDREN'S REACTIONS TO HOSPITALIZATION AND ILLNESS

The emotional reactions of children to illness and hospitalization depends on the type and quantity of the stress or tension produced by the illness, by the hospitalization and by the fantasies—either conscious or unconscious—that the child elaborates around both situations. The final outcome is, in any case, influenced by innumerable other variables as well: the child's age; his internal balance and level of development; his adaptive capacity; his ability to control—within reason—the fears and anxieties that are provoked by the illness; the type of hospitalization and accompanying procedures, either medical or surgical; the attitude and reactions of the parents; the attitude of the hospital's staff; the environmental conditions of the hospital, etc. All these factors can either facilitate or hinder the child's efforts at adaptation.

Thus, we ought to address ourselves first to the effects of the hospitalization and the illness themselves on the child. Then, we shall identify those influences (social and familial repercussions, etc.) that both events may exercise in the dynamics of the family and in the child's reaction.

EFFECTS OF SEPARATION

Let us start by considering children under the age of five. For them, one of the most vulnerable points in the hospitalization is the separation from the family, and particularly the mother. It results in the sequence described by Robertson (1958), Bowlby (1960), and others of a phase of protest followed by one of depression (these are, of course, easily observable in the young child). In contrast, for the child between the ages of five and ten the significant factor is the psychological and symbolic significance acquired by the hospitalization, the illness, and the treatment. For him, these are the sources of danger, just as the separation from the parents, and particularly the mother, was for the younger child.

For the hospitalized child, the fears, anticipations, fantasies, conflicts, and distortions centered around the hospitalization and illness are important, not only as the unavoidable psychological concomitants but also because they can directly influence and prolong the illness (Blom 1958). For example, a child who is highly excited and frightened before a surgical procedure may well need larger quantities of sedatives and anesthetics and be exposed to danger that such doses imply. Further, present day experience shows that hospitalizations—especially when certain types of precautions are not taken—can precipitate various types of emotional problems in some children. They can also influence the future emotional development and the personality of the child. Many factors can contribute to this outcome such as the separation from home and parents; surgical procedures; medical procedures of a traumatic painful nature (especially when they are repeated and the child has not had appropriate preparation for it); chronic illnesses of various types; the immobilization that is required in the case of some illnesses and procedures; the danger of death; the hospital visiting rules; the attitude and education of the hospital staff in relation to the emotional needs of children of various ages; the age of the child; the specific stage of development of the child in the various areas of his personality at that particular point in time; the resources available to him, for example on the side of the ego, such as his degree of comprehension; the previous experiences in the life of the child (including life in general and other contacts with doctors and hospitals in particular); the type of mother-child relationship; the general health and dynamic state of the family; the general emotional health of the family, etc. This list is incomplete and not intended to cover all the possible contributory facts, but it highlights the complexity of the subject.

In any case, what I want to emphasize is the importance of examining all of these variables from the point of view of the level of emotional development reached by any given child patient. Thus, separations resulting from hospitalizations are one leading cause of later disturbances. Yet, this is dependent on the age of the child and on the level of development that he has reached. The infant up to the age of two suffers intensely from "separation anxiety" because he is an integral part of a system, a biological unit formed by him and his mother. To this genetically determined biological unit psychological ties of an intense and primitive nature are added as the infant develops. It is for this reason that the separation of the child from his mother so early in life results in what can best be described as a biological type of vital anguish. (This anxiety, in my opinion, has survival value. Presumably it developed through millions of years in the evolution of the human species. This same separation-anxiety is clearly visible in many other animal species; it seems possible that the social and cultural superstructure that humans have developed may hide its enormous importance.) Separation anxiety reaches it acme some time between the tenth and eighteenth month in the life of the infant, but is is observable up to two and half years of age. After this it is a much less malignant phenomenon, though still capable of affecting children to different degrees up to the age of five. Between two and a half and five years the child's capacity to tolerate separations from his mother increases markedly. This capacity is enhanced if the separation is well planned and controlled. This increasing ability is due to the advances taking place in his ego development and in the area of object relationships. It allows him to accept, for limited periods of time, maternal substitutes when deprived of the maternal objects. (It is for this reason that the age for entry into nursery school is generally around two and a half or three years and rarely before. Children three and four years of age normaly have acquired the capacity to separate from the mother and accept maternal substitutes without undue anxiety.) Nevertheless, if the child is ill, running a termperature, in pain, frightened, or hurt, he will lose this capacity. As we know, under such conditions the child's behavior is regressive, and leads to functioning levels much more primitive and appropriate for younger children. This is so partly because the advances in the emotional development of the child, especially in the ego area, are still somewhat unstable and tentative. It takes a certain period of time for the mastery of the new skills to be established permanently, so that children are capable of successfully resisting the variety of types of stresses to which they are subjected.

For all the above reasons it is very fortunate indeed that hospitalizations nowadays tend to be much shorter than they were some years back. We have to be grateful for this to progress in medicine and surgery, to the antibiotics, to our present medical ability to prevent certain types of illnesses, such as poliomielitis, etc. In years past, extended separations from the mother during the first year of life resulted, on occasion, in the rather dramatic clinical picture of marasmus. This condition led children to die slowly without any apparent reason for it. It was Dr. Spitz (1945, 1946) who convincingly showed how the separation from the mother, under certain conditions, led to the clinical pictures that he described as hospitalism and anaclytic depressions. Even more important, Anna Freud (1952), Provence and Lipton (1962) and many others have shown that a child up to the age of eighteen months, if deprived of the presence of his mother—and of the stimulation that she provides—is a child whose biological maturation is significantly delayed. Thus, for example, he won't be able to hold up his head at three months of age, he won't be capable of sitting at around the sixth month of age, and walking and language are significantly delayed. We know, too, that if this separation is prolonged, irreversible damage to the cognitive and the intellectual function of the child takes place. In fact, it might happen that this IQ will be affected; the child may never reach the potential with which he was originally endowed. The stimulation that the mother provides during the course of her ministrations to her infant seems to activate biological processes that favor the maturational processes of the brain, that is, the rate of myelinization in the nervous pathways, the increase of vascularization in certain areas of the brain, the amount of dendritization that takes place, and so on. In other words, it seems to promote the maturation of the central nervous system in such a way that under ideal conditions the degree of development finally reached approximates the genetic potential with which the child had been endowed. I discuss these problems in more detail in chapter 17. I have tried to underline those consequences of the separation through hospitalization in the small child to highlight what might occur beyond the effects that this experience might possibly have in the course of the illness itself, or of surgical procedures, or the difficulties in managing the child in the hospital ward, or the consequences that this could have for his emotional development or possible later neurosis. The child is thus in the middle of developmental processes that require a "minimum of conditions" so that development can proceed in as ideal a form as possible. Interferences with these conditions such as long-term separations, especially when poorly planned, can and will affect development on a permanent basis and in negative ways. It should be clear that after the fifth year of life, hospitalizations do not interfere with the processes just described. The separation is not by then the dangerous factor, except in situations that are excessively traumatic and unfavorable.

Early in life, certain close interactions between biological and psychological processes are required to mobilize the development of the various aspects of the child's personality. It is essential, then, that the hospitalization of children be considered from all angles, in order to avoid severe interferences with the child's developmental processes. If separations are inevitable, one must try to minimize possible damage resulting from it. I have referred to the level and quality of the object relationships reached at different ages and to how hospitalizations are capable of interfering with this line of development. A precise knowledge of these various processes is necessary for planning a hospitalization intelligently—one that will minimize, or perhaps avoid altogether, the possible negative repercusions.

CHILDREN'S CONCEPTS OF ILLNESS

It is for this reason that it is essential to have some familiarity with the characteristics of the mental and thought processes of children of different ages. The level of efficiency at which the ego functions at various ages is highly dependent on these factors.

Thus, for example, a child's capacity to comprehend such things as death and illness is extremely rudimentary and incomplete early on in life. Concepts such as these are closely associated for everyone, (including children) with hospitals, doctors, and hospitalizations. The concept of death is something that is acquired slowly and progressively during childhood. It is not usual for a child before eleven or twelve years of age to truly understand all the implications and consequences of such a phenomenon. It is partly for this reason that in the child's mind death is such a frightful event. He does not see it as a natural phenomenon but as a punishment, as an enforced separation from those human beings that he is attached to, like an exile from which there is no return. Death is seen, then, as an active rejection, an active exclusion, because the idea that one is no more is beyond the comprehension of a child younger than eleven or twelve years of age.

Exactly the same takes place in relation to the concepts of illness or sickness. The general tendency is to interpret these processes as a punishment, as a sadistic attack on them resulting from their bad behavior, their transgressions of the prohibitions set up by the parents, and so on. This confusion generally persists in children up to eight or ten years. Even then the degree of understanding of which they are capable, though it leads to a better and more realistic grasp of the situation, is still mixed with fantasies of this type. These fantasies have a universal character and are present in the unconscious mentation of all human beings. This includes adult human beings, who quite frequently tend to interpret, at some level, their own illnesses or those of close relatives as a form of punishment, divine or otherwise. If we add to this that many children have suffered losses of relatives during the course of a hospitalization, or that they may have heard accounts of the "terrible" things that take place in a hospital, we will be able to understand why these fantasies and anxieties proliferate in his mind. To this we must add the tendency of young children to think in very concrete terms. For this reason, they tend to understand in a very literal way all the accounts, real or fictitious, that they may have heard about hospitalizations. They apply such concrete thinking to their own potential experiences there. In this way distortions tend to populate the fantasies of the child. They are sometimes quite surprising in nature. It is these distortions that frequently explain the behavior disorders and the disturbed and anxious manner observable in children while in the hospital, well beyond what is reasonable to expect. In other words, illness, hospitalization and death always have tremendous symbolic meaning and significance, no matter what the present reality of the child's understanding may be like.

The same is true of the role that pain plays. In large measure that role is related to the symbolic and psychological significance that pain, and the fantasies that accompany it, acquire in the mind of the child. Given the special characteristics of the thought processes of children, the child that is in pain, for whatever reason, frequently feels mistreated, persecuted, punished, and threatened, as Anna Freud (1952) has pointed out. This is a quasi-universal norm for children, even in those cases in which the pain is not the result of external manipulations by medical personnel, but the product of the illness itself. This is due to the concretistic and animistic qualities of the thought processes typical for children at certain ages. Anna Freud has also pointed out that when the anxiety arising from the fantasies that accompany the pain is minimal, the children have a greater ability to tolerate the pain, and tend to forget the experience quickly. All the above should alert us to the importance of planning a hospitalization very carefully.

CHILDREN'S REACTIONS

Regression

Frequently, the negative reactions resulting from illness, medical procedures and hospitalizations are the result of traumas. The traumatic experience may be of major proportions or lesser in significance. In the latter case repetition may lead to a cumulative effect that will act then as a severe trauma. With careful planning, potentially traumatic situations can frequently be avoided or at least minimized. But this requires planning and preparation of the child and/or adolescent by means of appropriate information, always given in accordance with the age, stage, and degree of development of the child. A traumatic situation is a psychological state during which the ego loses the capacity to keep control over its function, and particularly over the amounts of anxiety that overwhelms it, as well as of the situation that is provoking it. As a result, the ego finds itself totally overwhelmed by anxiety, and either gets paralyzed or takes regressive steps, in terms of its level of function.

The type of reactions or clinical manifestations that are more frequently observable during a period of hospitalization include regressions in behavior and in the child's capacity to function in various ways. Regressive behaviors are at the top of the list of observable reactions. For example, the sudden appearance of symptoms such as enuresis and encopresis, or both, in children who had already acquired the capacity to control their sphincters. I mentioned already that ego skills of recent acquisition are the ones abandoned more rapidly. Sometimes, the regression lasts just for a few days, and on other occasions it may be for a period of several weeks, or even months at a time. In the most severe cases it may last for several years. The psychiatric treatment of such children is imperative, given the negative repercussions that such regressive symptoms can have on the future development of their personalities.

Another example is the case of children who have mastered language recently (be that in the form of spoken sentences or just simple words) that may abandon this function, reverting to more infantile types of language. The same is true of the capacity to walk, if it had been acquired recently. A contributing factor to this regression is that hospitalizations tend to place patients in a situation of passivity, infantilizing them to some degree. This is true of both children and adults. They are dressed, bathed, and fed.

Control is frequently taken of their eliminatory functions; special lights may be left on in their rooms, etc. In short, the hospital takes possession of the body of the patient.

Resentment

Anna Freud (1952) has shown that it is not only the adult patient who feels resentful of this invasion. On the contrary, children— and this includes very small children—are similarly resentful of this state of affairs. In the case of children it is the mother who is in charge of the management of their bodies. Suddenly, they find a totally unknown person usurping a function that in itself constitutes an essential element of the very intimate relation between mothers and children. This change is not generally welcomed by the infant. He experiences it like a massive interference in his relationship to his mother, so much so that he may actively resist the ministrations offered by the caretakers of the hospital. This problem is made more serious by the type of functions that many such people will carry out, such as the administration of shots and medicines.

The same situation applies with older children who have the capacity to manage their own body functions independently. These are children who feed themselves, can dress and take baths independently, and can look after their eliminatory functions. The loss of control that such an interference with these functions represents tends to provoke in them marked anxiety. Thus, this type of interference acts like a seductive process, encouraging regressive moves to more infantile levels of functioning, and constitutes a great threat to the ego of those children who have just recently mastered these different skills.

For similar reasons, nakedness that may be required during medical examinations is very frequently a source of anxiety and resentment. This is particularly so with children in the latency period (five to twelve years of age), since they have already acquired strong feelings of shame and modesty, and do not welcome being observed naked by strangers. It is hardly necessary to emphasize that all of these feelings must be taken into account and must be respected during the course of medical examinations and hospitalizations.

Some other forms of regressions observed in small children and infants are the return of thumbsucking (that they may have abandoned years earlier) or in the very young child a renewed interest in bottles (which they may have given up already).

An increase in demandingness, in terms of attention, is quite common. If frustrated this way, they may dissolve in tears and despair. Occasionally, these incidents develop into temper tantrums, similar to those typical for the second year of life.

It is possible as well to observe behaviors of a highly negative character, tinted by hostile or overtly aggressive acts.

Sleep Disturbances

Disturbances of sleep are quite common. For example, difficulties in falling asleep; clinging and demanding behavior, especially requesting the presence of adults; the onset of episodes of nightmares that awaken the child in a state of fright, etc. The content of such nightmares is related to the experiences of the day or of the previous days in the hospital, especially when involving medical or surgical procedures of a painful or frightening nature.

Rapid changes of humor that oscillate between a depressive tone and one of extreme excitement are common. They may be accompanied by unwelcome forms of behavior. This can occur, for example, around feeding time or around a given diet. In the latter case it may become a major management problem for the parents and for the hospital staff. Cases of juvenile diabetes are a notorious and typical example of these difficulties.

Tachycardia, palpitations, hyperventilation, diarrhea, etc., are frequent symptoms of children who remain in a state of anxiety while at the hospital.

Hysterical conversion reactions of various types are not uncommon either. They tend to affect the muscles or the sensory organs. It is of interest to note that some of the genuine symptoms of the physical illness are, at a later date, incorporated and/or frequently utilized as models for the hysterical conversion. This happens, for example, with vomiting, aphonia, disturbances of vision, disturbances of walking, and so on. The large majority of these hysterical conversions are of short duration, usually days or just a few weeks. They tend to disappear as soon as the child regains his emotional equilibrium and the excessive tension, due to the illness and the hospitalization, is diminished.

Occasionally, we can observe some types of responses somewhat more alarming than those mentioned above. I refer to various types of dissociation of the personality, reactive in character. Among them should be mentioned amnesias, and some pseudodelusional conditions. The latter are not always easy to differentiate from genuine delusions due to drugs, high temperatures, and the like.

SURGERY

Surgical interventions always have a significant impact on children. This is dependent, at least in part, on the level of psychological development that the child has reached. Surgical interventions tend to be a nodal point around which there is a tendency to activate, reactivate, organize, and rationalize such universal fantasies as that of being attacked, that of being subjugated, physically damaged, or castrated. As Anna Freud (1952) pointed out, these fantasies are an integral part of the common and normal content of the mind of children of many different ages. Thus, during the phallic-oedipal phase, the unconscious fear of castration is a typical manifestation of this, not necessarily expressed directly but in symbolic form. The fears of damage to the body, its parts or certain organs are a good example of this. It is for that reason that children between the ages of three and six show an extraordinary interest when they observe, for example, somebody limping, or somebody who has lost an arm, an ear, or a blind person. This interest is accompanied by quite apparent anxiety, and by a multiplicity of questions that are addressed to the parents. Behind all of this is the question, "Can this happen to me?" Surgical interventions are a good vehicle for such fantasies; hence, the special care and preparation required in the case of children who must be subjected to surgical interventions. In this manner, it is possible to avoid much of the potential psychological damage of which they are capable. We should note that such damage as may occur is hardly ever related to the seriousness or severity of the surgical intervention itself, but to their symbolic significance and to the type, intensity, and distortions of the fantasies that are associated with them in the child's mind.

Similar responses to those that take place in the hospital are possible at home in case of illness. Perhaps they are less frequent and less intense in nature, since children at home are not overburdened by the anxiety and the complications created by the separation always implicit in a hospitalization. Further, small children—and this includes the large majority of children between four and five years of age—need a certain perceptual constancy. They get easily disorganized in a perceptual milieu which is new to them; when they are not in those places that are familiar to them, such as home. In the absence of the parents this reaction is facilitated and takes place much quicker.

Another important factor to be considered is that children normally have a rather low threshold for the tolerance of pain, and certainly much lower than that of the adult. This low threshold for pain applies to both physical and psychological pain. This fact must be taken into account by all those professions handling children in such circumstances.

On the other hand, because the child lacks the necessary ego resources to maintain control when confronted with pain, fear, tension, or anxiety, he tends to get disorganized rapidly in their presence. As a consequence of that disorganization, he may produce responses that are maladaptive, negativistic, hostile, and occasionally destructive. Just as a high temperature is a physiological adaptation to an infectious process, the child also produces psychological adaptation in relation to the stress of the hospitalization and the illness. Consequently, many of the symptoms that are observed should be considered at least in some measure as reactive. This is true as well of the negativistic behaviors, tantrums and the like that tend to take place in the pediatric wards, events that are always an irritant to the staff responsible for the welfare of the children, both nurses and physicians alike. It follows that a great deal of tolerance and understanding are absolutely necessary before we try to eliminate, by different means, these so-called undesirable behaviors. As in the case of a high temperature, before we attempt to treat it we must know its etiology, the infectious process responsible for it. In the same manner we must understand the fantasies, conflicts, and anxieties responsible for the undesirable behaviors and symptoms. It is only in this way that we will be in a position to help the child control his excessive anxiety, as well as help him to utilize those means at his disposal with the highest adaptational value.

Many of the reactions described above are essentially the result of psychological unbalances, generally of a transitory nature. As such they tend to disappear in a few days or a few weeks. Though this is generally true for the large majority of cases, there is a limited number of them where the course of events is quite different. Child psychiatrists and pediatricians know how common it is for parents of children with severe emotional disturbances to ascribe the beginning of the disturbance to an illness or a hospitalization; hence the importance of the preventive measures.

PARENTAL AND FAMILY RESPONSES

It is also true that such experiences in early childhood are frequently responsible for the unconscious attitudes observed during adulthood toward illness, physicians, and hospitals. It should be obvious that if we are negligent with children, we are probably creating problems that will complicate the professional life of physicians who handle adults. It is said, not without good reason, that the quality of the early experiences in kindergarten have the capacity to destroy our interest in school, and in learning, for many years to come, and occasionally, for the rest of one's life. Similarly, these first experiences with physicians and hospitals will exercise a significant influence on the type and quality of the future patient-physician relationship. Experience shows that many parents who are difficult, and sometimes even irrational, when their children are in need of hospitalization or surgical interventions have themselves suffered from negative experiences with the medical profession and hospitals in their own infancies and childhood. Such parents can unconsciously influence in a negative manner the attitude of their children to physicians and to hospitals by passing to the child their own unconscious anxieties. Children are part of a social system constituted by the basic family unit. In that system illness, hospitalizations and so on, of necessity, create new dynamic situations capable of influencing the outcome in a positive or negative way. Serious illnesses in children have the potential to create very real difficulties and occasional crisis in the daily handling of the family. These crises are strongly tinted with emotional elements and it is not just parents who are affected but brothers, sisters, grandparents, uncles, aunts, etc.

Family responses are very variable. They need to be studied with care before deciding on the most valuable type of intervention in any particular case. Suffice it to say that the family reaction to the illness or hospitalization is capable of ignoring the emotional needs of the family member affected.

Prugh (1972) and Richmond (1958) have called our attention to a sequence commonly observed as part of the family's reaction, when in the presence of severe illness in one of the children. They have described a realistic preoccupation at the onset of the illness that is followed quickly by:

1. A phase of negation and incredulity that can last for several weeks or even months.

2. A phase of fear and frustration, usually accompanied by depressive feelings, guilt, recriminations, and marital discord, while the parents try to displace the guilt from one member of the family to the next one, or to the doctor, and so on.

3. The phase of acquisition of sound information, as well as of intelligent planning. This includes the necessity of learning to live with a certain degree of uncertainty.

RISK FACTORS

The following factors could be of clinical relevance when trying to evaluate the amount of risk involved in any given hospitalization, as well as the possible severity and length of the reactions to be observed.

First, there is the age and level of development of the child. Clearly, the younger the child, the greater the risk.

Second, children who have been previously identified as having psychiatric problems are liable to have stronger reactions.

Third, we should always try to determine if the child has acquired the capacity to separate from his mother and the capacity to accept a mother substitute. If not, the risk is high, and in such cases it would be quite appropriate to allow the mother to accompany the child during the hospitalization. It is then easy to conclude that all those hospitalizations, surgical interventions (elective in character), etc., should be postponed, if at all possible, to that time in the life of the child when he would have acquired these skills.

Fourth, it is useful to explore in general terms how much capacity the child has to express himself verbally, so that he is able to communicate his anxieties, fantasies, and misconceptions. The same should be done in terms of the capacity to react emotionally—to cry, to verbalize, or to express in any other reasonable form his hostility and anger. The greater the skills the child has in these various areas, the better protected he will be for the experiences that are to come.

Fifth, we should explore in general terms the child's reactions when facing new situations, especially those that carry with them a certain tenor of anxiety. Naturally, previous hospitalizations and medical manipulations are in this latter group of experiences. In this way, we can form a general idea of what is to be expected, while simultaneously taking any necessary special measures required in order to help and protect those children who tend to react excessively.

Sixth, if a child needs hospitalization, his capacity to relate to other children is an important consideration. It is well known that misery likes company. In any case, it is surprising how much support children can offer one another.

Seventh, it is important to determine the balance in the child's mind between a realistic understanding of his illness, the medical or surgical procedures to be employed, the hospitalization, and the fantasies and misconceptions that are associated with them. This balance must definitely be in favor of reality, at least for those children who have, by reasons of age, the capacity to understand.

PREPARING THE CHILD

The most significant part of the damage caused by these different experiences results from fantasies, misperceptions, and misconceptions, and not really from the reality of the situation. In short, the damage is largely due to the subjective interpretation given to these experiences. In order to obtain a good balance, we must rely heavily on parental cooperation so that the necessary information is communicated to the child. Unfortunately as we have mentioned, not all parents are capable of fulfilling this role. The pediatrician, the surgeon, and if necessary, the child psychiatrist will have to contribute more heavily to the preparation of the child in such cases. The type of preparation that is practically possible in most cases consists of:

First, the information to be conveyed should include a description of the procedures and what the child ought to expect. It must be given at a level that is appropriate for his "chronological age," and capacity to understand. The information must conform to reality and be given in a truthful spirit. It should be verbalized in a nonalarming, nontraumatic form. If pain is involved, this should be explained, with a careful description of all the efforts that would be made in order to reduce it to a minimum. It is helpful as well to discuss how the child can contribute to a successful examination or surgical intervention.

Of course, it is always easier to say than to do, a problem that is compounded because children cannot distinguish clearly between the suffering caused by the illness itself, and that caused by the various medical treatments that are utilized during the process of the illness. This is more so at certain ages. Further, since the large majority of children tend to interpret medical manipulations as punishment for their transgressions, disobediences, naughtiness, etc., this element will remain present to some degree. This will be so even in those cases where the reality of the situation has been confronted and explained as extensively and truthfuly as is possible. Perhaps the most important thing to realize is that we are trying to avoid traumatizing the child, if at all possible, but at the very least trying to minimize it. This can be achieved by offering the child as many opportunities as possible to verbalize and face his fears, his anxieties, his fantasies, and to understand the pain that will be associated with the different procedures required during the hospitalization. Given the many limitations of children at different ages, it is not always possible to do this in an ideal manner.

Second, the information should be offered with reasonable anticipation, so that he can have some time to prepare for it. A period of five to eight days is generally reasonable. The child may pose a number of questions during this time. It is important that he be answered accurately, without distortions or lies. Of course, this ought to be done with sensibility, care, and in an appropriate language.

Third, a short visit to the hospital previous to the hospitalization may prove of enormous value.

Fourth, it is essential for pediatric hospitals to have liberal hours for visitation. If necessary, it is desirable to make special arrangements for the mother to stay with the child on a day-to-day, or perhaps even permanent basis. Nowadays this is a common policy in many such settings and, of course, it is a practice that ought to be encouraged. In the preantibiotic era, the fear of possible contaminations or infections was a serious obstacle in this regard.

Fifth, it is important, especially in the case of small children that they be allowed to take some object from the home to the hospital; for example, one or more toys that the child is particularly fond of. Those children who still have a "transitional object" such as a blanket or a teddy bear should be allowed to take it to the hospital. Transitional objects are enormously supportive to the child, facilitating the maintenance of some degree of control over his emotions and fears and helping with his ego functioning in general. In the child's mind such objects constitute a symbolic tie of great significance with the home and with the parents.

Sixth, phone calls for those children of an appropriate age are useful and desirable. They contribute to the morale of the child by allowing him to maintain a certain degree of contact with the parents and the home. They help, too, to counteract some of the unconscious fantasies of desertion and abandonment that tend to inhabit the mind of the hospitalized child.

Seventh, it is essential that physicians and nurses take some time to carefully explain to the child those procedures to which he is going to be subjected, and the type and amount of pain that may be involved in the procedures. Naturally, the child should be of an age at which he can have an understanding of what is explained. In any case, this is generally possible even if only in a limited manner. Frequently, physicians and nurses try to hide from the child the procedures to which they are going to subject him. In this way they alarm the child—who becomes negativistic, terrified, uncooperative, cries, and may become violent. Unfortunately, this type of reaction can be seen on occasion, for a variety of reasons, even when the steps outlined have been followed. Nevertheless, the appropriate preparation of the child, though it may be somewhat inconvenient for the staff, can in most cases significantly reduce the traumatic potential of many of the child's experiences during the hospitalization. This preparation is indeed essential in cases involving medical procedures that cause pain, or that represent for the child an assault on his physical integrity. But we must accept that in many of these situations there is no ideal manner of handling the problem. We must thus be contented with the lesser evil possible.

It is of some help if, at the same time that we explain the situation to the child, we allow him to play with or manipulate some of the instruments that are going to be used in his treatment or medical procedures; for example, the mask in an anesthetic situation. In an attempt to capture his imagination, we can compare such a mask to those used by pilots or astronauts. The same is true in relation to stethoscopes, syringes, and the like.

Eighth, in the case of surgical interventions, especially in small children and with children of any age who happen to suffer from severe psychiatric disturbances, we strongly recommend allowing the mother to be present during the preoperative procedures. It is recommended, too, to allow her to accompany the child to the surgical room. It is important to have the mother present at the moment that the child will wake from the anesthetic. This is a time of great confusion and anxiety and to wake up in pain, and among strangers, is distressing to the child and potentially traumatic.

Ninth, restrictions of the child's movements are frequently necessary. Yet, these procedures should be reduced to whatever is absolutely necessary, both while the child is in the hospital or at home. Restriction of mobility blocks one of the best discharge channels of anger available to children, and particularly so of aggressive tension. Naturally, there are times in which this is unavoidable for orthopedic, surgical, or medical reasons.

When such limitations are imposed—and we all know how difficult they are to enforce—we frequently observe a marked increase in aggressive outbursts in the behavior of children. This increase in hostility and aggressive manifestations coincides not only with the restrictive period, but sometimes continues once the restriction has been ended. Benign forms of expression of this increase in aggression can be seen in a state of generalized negativism, and in increases in the usage of dirty words, dirty expressions, and offensive language.

Tenth, recreational and activities programs for children of various ages are a great asset to have in a pediatric ward. These programs should be run by professionals with a good awareness of the developmental needs of children and the peculiarities of their psychological processes. Such professions should be selected on the basis of their ability to motivate children and their ability to earn a child's trust. Well-equipped play rooms are essential. These ought to provide toys for children of different ages and with different levels of skills, and should include a fair representation of medical types of toys. The importance of the latter becomes apparent, if we understand that children use toys and play as activities that help them not only in gaining understanding, but in actively mastering many situations that otherwise would lead to anxiety. You will have observed children who, after a frightening visit to a physician, to a dentist, and so on, may adopt in play the role of the professional in relation to siblings, friends, or toys. This type of game, where he pulls teeth or gives shots to other children, tends to repeat itself ad infinitum. This repetition stops at the point where the child acquires sufficient mastery over the anxiety provoked by the experience. This type of defense mechanism is very favored by children, and of great service to them. We refer to it as "turning passive into active." Naturally, that is an enormous help when the staff is well acquainted with such defense mechanisms, especially if they are capable of eliciting them. In this way, they can facilitate the process of adaptation to the hospital, as well as the resolution of many of the anxieties of the child. For older children, educational programs are essential. This is particularly important in the case of long-term hospitalization. Such programs help the child to keep his mind occupied in constructive and positive activities and as such away from ruminations and fantasies of a negative or destructive character.

Eleventh, some pediatric hospitals are now experimenting with weekly meetings, usually organized by a social worker or a child psychiatrist. In these meetings the staff nurses, pediatricians, and so on get together. The purpose is to help children to control the anxieties provoked by the hospitalization, medical procedures, etc. Such meetings have as well a supportive and educative function for nurses and other staff, and as such tend to improve the climate in terms of relations between children and staff. As one of our colleagues, Dr. Poznanski, remarks (1975), "This tendency may well become the rule for the future."

References

Blom, G.E. (1958). Emotional reactions of hospitalized children to illness. *Pediatrics* 22:590-600.

Bowlby, J. (1960). Grief and mourning in infancy and early childhood. *Psychoanalytic Study of the Child* 15:9-520.

Freud, A. (1952). The role of bodily illness in the mental life of the child. *Psychoanalytic Study of the Child* 7:69-81.

Poznanski, E.O. (1975). Special therapeutic considerations: the hospitalized child. Unpublished paper.

Provence, S., and Lipton, R.C. (1962). *Infants in Institutions.* New York: International Universities Press.

Prugh, D.G. (1972). Children's reaction to illness, hospitalization, and surgery. *The Child* 1:177-193.

Richmond, J.B. (1958). The pediatric patient in illness. In *The Psychology of Medical Practice.* Philadelphia: Saunders.

Robertson, J. (1958). *Young Children in Hospitals.* New York: Basic Books.

Spitz, R.A. (1945). Hospitalism: an inquiry into the genesis of psychiatric conditions in early childhood. *Psychoanalytic Study of the Child* 1:53-74.

——— (1946). Hospitalism: a follow-up report. *Psychoanalytic Study of the Child* 2:113-117.

Chapter Seventeen

DAY-CARE CENTERS

The negative impact of poorly conceived day-care centers on the intellectual, emotional, and psychological development of children is so potentially great that an examination of some of the factors involved is imperative.

Obviously, the nature of the impact will be different according to a number of variables, such as the "quality" of the "care" provided in in any such given institution, the amount of time that the child remains in the day-care setting every day, the type of relationship between the child or infant and his parents, especially the amount of interaction between mother and child after he comes back from the day-care center to his home every day, and, most important, the age of the child.

In my view, the greatest potential danger concerns infants ranging in age from a few days or weeks to one and a half years of age. The second most endangered group (but less fundamentally so than the earlier age range) is those children between one and a half and two and a half or three years of age. The potential damage that can accrue to children outside these groups is so significantly reduced that we will not discuss here the problems involved for them (though there are some).

If we consider first the dangers involved for children in the age group of up to one and a half years of age, we have to examine at least three distinct sets of variables. Each of them plays a fundamental role in the healthy development of the infant (not only physical health but also good intellectual, emotional, and psychological development). The first set of variables comes from the child himself. The second comes from the type of environment in which the child lives, including those human objects responsible for his care. The third is the resultant of the interaction between the endowment (the genetic makeup of all humans as a species and that peculiar to each individual) and the environment (including the human objects).

BRAIN DEVELOPMENT

Those variables that concern the infant himself are in part genetically determined and are essential to certain characteristics specific for the development of the human brain. Thus, comparatively speaking, the human infant is born with an extremely immature, unfinished brain—it takes one and a half to two years after birth to reach the level of maturity that is typical at the time of birth in other mammal species. Embryological maturational forces push brain development in the anatomo-physiological sense to its completion. Such forces, though genetically determined, need, in order to complete their tasks, *the collaboration of specific forms of environmental stimulation.* In other words, the genetic developmental embryological forces cannot unfold the anatomo-physiological blueprint of the brain to its ideal potential without the essential contribution of environmental factors. This environmental contribution is in the nature of a diversity of stimuli that must reach the brain. The function of these stimuli is to trigger off and stimulate those genetic embryological mechanisms to complete its task.

Admittedly, this is still an obscure area, but the evidence available nowadays is at least quite suggestive, if not conclusive. Different forms of external stimulation (usually contained in the multiplicity of interactions of the mother with her baby) seem to influence the internal, anatomical-maturational processes by at least three different types of mechanisms:

1. *It seems to favour significant increases in a progressive and more complex arborization of dendrites during the first few months of life.* The importance of this phenomenon should be clearly understood. More dendrites mean increased and more complex pathways in the brain. More pathways mean more functional capabilities and better possibilities for that brain.

Conel's studies of the cerebral cortex of babies (1939) have demonstrated that though the number of cells (neurons) in the cortex is fixed at birth, complex morphological changes continue to occur for long periods of time. Thus he found progressive arborization of dendritic processes during the few months following birth without quantitative cellular increase. The situation here would be similar to a sophisticated piece of electronic equipment that has been poorly wired, where there are not as many connections between the systems as there could have been. Naturally, such a situation will unnecessarily restrict the functional capabilities of the total equipment. Richmond and Lipton (1959) stated that "since it is now accepted generally that neurons are connected in a network and not merely in a linear series, and that nerve impulses pass about the connections in a circular, more or less continuing fashion, the potential significance of this growing arborization of dendrites for the development of the infant may be appreciated" (p. 80). Possibly then, understimulation of the brain during the first few months of life, as is bound to happen in a day-care center situation (the reasons for this will be discussed later) may well lead to an inferior quality of brain structure (less dendritization, fewer connections and fewer functional pathways). Furthermore, such developmental maturational processes as lead to appropriate dendritization can only occur during a limited time after birth. If they do not take place then, during that critical period, they cannot be brought about at a later date. The damage, in the sense of loss of capabilities and function, is permanent.

2. *By increasing the degree of vascularization in certain anatomical structures of the brain.* The relationship between function, functional capacity, and the degree of vascularization of an organ

(implying here the amount of oxygen available to the organ) is a well-established medical fact. If the heart's vascular system deteriorates with aging and through arteriosclerosis, the organ-functional capabilities are seriously reduced—angina symptoms appear, a heart attack may follow, etc., imposing marked restrictions in the functional capacities of the patient. Similarly, an arteriosclerotic brain interferes with brain function; memory suffers and the quality of the thought process is affected. In extreme cases a senile dementia ensues.

Comparative anatomical studies of the brain of different species clearly show the relation between the excellence of a function in a given species and the degree of vascularization of the area of the brain controlling that function. Craigie (1955), for example, found that the "more acute sense of hearing of snakes probably is reflected in vascularity of the cochlear nucleus notably in excess of that in other reptiles, and the mobility of the tongue is suggested by a capillary supply in the hypoglossal nucleus about twice as rich in snakes and lizards as in the turtle and the alligator" (p. 28). The extreme importance of these findings for child development is highlighted when we consider that the process of vascularization of much of the brain is far from finished at birth. In various species it seems to take several months after birth to complete itself; moreover there seems to be a direct correlation between external stimulation of specific areas of the brain (after birth) and the final degree of vascularization that such areas will obtain. Thus, for example, Rao (quoted in Craigie 1955) removed the eyes of rats at birth and when they reached maturity proceeded to study the capillary beds in the visual centres. He concluded that there was a marked retardation of development of the contained blood vessels as the result of the removal of the eyes some time before they would have normally begun to function. He thought it "due to the absence of that portion of the functional activity in visual correlation centres of the brain which would normally have been stimulated by impulses coming through the optic nerves" (had he not removed the eyes). The same seems to be true of human babies according to Mali and Raiha (cited in Craigie 1955). These authors examined premature infants at birth and concluded that the density of the meshes in the cerebral capillary beds is considerably less at birth than in later life.

3. *By favoring the process of myelinization.* Myelinization and function are very closely related. Here again, there is hard evidence from animal experimentation suggesting clearly that environmental stimulation has significant effects upon ultimate structure and function.

For example, Langworthy's studies of kittens (1933) showed that myelinization is significantly influenced by neuronal function, i.e. light stimulation. By blindfolding kittens from birth, he demonstrated histologically that the optic nerve of the blindfolded eye shows less myelinization than the contralateral *stimulated eye.*

Sontag (1941) has stated that "animal experimentation suggests that the myelinization of specific nerves can be accelerated by stimulation of the nerves, and there is, of course, considerable relationship between the function of nerve fibre and its state of myelinization" (p.1001). Kennard (1948) has apparently made similar findings in human infants. Premature human babies whose eyes were exposed to light since birth show more mature optic nerve development than other full-term infants of an equivalent age at their time of death.

Richmond and Lipton (1959) concluded that these "types of studies seem to give support to the contention that, even after the foetal stage, environmental stimulation (or lack thereof) can modify developing structure in the central nervous system" (p. 82).[1]

1. More recently Cragg (1968) has stated: "The effects of function on neuronal structure are of fundamental importance to the problem of how neurons acquire the right connections in the developing brain, and how the function of the brain matures. In recent years there has been a great advance in detecting morphological correlates of more sophisticated 'educational' influences as well as the cruder effects of neuronal damage. . . . In the visual system it is possible to apply some degree of sensory deprivation without the use of neuronal damage, and to study the effects upon the morphology of successive orders of visual neurons. It must be admitted that there is no physiological evidence that depriving the eyes of light reduces the rate of firing in the optic nerve, yet this procedure has been shown to be effective in reducing the amount of AChE in the retina, in retarding the myelinization of the optic nerve, in reducing the RNA content and size of retinal ganglion cells, and in stopping the growth of neurons in the lateral geniculate nucleus post-synaptic geniculate neurons project to the visual cortex, and here a reduced nuclear diameter, a reduction of the internuclear material (cytoplasm, axons, dendrites and glia) and a

Thus far I have referred to observable anatomical changes. More recent studies suggest that maternal deprivation (in the pup rat for example) creates biochemical imbalances that alter some enzymatic and hormonal systems. Butler, Suskind, and Shanberg (1978) described how pup rats separated from their mothers and placed in an incubator for periods of one hour or more showed a reduction of 50 percent of ornithine decarboxylase (ODC) in their brains and hearts. ODC is the first step in the synthesis of polyamines and is generally increased in those tissues undergoing rapid growth and differentiation. This enzyme activity reaches an acme in the periods of maximum synthesis of DNA and RNA and goes to lower levels when the period of rapid growth in the rat comes to an end.

That the diminution of ODC in maternally deprived pup rats is not linked to the lack of nutriment was demonstrated by allowing the pup rats to interact with a lactating adult rat whose breast glands were ligated. Under this condition there is no diminution in the brain of ODC, a fact that, as the authors suggest, seems to demonstrate that ODC diminution is not caused by lack of nutriment nor does it seem to be mediated by the adrenal hormone. On the contrary, the studies seem to suggest that it is the active interaction of the pup rats with their mothers that is necessary to maintain polyamine metabolism within normal limits in the brain of the pup rat during rapid development.

Kuhn, Butler, and Shanberg (1978) described how an interruption in the mother-child relationship constitutes a "stress" situation with adverse results for the pup rats from the biochemical,

---

reduction in the density of blood capillaries has been detected. Conversely a visually enriched environment combined with training in visual problems has been claimed to result in an increased thickness of visual cortex in rats, an increased cortical content of AChE, an increase in dendritic branching, and an increased number of glial cells.

More subtle changes in neuronal connexions as the result of disuse have been detected by electrophysiology, but cannot as yet be approached by neuroanatomy. Thus if cats are reared from birth with one eye closed and tested at three months, the closed eye is found to have lost the ability to alter the firing rate of the majority of cells in the visual cortex. When both eyes are deprived of light, the effects are less severe, so that competition for neuronal connections appears to be involved. When the eyes are prevented from working together by alternating an opaque occluder between them or by artificially deviating one of them to produce a squint, the majority of cells in the visual cortex are driven by one eye or the other only, and not by both as in normal cats" (pp. 30-34).

physiological, and behavioral points of view. Shanberg and Butler were able to ascertain that ornithine decarboxylase is markedly reduced as rapidly as an hour after the maternal deprivation. It increases rapidly again where the contact is reestablished. They concluded that the changes in ODC are directly associated with the presence or absence of maternal ministrations. They concluded as well that ODC diminution is mediated by variations in serum concentration of other hormones. Their reports suggest that a diminution in secretion of one or more of the hormones of the anterior pituitary is involved in the biochemical sequelae that follow the stress of the maternal deprivation. With this in mind they measured the concentration of the growth hormone in the pup rats deprived of their mothers, finding that it was much less than in the control rats.

Their experiments support the hypothesis that maternal deprivation determines a neuroendocrine reaction that includes a diminution in serum of the level of the growth hormone and that this in turn is responsible for the diminution of ODC in the brain.

This information is consistent with clinical studies on human subjects indicating a reduced response of the growth hormone to the ARGININA stimulation test when administered during maternal deprivation. According to Shanberg and Butler, this could be the mechanism implicated in the lack of development observable in the maternal deprivation syndrome in human beings.

The similarities in the neuroendocrine response to maternal deprivation in pup rats before weaning, to the neuroendocrine profile observed in cases of failure to thrive in the human baby, suggests that the separation of pup rats from their mother may be an appropriate model for this human disorder.

Cummins, Livesey, and Evans (1977) concluded that the differences in the brain development of rats, achieved by means of an enrichment or an impoverishment of sensory stimulation, represents a retardation or insufficiency in the development of their neurons, a development that is dependent in the amount of sensory stimulation provided by the environment.

If pup rats are separated after weaning and placed in a sensorily enriched environment or an impoverished one, the rats in the enriched environment acquire brain cortices larger and more complex than those of the deprived rats. This greater development in the cortex is represented by a greater depth of the cortex, more dendritic branches, and more glial cells. These authors propose that this increase in development is due to social interactions and to the richness of stimulation provided by the objects available for exploration; all of this seems to stimulate in a nonspecific manner the cortical elements, and gets finally translated into a biosynthetic activity. These authors believe that during autogenesis the development of some neurons can be described as dependent on the environment, or that, in other words, they develop optimally only if they receive the necessary amount of stimulation from it.

The possible significance of all this for human development is evident. Research in this area is imperative, as it very likely holds the key to the secrets not only of many aspects of human development, but perhaps also of various types of mental illness.

Given that the adult brain weighs 1200-1300 grams and that at birth it weighs only 300-350 grams, we can understand the enormous importance of the mother-child interaction (as the provider of essential stimulation) during the earliest stages. Significantly, by two years the child's brain would have trebled its weight. In other words, it would have reached 900-1050 grams of its total weight and much of its anatomical, histological, and biochemical immaturity will be coming to a close.

Since the first two years of life seem to be the critical period for all these developments to take place, it follows that if the right kind of stimulation is not provided during this phase, the result may be a structure that, though not necessarily "damaged" (in the sense of brain damage), has certainly not developed to its full potential.

If we take into account the possibility of cumulative effects of this type, leading to inferior development in multiple areas of the brain, it is conceivable that the finished brain is one of "inferior quality" for those unfortunate children whose fate it will be to grow, during their first two years of life, under conditions of deprivation and understimulation. Such conditions are typical of a variety of environments, including, in my view, most of the existing day-care centers and no doubt those numbered in the thousands that are to be created.

Students of child development and child psychoanalysts have known for many years that raising human infants outside the family model, in such institutions as orphanages, foundling homes, etc., leads to disastrous results. Observation over observation, and study after study by a large number of workers in the field, have clearly demonstrated this. Naturally, poor family situations lead to similar results. One of the problems here is the balance between the time the child spends in the day-care centers, very frequently understimulated, and the time the child spends at home receiving adequate stimulation. First, we know nothing of how many hours a child can survive in an understimulated environment and still do well developmentally, always assuming that he will receive what he needs at some point during his daily waking life. Second, many people are demanding day-care center services around the clock. If they are available many children will no doubt be deposited for many days at a time in day-care centers; sometimes legitimately, as in the case of severe parental illness with no possible alternative arrangement for the care of the child, but at other times just for convenience and disregarding the child's needs and best interests, for example, parents who go on long vacations and do not want to take their child with them. Still, in many other cases children will be left in day-care centers simply because they have become burdensome to many of the new generation of parents. Third, there are many day-care centers whose service extends from 6:30 A.M. to 6:30 P.M., i.e. a block of twelve solid hours. During this time, there will be at least two shifts of staff and this raises the problem of multiple caretakers for the child and its complications. Further, even if children are picked up by their working mothers, at (let us say) 5:30 P.M., many of these women will still have to look after their homes, husbands, and perhaps other children, as well as having meals to prepare and needing recreation for themselves, etc. It seems quite unlikely that such mothers, apart from having had a long and wearing day at work or school, will have much time to devote to their infants.

These are, I think, far from the ideal conditions under which appropriate stimulation will take place.

As I mentioned in another publication Nagera (1972), Spitz (1945) has quite clearly demonstrated the tremendous developmental differences between the children of professionals, growing up in their parental homes (family model), and children raised in institutions. The first group (children of professionals growing up at home) showed a developmental quotient of 133 as the average for the first four months of life, and that average was maintained toward the end of the first year of life. The children raised in the foundling home showed an initial developmental quotient of 124 as the average for the first four months of life (similar to the first group) but, in sharp contrast with the first group, that average of 124 deteriorated markedly to 72 by the end of their first year of life. Spitz's follow-up studies, though limited in nature, tended to show that this drop in developmental quotient and its behavioral manifestations are irreversible once a certain amount of time has elapsed.

Similarly, Provence and Lipton (1962) have clearly demonstrated, by means of direct observation of infants, the appalling damage to the personality and more especially to ego and intellectual development resulting from growing up under conditions of deprivation and understimulation, i.e. by lack of sufficient human contact and interaction during the early stage of the child's development.

Some of these developmental lags can be "undone" by placing such children in a more suitable environment (a good foster home, for example), at the appropriate time. As I have written elsewhere (Nagera 1972), it seems to me that in another sense many such children are irreversibly and permanently damaged. I mean now that though they will catch up to the levels of the normal, at least in many gross areas such as language and motility, normality has such wide variations that we may have a "normal" human being who is permanently condemned to perform in terms of his intelligence, at the lower end of normality. To be graphic, it is the difference between somebody digging holes in a road and somebody with intelligence necessary for a university education. Thus, though "normal," our deprivational child-rearing practices may have blunted his original genetic potential to such a point that his best is an IQ of 80, while genetically, and given more favorable circumstances in babyhood, he might have reached an IQ of 120. (p. 186)

Clearly, no sensible society can afford to damage hundreds of thousands of its children by mass-producing and officially condoning, institutionalizing and supporting child-rearing practices known to produce such disastrous results.

Observations such as those described by Provence and Lipton (1962), Spitz (1945), Bowlby (1960, 1961), Ribble (1943, 1944), Burlingham and Freud (1942, 1944), Caldwell (1967), Escalona (1967), Harlow (1959), Pavenstedt (1967), Robertson (1952), Robertson and Robertson (1967, 1968, 1969), Tynes (1967), and Winnicott (1965) were essentially explained as the result of the lack of sufficient human contacts and interactions. The children observed were in reasonably good physical surroundings and their basic needs for food, cleanliness, hygiene, etc. were well provided for. Essentially these authors' assumption was correct, though they had not clearly made the link between lack of stimulation and poorer physiological development of the brain structure.

Clearly, then, the first step that we must ensure developmentally is that the internal maturational embryological forces unfold as ideally as possible, That, as we have shown, requires external stimulation of the kind and quality contained "usually" in the mother-child relationship. This will ensure the best basic equipment in the form of the best brain that the child's endowment has provided him with. But that condition, essential as it obviously is, is not enough in the human species. Most human behavior and controls are learned—a most significant difference from that of all other species. In the latter, most behavior is controlled instinctually. In other words, it is controlled automatically by innate mechanisms in the brain that trigger off adaptive responses after the reception of the significant signals and stimuli from the environment. Self-preservation, mating behavior, preservation of the species, food gathering, etc. are frequently regulated in this manner. No so with the human infant.

To start with, his brain is enormously superior in functional capabilities to that of any other species. Evolution has not provided him with the type of instinctual patterns of behavior described above and observed in other species. He must, when the time comes—since he is helpless and dependent on parental care and teaching for an inordinately long time—use his intelligence to deal with his environment, with dangers, with other people. His specially developed brain has provided him with the capacity to learn to solve problems in a variety of ways. In other words, he can choose "intelligently" from several alternatives, the most adaptive response in a given set of circumstances. He is not restricted, like other species, to a single stereotyped solution. He has the capacity for language development as a tool of communication. He can, and indeed has, established innumerable forms of social organization and culture. He can store and teach his descendants that culture. He can modify his environment to suit his needs and for this reason he has to a large extent the greatest capacity for survival, in terms of evolution, of any species known. By the same token, he possesses the greatest capacity for destruction, both intraspecies, and of his environment.

All these differences clearly demonstrate that he must start learning from birth, and at incredible pace, if he is going to join in an adaptive healthy manner his social group and its organization. This learning is predicated on an active and constant interaction *from birth onward* with human objects. The intensity of the contact needed to achieve this aim *is generally lacking under the institutional conditions* of foundling homes, orphanages and most likely in ill-advised day-care centers. To use a comparison, it is not enough to have acquired the best computer possible (the best brain possible for a given child); it is also necessary to programme it wisely and efficiently. The best computer, if mishandled and badly programmed, will be an inefficient piece of equipment.

We have enough evidence in the field of human development to know that the best programmer of the human brain and, as such, of human behavior is a good mother-child interaction in the first few years of life. Once that basic and early programming has been achieved, many others (in the forms of teachers, etc.) can participate successfully in the further programming of the human brain.[2]

One essential factor in this regard is the constancy of the object; the constancy of care of the object ministering to the child. The child's brain, at the same time that it is developing and acquiring more complex capabilities, must be exercised. It must be exposed to innumerable experiences, not only so that it will receive essential stimuli and continue to grow, but also so that it may organize itself, learning slowly to distinguish (given its capacity to think) inside from outside, self from object, and the body parts under its control and command, as that control is progressively acquired. Similarly, the child must go successfully (if normality is to be achieved) through the process of separation-individuation and must learn to use his ego apparatuses as these become structured as well as understand the innumerable complexities of its environment. Most important, he must learn very early to establish controls over his own primitive reactions and feelings. To further complicate the problem, all these developments must take place in a situation where the infant is not excessively subjected to undesirable forms of stimuli either. Thus, in the earliest stages, it is imperative that the child (the child's brain) not be subjected to overwhelming, traumatic forms of experiences that it cannot handle and that are enormously disruptive in terms of personality organization. Such stimuli, capable of overwhelming the necessary homeostatic equilibrium in the child, can come from outside; for example, excessive handling or mishandling, excessive cold or heat, multiple sources of unorganized sounds and other undesirable stimuli impinging on the baby for prolonged periods of time, enforced separations, etc. It can come from the inside when the baby is left to suffer unduly from hunger or pain.

CONSTANCY OF OBJECTS

Granted the ideal background for human and brain development, i.e. *neither too excessive nor insufficient stimuli* but the

2. None of this should be taken literally. Programming is a graphic word of some explanatory value, but as a term it possesses connotations that are inappropriate and insufficient to describe human development. Still, it expresses graphically some of the problems at hand.

happy medium, the child still needs some *constancy of objects* to organize its experiences, to understand its world. An example may clarify this. When a newborn baby is sufficiently hungry his pleasure-pain equilibrium—his homeostatic equilibrium—is disturbed. A disturbing feeling interferes with his well-being. This automatically leads to clear signs of distress which are picked up by the mother. This, in turn, activates the behavior of the healthy mother, who immediately relates to the baby's needs. Usually, the mother has a very ritualized, stereotyped procedure while going about getting ready to satisfy the baby's hunger and thus alleviate or remove his distress. She might go and see her baby, talk to him, manipulate him to ascertain the cause of the cry or other signals released by the infant (he might be wet or uncomfortable for a variety of reasons). Then she may go to the kitchen to fetch bottles and prepare the baby's milk. All this time the child is receiving a variety of sensory stimulation: the steps of the mother while she moves about, her voice if she talks to him (this tends to be stereotyped too), opening the refrigerator, closing it, sounds produced by the handling of bottles, glasses, spoons, pans, etc. The baby that must have been quite disturbed by his first few and new experiences of hunger learns that, after all the stimuli that reach him, satisfaction arrives and his hunger and distress disappear.

Naturally, once he has established these links in his mind (after a few good experiences of satisfaction) one can observe how his crying stops automatically as soon as he can hear the noises of his mother's activity in the preparation of his food. Thus, at this point, the internal distress is not a frightening, disturbing experience of discomfort, but one that is associated with relief and satisfaction. In short, despair becomes hope. Further, he has made, in a primitive form, the first connections between cause and effect, has learned that control pays, that waiting and being attentive can bring rewards, etc. Obviously, *these first steps in the organization of the mind and of the inner world* of feelings and affects, of learning and knowing something for the first time, are possible— or more feasible and easier—if the object who ministers to the child is constant. Her stereotyped, routine behavior and the sameness of this behavior allow the baby to find his bearings, to know the situation, or rather to identify it as similar to previous experiences and consequently to predict the outcome. A constant change of caretakers, with different ways and different manners of ministering to the baby—in short, the lack of sameness at the appropriate times—will, I think, make it much more difficult for him to find his bearings, to learn about the situation, to predict the outcome, to acquire early control structures, to be confident and relaxed in the face of the internal distress. Clearly, sameness, familiarity, and the repetition of similar experiences lead to learning, *to primitive understanding, and to organization, in the mind.* Without this early and primitive process of organization and integration, later learning becomes difficult. Constantly changing the system by means of which we attempt to teach the child something is disruptive and makes the mastery of the tasks more difficult, confusing, and hopeless.

This simplified example, relating to feeding and its significance for mental organization and structuring, can be multiplied ad infinitum in terms of what is happening constantly in the context of the mother-child interaction. It is for these reasons that I believe that in early stages *of the process of the organization of the mind* the existence of essentially one caretaker for the child—the existence of sameness in certain experiences, though not in all—is of enormous significance. After some time, i.e. after the ego structure has achieved a certain level of organization, the child is able to deal with more complex tasks even if some of the variables involved are changed frequently. The need for constancy of the caretaker still exists at somewhat later stages but that need is then based on factors other than the need for organization in the mind and for the organization of our first mental processes. These new factors concern the development of object-relatedness, its quality and the special dependence that is thus created between infant and mother.

Day-care situations will of necessity introduce a multiplicity of different caretakers to deal with the basic needs of the very young baby, precisely at the very time when he or she is in the greatest need of sameness of certain experiences. This problem will be discussed later on in this chapter.

The interesting electroencephalographic findings during the first three months of life seem to throw some light on the peculiar developmental processes of this period and on the enormous importance of the presence of an empathic mother during this time. As we know, the electroencephalographic pattern characteristic for most of the first three months is the delta waves, which, in the adult, correspond to a state of marked somnolence. These delta waves disappear only at moments when the baby becomes attentive in a special fashion (more frequently during the second and third months), at which points the functional capacity is heightened and alpha waves replace the delta waves.[3] The type of stimuli that causes the very young infant to emerge from his usually somnolent state can be presumed to be an increase of his internal needs, or some form of discomfort. At this point an empathic mother will come to her baby. The communication and interaction between mother and infant thus take place during a stage of heightened alertness and functional capacity on the infant's part. It seems plausible that the baby's experiences under these very special functional conditions are of special significance and that the contacts and interactions between the baby and his mother at such points (when the apha wave displaces the delta pattern) not only facilitate and encourage the child's ego development but also mark the beginning of an increasing awareness of the object.

I think it is most significant that the institutionalized child and the child at a day-care center will frequently miss this opportunity for contact and interaction with another human being when they are in a state of increased functional alertness. One reason for this is that such states are of very short duration, especially if no appropriate interaction follows. Also, they are quite likely to go unnoticed by a staff responsible for a large number of babies and who consequently must devote most of their time to coping with feeding, changing, etc. Further, these occasional states of alertness

3. Oswald (1966) remarked that "the alpha rhythm is an indication that the brain is functioning at one particular level of efficiency, alertness or 'vigilance'.... When the alpha rhythm is lost in drowsiness, the brain is functioning at a lower level of effectiveness" (p. 21).

during the first few weeks of life usually charm mothers, who respond intensely and in kind to the child, as all those who have had the opportunity to observe babies and their mothers will confirm. Interestingly enough, this response is not likely to be elicited in anybody else but the child's mother.[4]

I believe that this type of interaction has a chain effect: such states of alertness tend to arise more frequently when the child is responded to. Thus the mother's response leads to increased alertness and to the wish for more contact.

It seems too that by the second and third months specific aspects of the mother's behavior—certain types of stimulation and play— will have an arousing capacity similar to that of the internal needs of the baby. Conversely, a lack of response to these early occasional states of alertness in the institutionalized child probably contributes to, and perhaps determines, his later more withdrawn attitude, lack of alertness, etc.

Though I have highlighted the special value, during the first three months of life, of the infant-mother interaction during the states of alertness, the value of the ministrations of the mother at other times should not be underestimated. Many such ministrations take place when the functional condition of the baby's brain is of the somnolent type (delta-wave pattern).[5] Naturally, their impact on the baby is of a different quality. At this time things happen to him when he is not alloplastically orientated (as in the state of alertness). Nevertheless, the ministrations of the mother under the delta-wave conditions do provide him with a wide range of new sensory stimulation that makes contributions to the functional awakening and the gradual development of different ego apparatuses and structures and, at the beginning, perhaps more

4. After all, mothers gain as much pleasure as the child does from these interactions. A healthy, empathic mother takes enormous pride in her infant, in what she does for him, in his little achievements as they occur and radiates back this pleasure and warmth to the child. It is of course not possible to expect that quality and warmth in the communications between a stranger and an infant. After all, the mother has been prepared for this response biologically and psychologically by her nine months of pregnancy. That pregnancy and that infant have an emotional and psychological value to her (in a normal situation) that is unique and cannot easily be replicated by somebody who is "doing a job" and is dealing with many infants simultaneously.

5. Feeding of very young infants often takes place under this condition.

especially the perceptual one. Through these ministrations the mother manages to provide much of the necessary and basic conditions of minimum comfort and well-being, without which ego development will not proceed normally.

SEPARATION

One could discuss too the implications that the day-care centers will have at different developmental stages, i.e. the possibility of delays in the typical developmental milestones, smiling, hand-eye and ego integration, holding the head, babbling, sitting, crawling, walking, talking, etc. and the impact that such early developmental delays (and what they signify) might have in the final organization of the personality and on its quality. However, such a task will lead us too far afield. Furthermore, the paucity of our knowledge in this regard may make the effort unrewarding at this time. Think, for example, of the phenomenon of the stranger anxiety that appears about the tenth month of life, sometimes earlier, sometimes later. We can say with certainty that the child at such a time is distressed at the recognition or approach of a stranger, partly because it highlights his own mother's absence. Babies' distress in this situation varies greatly, but some do become markedly upset and disturbed if handed to a stranger, or if a stranger forces his presence on them. One cannot but wonder what the day-care situation does to babies suffering acutely from stranger anxiety, since many strangers will not only approach them but force their ministrations upon them. In this case, as in many others, we are not in a position to give definite answers as to the possible implications for the child's development of this type of mismanagement. Yet it seems, at the very least, unwise to force on the baby something against which his whole nature revolts, just because we are not aware of the possible consequences of this practice. What if we were to find in retrospect that it has undesirable effects on the child's development and mental health at a point at which we may have already subjected hundreds of thousands of babies to this experience?

By the time the child is approaching what Anna Freud has referred to as object constancy, the quality of the toddler relationship to the mother makes him extremely dependent on her, at a point when his ego development is so limited, that we know that he cannot handle separations from his mother (or his primary objects) without in most cases being overwhelmed by anxiety of traumatic proportions. Repeated experiences of this type, especially if they have traumatic proportions, are well known to have damaging effects on the child's personality and mental health. This reaction of young children is so well known in the field of mental health that we have coined the term "separation anxiety" to describe it. The term refers to the biological unity that exists between the mother and her infant, a unity that, if disturbed, leads in some cases to very unwelcome results in the development of the child. It must be clear that in this case we are not referring only to permanent separations but to transitory ones as well; separations that may last just a few hours at a time. Furthermore, we have sufficient clinical evidence to assume that, though separations from his biological object are always unwelcome to the very young infant, there is a particularly vulnerable and critical period in this regard in the early part of the second year of life. From all we know, it must be said that special efforts must be made not to expose the child to unnecessary separations during this especially critical period. At this time and for developmental reasons the child has little tolerance for the absence of his object. This is feared per se, but, further, when the child is confronted with the mother's absence his *automatic response is an anxiety state* that on many occasions reaches overwhelming proportions. Repeated traumas of this type in especially susceptible children will not fail to have serious consequences for their later development.

The reasons for this phenomenon are not difficult to understand. They are based on a normal relative imbalance that exists in three fundamental lines of development during the second year of life. The first concerns the ego, i.e. the degree of ego development reached or, more generally speaking, the child's capacity (or lack of it) to understand the happenings in the world around him, the quality and level of his thought processes, the child's ego capacity to bind and to cope with anxiety as it arises, the existence of an early capacity for introjection, etc.

The second reason concerns the line of development of object relations and reflects the level and quality that object relations have reached at this point in life. There has been a gradual development from the stage of need satisfaction, i.e. that stage when what is most important is the satisfaction of the baby's basic needs—somewhat irrespective of which object satisfies them—to that of object constancy. When the infant reaches the stage of object constancy it is no longer the child's needs or the object's need-fulfilling functions that are important. Instead, *the object,* independently of its need-fulfilling functions, has become the child's primary concern. As we know, the transition from the phase of need satisfaction to that of object constancy happens very gradually. It starts during the third or fourth month of life, gaining momentum during the second half of the first year and is usually well established (object constancy) in the second year, more frequently towards the end of the first half of the second year.

At this time, the child's interests are centered on his mother. His feeling secure and safe is predicated on the mother's presence. His reaction to separation is based on this simple fact, coupled with the ego's inability to distinguish as yet between temporary absence and complete disappearance, or even the capacity to link absence with the subsequent return of the object. It is no wonder, then, that he reacts with anxiety when the mother is not around. A child of this age has no concept of time either. From his egocentric position, and given that he feels most secure when with his mother, especially in situations of fear, distress and anger, he cannot understand that the mother is not there when he requires her presence.[6] Her absence, especially in situations of distress, fear, pain or danger, provokes an automatic anxiety response and, since the child's ego is very easily put out of action by anxiety during the second year of life, it follows that he cannot make use of the scarce resources that he has available in any attempts at understanding,

6. Here he is not different behaviorally from many other species of animals. For as long as they are too immature to have acquired independence, safety only exists in the pack and by the side of the mother.

coping, and binding the anxiety, the terror, that overwhelms him on such occasions.[7] He has not yet sufficiently developed the capacity to delay his affective response, to *pause and consider the meaning of, and the reasons for the mother's absence.* Parenthetically, I should say that no other animal species will subject their infants to experiences they are not endowed to cope with, except the human animal.

A few months later, this imbalance between the extreme fixation to the mother and the ego's inability to process information and delay anxiety is altered. The ego's further development makes the child's response to the same events quite different. Thus, we have observed children who in the first part of their second year of life are overwhelmed by their mother's absence while in the second part of the same year they were quite able to cope with the same experience without being overcome by fear. One child I have in mind, as an example, woke up during the night and went searching for his mother. His grandmother told him that mommy had gone out, as he knew, but had left the message for him that she was going to be back soon. The small infant turned around, walked to his bed while saying to himself several times, "Mommy will be back soon," adding, "Mommy gone to the movies." In contrast with a few months earlier when he would have been in a panic, he fell asleep again without any difficulty or distress. He could now master the meaning of her absence as his own explanatory addition to the mother's message "gone to the movies" demonstrates. It is of interest that he is able now to bind the anxiety which otherwise, as in the past, would have overwhelmed him, by means of meaningful thought processes. Note that at this time "movie" was for him a place where mother went on occasion and from which she returned soon. He did not really know the actual and concrete meaning of the word "movie." Anny Katan (1961) has shown how the ego's capacity to tolerate and to bind anxiety increases markedly during the second year because of the beginning of language development, which is no doubt correlated with an increased capacity to think conceptually.

Day-care centers will presumably accept toddlers during this

7. Adults, too, cannot think clearly when overcome by fear or when in a panic.

critical stage, something that ideally does not seem desirable. How to screen such children in their admissions procedure, how to minimize the distress of the child when powerful reasons force its admission, etc., are questions in urgent need of answers.

It is of course true that, in spite of the close tie of the toddler to his mother, he takes notice of and relates to other familiar persons, especially when they make efforts to earn the toddler's sympathy. Fathers, grandparents, older siblings and others become part of the toddler's enlarging world. Yet it should be clearly realized that these other relations take place only under the shadow of the relationship to the mother. The two-year-old child can spend much time playing with grandparents and others away from the mother (if these people can appeal to the toddler's interest), secure in his knowledge that the mother is around in the house, though not necessarily in sight. To assume that this behavior suggests the toddler's independence from his mother is quite mistaken. If she leaves the house, the toddler immediately demands to go with her and refuses to continue playing; if left behind he breaks down in tears and anxiety. By the same token, there are times and activities that as far as the toddler is concerned belong exclusively in the context of his relationship to his mother. At such points he will demand her presence and refuse substitutes, even those with whom he has a good relationship generally speaking. Bedtime, feeding time, when the child wakes from his sleep, when he is unwell, has been hurt, is frightened, etc. are good samples of such situations. All this shows, I believe, some of the violence that is introduced into the developmental patterns of the young baby and toddler by a day-care situation. The results of such violence to the system are not easily predictable, since children vary in their capacity to adapt to and tolerate stresses. The cumulative nature of the stresses introduced makes one fear the final outcome if such child-rearing practices become widespread. One thing seems clear: we will produce a different type of child and for all we know one that is liable to multiple handicaps for adaptation given our social organization and needs.

We know too that by the time the child is two and a half or three years of age he not only can separate for long periods of time, but can readily accept mother substitutes or surrogates during that time in the form of teachers, for example, in a good nursery school setting. Further, in a favorable setting (nursery school) he will be capable of profiting from the experience and of making significant developmental gains. Yet even then, we are familiar with the fact that if the child feels unwell, gets hurt, or is frightened, he will cry bitterly for the presence of the mother, in spite of his increased capacity to tolerate her absence and accept substitutes.

There are many other areas where a good mother-child interaction is significant. To mention just one example, Moore and Ucko (1957) found that *for most children an adequate amount of interplay with the mother is an important factor conducive to the establishment of an appropriate sleep rhythm.* They called this form of contact "excess nursing," i.e. a measure of the time given by the mother to the baby *for contact and play over and above what he may need for feeding.* Those babies who in their samples received the least excess nursing time had the greatest tendency to wake, while those who had ten to twenty minutes in addition to the feeding time settled best in their sleep patterns. Here again, it is difficult to see how a day-care arrangement, with a large ratio of babies to staff can fulfill such requirements. Theoretically, if Moore and Ucko's observations are correct, there is potential for sleep disturbances in these babies, with frequent waking up in the evening. One cannot but wonder what this will do to the mother-child relationship, especially in the case of mothers who have a busy day for reasons of work, studies, etc. and badly need their sleep.

PHYSICAL FACILITIES

Day-care center physical facilities should provide a suitable environment for a population of children that ranges widely in age (see Robinson 1967). For our purposes we are restricting the discussion to children up to two and a half years of age. A hygienic and safe environment; adequate lighting and ventilation; sufficient space for each age group needs; flexibility for separation of children according to their ages (since the needs of a three-month-old are enormously different from those of a toddler); rooms for resting; appropriate space and provision to deal with the feeding situation; flexible, multipurpose utilitarian furniture; appropriate bathroom facilities to include toilets of suitable size for a toddler; potties for the younger toddler; appropriate washing facilities for babies; an isolation room for sick children (especially important in cases of contagious diseases in order to avoid small epidemics); first-class facilities for the preparation of food; suitable playground facilities; a good provision of adequate and stimulating toys selected for their appropriateness according to age and their ability to promote perceptual, cognitive, motoric, and conceptual development; good first-aid facilities; easy access to nurses' services and pediatricians; a good provision of appropriate milk, food, bottles, and other utensils, as well as easy access to emergency services; facilities for the sterilization of bottles, etc. are some of the essential requirements. This is by no means a comprehensive list of basic needs for a setting where a large number of small children are going to be looked after for substantial periods of time on a daily basis. Nevertheless, it is easy to see that present ordinances regulating day-care facilities leave much to be desired and do not ensure at all that a reasonable environment and reasonable care be provided for the children. Many day-care centers as they now exist are about the most inappropriate lodgings one can think of, such as damp, dark, not sufficiently heated church basements, and the like. This is not only prejudicial to the children but demoralizing to a staff on whom extraordinary demands are going to be placed. Overcrowded conditions in the centres will be self-defeating. Not only will they interfere with safety and create dangerous conditions for the spread of many potentially dangerous infectious diseases of childhood but they will create a chaotic environment, with multiple sources of loud noises, occuring simultaneously all the time—a situation that makes adults tired and inefficient rather quickly and proves extremely disrupting to babies and toddlers. It is true that babies have (especially early on) a high threshold for sound. Yet this means mostly one type of loud sound. A multiplicity of sources of loud sounds is a different problem—one, in fact, that at the early stages negatively affects the development of the mind, interfering with the development of perceptual-cognitive discrimination, orientation in the world, establishment of cause and effect connections, etc.—as our multiple clinical observations demonstrate. Further, crowded conditions will interfere to some degree with motor development and the necessary exploration of the world around that goes with it. Under such conditions babies will have little opportunity, for example, for crawling and consequently for exploring, learning and exercising their already acquired new skills, etc. Much the same will apply to the toddlers, let alone the fact that toddlers are naturally uncomfortable in a limited space and overcrowded conditions. In the toddler's case one has further to consider their normal need to be frequently on the move as well as the fact that they do not normally engage in constructive play with other children and toddlers (that would somewhat reduce the need for space and equipment). As we know, there is only essentially parallel play in a toddler's organization, a fact that increase the need for space so that they do not clash or interfere unnecessarily with one another, and so that the more aggressive toddlers are not constantly hitting and attacking other less aggressive or smaller toddlers or snatching and grabbing away their toys. Such a situation will only terrify the less aggressive, more passive toddler, who already feels more or less fearful because of the absence of his familiar object, the mother. For the more aggressive toddler this environment will unduly reinforce his aggressive tendencies, making it all the more difficult (and more conflictual) for him to acquire the necessary controls over his aggression as well as the ability to impose the necessary restrictions over it. Observations of children demonstrate quite clearly that this type of toddler, with an excess of motoric and aggressive energy, needs special handling if he is not to find himself later on in serious difficulties with his aggression, with others and with himself.

STAFF

If we consider now who is going to staff the day-care centers we find that present provisions in law for the regulation of centers leave much to be desired. For example, in the State of Michigan the only qualification required for the director's position is *any college degree*. Most college degrees offer little, if any, information regarding the developmental needs of children especially in the age group from birth to two and a half years of age. The qualifications of other staff is totally unspecified; this implies that day-care centers will help to alleviate in some measure the unemployment situation. I seriously doubt that being unemployed is a sufficient criterion for entrusting anybody with the most precious and delicate possession of our society, our very young infants. Clearly some screening procedure is essential here to ensure that the disturbed, the unsympathetic and the cruel to children will not assume caretaking positions in day-care centers for the very young, nor indeed for any age group. Some experience with infants, some form of training and some natural maternal qualities are highly desirable qualities for these positions. Obviously, too, a minimum of training regarding infants' needs and ideal conditions for their development should be a sine qua non. Similarly, highly informative and simple courses on the major causes of accidents in babies and toddlers are required if many unnecessary tragedies are ot be averted. We have only to consider that the toddler group has an enormous incidence of fatal or very serious accidents, frequently by the ingestion of toxic substances. The toddler, as we know, tends to ingest the contents of whatever is within his reach. Similar dangers exist in relation to electrical appliances, unsafe toys, etc. Effective prevention of serious accidents has to be based on appropriate supervision, vigilance, and an increased awareness of the major causes of accidents for the age group. These considerations refer mostly to the very minimum of "quality" required of the staff. Another essential consideration concerns the quantity of staff required. In this regard the ratio of staff to children should be much greater in the case of young infants than of older age groups.

Since a large number of children will spend no less than eight hours a day at the centre, we must ensure that there is sufficient interaction with babies so that they receive the necessary stimulation. That interaction, as we have pointed out earlier, is more effective at certain times than others. The staff must be alerted to this so that they are ready to go to the baby at the right itme. The interaction should not be reduced to the time of feeding, cleaning or changing. It is obvious that if the ratio of staff to babies is not high enough, they will be reduced to performing the minimal functions of changing and feeding. Babies will be left to suffer from hunger and other undesirable stimuli simply because the staff cannot get to them within reasonable time, if they have to handle an excessive number of babies. Babies place enormous demands on their caretakers, particularly at certain stages. Babies within the first few weeks of life spend much time sleeping, but especially after six months and onward they require a great deal of attention, handling, and human interaction. Naturally they should be held and carried around sufficiently. They should be played with, otherwise there will be retardations in their developmental milestones, speech development, etc. Ideally, then, there should be one caretaker for three babies (at the most) in this age group. As mentioned in the first part of this chapter, it is most important that, so far as possible, the same caretaker is responsible for the same group of babies in a consistent manner. This may be very difficult to accomplish because of holidays, sickness, days off, etc., more especially in centers that are open for more than five days a week.

Another complicating factor is the number of shifts of staff during the working hours of the center. We know of day-care centers that are open from 6:30 A.M. to 6:30 P.M. and there are demands for services around the clock. The directors of many day-care centers feel that shifts of six hours are about as much as staff can reasonable handle. The question introduces the problem of multiplicity of handlers and caretakers for babies, i.e. lack of constancy of objects, the importance of which has been discussed earlier. We must take into account that even in the case of those centers that try to provide constancy of objects, the babies are, of necessity, handled by at least two staff plus the mother. The development of the baby's capacity for suitable object relationships later on in life is very much dependent on the nature and quality of these early experiences. What we have described earlier as the stage of object constancy in children—which incidentally is essential developmentally if a "normal" personality is to achieve a good capacity for object relations and otherwise—is somewhat similar to the process of imprinting in other animal species. One essential difference is that the "imprinting" to an adult human is a much slower process than in other species. For this attachment to take place, a multiplicity of interactions with the same object, during at least a year, is necessary. This type of attachment reaches its summit when object constancy is fully established.

This is in sharp contrast with the same process in, for example, geese, where attachment behavior (imprinting) takes place instantly and immediately after hatching.[8] Without wanting to stretch the similarities too much between human and animal attachment behavior and imprinting, the fact still remains that, in both cases, such processes are essential for the normal development of object relationships with members of the species. In the human, basic faults in the capacity to attach oneself to other humans lead to catastrophic results in extreme cases, and to very undesirable outcomes in less extreme cases.

On the basis of the information available regarding different types of child-rearing practices and their known outcomes, as well as our current knowledge of the basic needs of the human infant to develop normally and ideally, I cannot but seriously question the advisability for establishing day-care centers (for the age group I have been referring to) on the grand scale that the United States in now planning. I fear that the widespread and indiscriminate use of such facilities, for infants in the age range between birth and two and a half years of age, may result in the United States mass-producing large numbers of children with serious emotional problems and psychopathology. Furthermore, we may mass-produce large numbers of low achievement, low IQ youngsters, babies whose brains are understimulated and mismanaged and whose emotional development has been interfered with by inappropriate

8. In other higher species, such as dogs and other mammals, the procedure is not as simples as in geese. There is an ideal time during which it takes place, usually not immediately after birth, requiring certain types of interaction during more prolonged periods of time. After this, the attachment behavior is established and the imprinting process completed.

day-care center practices. These children will later on need Head Start programs and special remedial classes in school, and will probably continue to be in general and, in spite of every effort, low achievers. We are all painfully aware of the small return that Head Start program has brought to those unfortunate children whose fate it was to grow under poor environmental conditions in early life. This painful awareness has led to the realization that programs such as Head Start reach the child far too late to be effective. Hence the move toward identifying the "problem family" earlier, thus helping to prevent the damage to their children during babyhood and the toddler stage. This is a much more sensible approach since the disturbances that Head Start program try to remedy have their origin in early life.

From the considerations in this paper it seems likely that day-care center facilities for children (in the age group we have been discussing) is, to say the least, pregnant with dangers. They can be minimized and even averted if we devote a substantial amount of time, money, and research effort to understand and then to supply those ingredients that make for healthy development to children in day-care settings. At present, we are far from able to do this efficiently and with certainty. Careful design of day-care centers and extensive and sound training of their staff may go a long way in the right direction. Anna Freud (1967) recently restated what she said 40 or 45 years ago; that is:

> In this field [child care] we proceed to action without inquiring into the quality of the material with which we deal.... Work with metal, and ideas about what can be constructed from it, are based on the quality of this particular material. Whatever plans are made for it are made on the basis of the knowledge of these qualities—whether you can bend it, heat it, etc.
>
> But it has not been so with work with children. This has been determined by extraneous factors—by feelings about them, financial possibilities, social opportunities, religious motives, or the very personal motives of a child worker. I think that many of the unexpected outcomes and many failures have been simply due to the fact that the handling of children has not been based on knowledge of their nature ... I think very seldom has a conference [at the Child

Study Centre of Yale University in 1966] expressed as clearly as this one that we should start with the developmental needs of children, and that plans for children should be based on detailed knowledge about their needs and the possibility of meeting those needs. [(pp. 227-228)]

I admit readily that many families and mothers do not or cannot give their infants the time and attention that they so essentially require. There are many reasons for this. Sometimes they just have too many children, or have physical or emotional incapacities, or obligations outside the home such as working to meet the basic needs of food and shelter, etc. With others it is the appalling socioeconomic conditions under which they live that have led to emotional despair and apathy. A day-care center may be a welcome addition to the lives of these unfortunate children, providing much of what is missing at home in the form of stimulation, enrichment of the environment, adequate diet, a minimum of structure, adequate medical care, etc. There can be no question that some children would be better off fostered, in residential care, or in day-care centers, than they are at home. Indeed, the lives of some children, let alone their emotional health, can be in jeopardy if they remain with their parents, as the increasing instances of battered and murdered children demonstrate. Nevertheless, in my view, day-care centers should for the time being strictly restrict admissions to the group of children described above, and only after being well satisfied that no suitable alternative methods can be implemented to improve the home situation. Anna Freud (1967) has rightly remarked that if we really believe in the superior advantage of family care to any other form of care, much effort should be concentrated on helping home life to fulfill children's needs. We should provide financial support, advice, and guidance, with supplementation of home care by intensive day care geared to correct the lack of family care only when no other alternative is available. She questions whether the authorities really do everything possible to promote family care and make it financially possible. She points out that many children are deserted or become unwanted burdens to their unmarried mothers—children that in many cases could be kept by the mother or relatives and at less cost to society if support were forthcoming. But we should not turn what is a tragedy of certain socioeconomic, lower-class groups into an institutionalized norm for all children, condoned and supported by the state. After all, neglect in this area is not simply a job not done with the possibility of making up for it later. It is a wrong that connot be redressed.

There are as well, of course, other genuine conflicts between the best interests of the infant and of many young mothers still at college or university, not to mention high school, that seem to make day-care centers desirable. Here innovative solutions are required and some have been produced. I recall a television program showing a special class for unmarried high school mothers where they were allowed to take their babies and minister to them while being instructed. Similarly, we could provide videotaped versions of the courses that young mothers could watch at home. A videotaped lecture can be interrupted at any time, while the mother attends to her baby's needs, and be continued afterwards at leisure. They can be watched while young babies sleep, etc.

It is most unfortunate that many spurious issues have become attached to the question of day-care centers—for example, women's liberation movements that, in their legitimate search for equality of rights and opportunities, make blind demands for day-care facilities without considering *the equal rights of the child to develop intellectually and emotionally as fully as possible.* I am aware that it is only a small minority of extremists in this movement that will be unwilling to examine rationally the implications of some of these demands. Nevertheless, since they tend to be the most vocal and outspoken group we have an obligation to educate and alert all women—especially those who have reached motherhood—to the possible dangers for their infants involved in this demand. Bettye Caldwell (1971) remarks that at the 1970 White House Conference on Children, delegates of various women's groups were among the most vocal demanding that day-care services be made available around the clock, year in year out, for all who want it (p. 48). I want to make it quite clear that I have no objection whatsoever to women's legitimate rights for equality of opportunities in education and the like. But I do have, as I state elsewhere (Nagera 1972), the strongest objection to neglecting the similarly legitimate rights of infants, especially since they cannot speak up for themselves and cannot look after their best interests.

Another spurious issue that has attached itself to the day-care center is a political one. The liberal-minded person and politician see in this development a highly desirable aim. They are, of course, considering the issue essentially in the sociopolitical, philosophical sense. For the conservative-minded this development has the unpleasant flavor of a movement in the direction of an unlimited, unrestricted, and unqualified social-welfare organization. They, too, are taking a sociopolitical, philosophical point of view. I want to suggest that both approaches are incorrect and neither of them should decide this issue. The issue should be decided by a rational and professional examination of the factors involved, based on sound knowledge of the developmental needs and best interests of the child under present societal conditions. It will be ironic if the noble intentions of the liberal-minded citizen support a plan, in the hope of bettering social conditions, that in the end does not contribute to the welfare of the child, parents, or society at large; but just the opposite. It would be similarly ironic if the conservative-minded were successful in defeating a plan, out of sociopolitical considerations, that could greatly benefit large numbers of children and their families. Clearly, if made into a political issue the outcome could be disastrous.

Finally, it is perhaps not widely known that day-care center programs of the type we are now considering were widely implemented at the end of the war in several of the Iron Curtain countries. The rationale in their case was their desire to transform what were essentially agricultural economies into industrialized countries. For this purpose they needed more manpower (in this case womanpower) and in order to free women to work in industry they embarked in wide programs of day-care run by the state. Meers (1971) has studied this and visited these countries recently. I have been told by Meers that after some twenty-five years of experience these different countries are quickly changing and modifying this practice. Apparently, many of the children under such care have become severe social casualties, burdens to themselves and to society, to the point that the human losses thus incurred far outweigh the gains that were hoped for initially.

References

Bowlby, J. (1960). Grief and mourning in infancy and early childhood. *Psychoanalytic Study of the Child* 15:9-52.

——— (1961). Processess of mourning. *International Journal of Psychoanalysis* 42:317-340.

Burlingham, D., and Freud, A. (1942). *Young Children in War-Time.* London: Allen and Unwin.

——— *(1944). Infants Without Families.* London: Allen and Unwin.

Butler, S. R., Suskind, M. R. and Shanberg, S. M. (1978). Maternal behavior as a regulator of polyamine biosynthesis in brain and heart of the developing rat pup. *Science* 199:445-447.

Caldwell, B. M. (1967). A day-care programme for fostering cognitive development. In *On Rearing Infants and Young Children in Institutions,* ed. H. L. Witmer. Washington, D. C.: U.S. Government Printing Office.

——— (1971). A timid giant grows bolder. *Saturday Review,* February 20, p. 47.

Cragg, B. G. (1968). Gross, microscopial and ultramicroscopial anatomy of the adult nervous system. In *Applied Neurochemistry,* ed. A. N. Davidson. Philadelphia: Davis.

Craigie, E. H. (1955). Vascular patterns of the developing nervous system. In *Biochemistry of the Developing Nervous System,* ed. E. Walsh. New York: Academic Press.

Cummins, R. A., Livesey, P. J., and Evans, J. G. M. (1977). A developmental theory of environmental enrichment. *Science* 197:692-694.

Escalona, S. K. (1967). Developmental needs of children under two-and-a-half years old. In *On Rearing Infants and Young Children in Institutions,* ed. H. L. Witmer. Washington, D.C.: U.S. Government Printing Office.

Freud, A. (1967). Residential vs. foster care. In *The Writings of Anna Freud,* vol. 7. New York: International Universities Press.

Gavrin, L. (1967). An institution for young children. In *On Rearing Infants and Young Children in Institutions,* ed. H. L. Witmer. Washington, D.C.: U.S. Government Printing Office.

Harlow, H. F. (1959). Love in infant monkeys. *Scientific American*, vol. 20, no. 6, pp. 68-74.

Katan, A. (1961). Some thoughts about the role of verbalization in early childhood. *Psychoanalytic Study of the Child* 16:84-188.

Kennard, M. H. (1948). Myelinization of the central nervous system in relation to functions. In *Problems of Early Infancy*, ed. M.J.E. Senn. New York: Josiah Macy, Jr. Foundation.

Kuhn, C. M., Butler, S. R., and Schanberg, S. M. (1978). Selective depression of serum growth hormone during maternal deprivation in rat pups. *Science* 201:1034-1036.

Langworthy, O. H. (1933). Development of behaviour patterns and myelinization of the nervous system in the human foetus and infant. Carnegie Institution. *Publications* 139-143.

Meers, D. R. (1971). International day care: a selective review and psychoanalytic critique. In *Day Care: Resources for Decision*. Office of Economic Opportunity.

Moore, T., and Ucko, L. E. (1957). Night waking in early infancy. *Archives of Diseases in Childhood* 32:333-342.

Nagera, H. (1966). *Early Childhood Disturbances, the Infantile Neuroses and the Adulthood Disturbance*. New York: International Universities Press.

Oswald, I. (1966). *Sleep*. London: Penguin Books.

Pavenstedt, E. (1967). Some characteristics and needs of children two and a half to five. In *On Rearing Infants and Young Children in Institutions*, ed. H. L. Witmer. Washington, D.C.: U.S. Government Printing Office.

Provence, S., and Lipton, R. C. (1962). *Infants in Institutions*. New York: International Universities Press.

Ribble, M. A. (1943). *The Rights of Infants*. New York: Columbia University Press.

——— (1944). Infantile experience in relation to personality development. In *Personality and Behaviour Disorders*, vol. 2, ed. J. McV. Hunt. New York: Ronald Press.

Richmond, J. B., and Lipton, E. (1959). Some aspects of the neurophysiology of the newborn and their implications for child development. In *Dynamic Psychopathology in Childhood*, ed. L. Jessner and E. Pavenstedt. New York: Grune and Stratton.

Robertson, J. (1953). *A Two-year Old Goes to Hospital*. New York: New York University Film Library.

Robertson, J., and Robertson, J. (1967). *Kate, Two Years Five Months, In*

Foster Care for Twenty-Seven Days. New York: New York University Film Library.

——— (1968). *Jane, Seventeen Months, in Foster Care for Ten Days.* New York: New York University Film Library.

Robinson, H. (1967). A proposed day care experiment and its physical plant. In *On Rearing Infants and Young Children in Institutions*, ed. H. L. Witmer. Washington, D.C.: U.S. Government Printing Office.

Sontag, W. L. (1941). The significance of foetal environmental differences. *American Journal of Obstetrics and Gynecology* 42: 996-1003.

Spitz, R. A. (1945) Hospitalism. *Psychoanalytic Study of the Child* 1:53-74.

Spitz, R. A. and Cobliner, W. G. (1965). *The First Year of Life.* New York: International Universities Press.

Tynes, H. (1967). A residential nursery for very young babies. In *On Rearing Infants and Young Children in Institutions*, ed. H. L. Witmer. Washington, D.C.: U. S. Government Printing Office.

Winnicott, D. W. (1965). *The Maturational Process and the Facilitating Environment.* New York: International Universities Press.

Chapter Eighteen

THE PRIMARY CARETAKER SYSTEM: A METHOD FOR RUNNING INPATIENT UNITS FOR CHILDREN

In September of 1974 the Children's Psychiatric Hospital initiated a new functional structure in its inpatient services for children, a structure based, on the type of relationship we considered necessary, indeed essential, between the children and the ward staff if a therapeutic climate was to prevail. It gradually came to be known as the Primary Caretaker System, a term that refers to the fact that two children are assigned to the care of one senior staff on a permanent basis. The role of the primary caretaker in the life of the children on the ward is based on the one hand on the family model, and on the other on considerations of the developmental rights and developmental needs of children. Obviously, every attempt must be made to meet these different rights and needs in the somewhat "abnormal" situation of an inpatient ward. The primary caretaker is completely responsible for the behavior and welfare of these two children. This arrangement also attempts to take into account the fact that the removal of a child from his family and into an institution poses many dangers for the normal unfolding of the child's developmental potential. These dangers are twofold, some come form the separation itself, and others are related to the experiences the child may be exposed to in an institution. Thus, we have to consider the contradictory situation that while we are attempting to "cure" the child of various types of "psychopathology," "abnormal behaviors," etc., we might be contributing to the development of problems in the child as serious, if not more serious than the ones that brought him to us originally.

THE PRIMARY CARETAKER SYSTEM RATIONALE

In the new system the primary caretaker is assigned responsibility for two children and two children only. He or she is expected to play the role of a parent surrogate for the two children for as long as the children are in the service. Each primary caretaker and his or her two children are conceived of as a small "family unit" within the ward. Since there are as many as 18 children per ward there are as many as nine different family units on each ward. It is to be expected that no two of these families are alike, just as in the real world. Each family thus is a unique organization that must make the necessary adjustments to each others' personalities, character, likes and dislikes, etc. as well as to the specific behavioral abnormalities and psychopathologies of the children. Yet at the same time and within as much behavioral and adaptational flexibility as each family must provide for each of its members, they must set a number of appropriate limits. This is necessary in order to have a smooth and healthy relationship within the family itself as well as with every other family and their members. Similarly, all the families belong in a larger social system, the ward. Like all societies, the wards require certain regulations to ensure the welfare of all of its members. These must be kept not only by the families as families, but by each one of the members of each family as part of the larger society. The golden rule here is that the rights of any one child (or family) end at the point when they interfere inappropriately with the rights of the other children (or families), the staff generally, and/or the institution.

In this way the wards reproduce to a reasonable degree the structure and organization of society at large. They are a sort of experimental model of it. More important, this structure offers an excellent opportunity to observe, study, handle, and teach the child the adaptational and interactional skills that he may not have. The lack may be the result on the one hand of inappropriate early experiences, lack of opportunity, lack of education, the disturbed or abnormal family patterns of interaction, the psychopathology of the family as a group, or the psychopathology of the parents. On the other hand, the child's lack may be due to the nature of his own psychological conflicts and needs, the nature of his psychopathology, his developmental conflicts, his developmental stage, etc.

In this "experimental society" of the ward the child is afforded plenty of opportunity to be educated in social manners and social interactions. This educative aspect should not be demeaned on the basis that that is not "treatment". In fact, this is indeed an essential and integral part of the treatment of the child. They are an important part of raising children, which in this context means using appropriate educational means that help to unfold those developmental processes in the child that hopefully lead to a well-balanced, mature adult. Thus, children have the opportunity to learn that there are many other styles of behavior and interaction than those to which they have been exposed so far in their own families, or in their own social groups. Many of our children come from backgrounds (familial and societal) that do not give much opportunity to learn these skills and thereby to produce positive ego-building identifications and ideals that promote human growth, favor the avoidance and/or resolution of conflicts, and help to control behavior. Further, the children can see in actual life the positive benefits to be derived from the use of the alternative styles. They can soon identify those modes of behavior and interactional styles that not only give the most pleasure, but yield the most positive results in terms of their own well-being and welfare. In this context too there are many opportunities for corrective emotional experiences that tend to favor positive internalizations and constructive identifications that enrich the personality and facilitate adaptation to society.

Other children's interactional difficulties and behaviors result from specific conflicts, and are the natural outcome of their psychopathology. For them, our setting highlights the causative factors. Thus sibling rivalry, envy, jealousy, anal-sadistic interactions, oedipal conflicts, superego defects, etc. are offered a context for reasonable and controlled expression. Furthermore, the setting allows the parent surrogate to directly and constantly observe over extended periods of time how the abnormal behavior triggers itself off, or evolves around various incidents. Such observations are invaluable as communications to the child therapist who can gain much insight by coupling it with the productions of the child during therapy. He or she is thus in a much better position to understand and interpret the behavior and problems of the child.

The obvious advantage of the primary caretaker system in this area is that the primary caretaker only has to attend to and interact with his or her two children. Though there is a "milieu" and, in my view, a very "therapeutic" one, it is not a situation where all the members of the milieu tend to take care of and interact with any one of the children for brief periods of time, in an indiscriminate manner, or according to need. In my view the latter system is less efficient for getting to know the children intimately, providing the kind of emotional climate necessary for the "milieu" to be therapeutic, or providing therapists with consistent, long-term, meaningful observations of a specific child.

The Primary Caretaker's Relation to His Wards

The primary caretaker is a permanent member of the staff, generally either a psychiatric nurse or a psychiatric care worker. Attempts should always be made to find a primary caretaker whose personality and character fits the specific children well. Similarly, appropriate "matching" of the two siblings is highly desirable. All this requires an extensive and detailed clinical evaluation of the children and a good working knowledge of the personality, skills, and lags of those performing the role of primary caretakers.

Usually the head nurse and the chief of the unit have best working knowledge of the assets and shortcomings of any given staff. The child's assignments to the primary caretaker should generally be a "team decision" after careful consideration of all the factors and information available. The assigned "therapist" of the child (and his or her supervisor if there is one) would naturally be involved in the decision making as well.

The primary caretaker function is very much that of a parent surrogate. He organizes the child's day, sets the limits, controls the behavior, and offers the rewards. Like any parent he is concerned with the behavior and welfare of the child not only during the hours he or she actually spends with the child, but is concerned about the child's behavior at school, school lunch hour, as well as with his clothing, toys, and general health, etc. If any restrictions of privileges or "punishments" are required, he will determine what these are to be, length of time, and so on. Thus he functiions as an ego auxiliary when necessary and plays the role of an ego and superego ideal. Like any parent, he or she also holds the power of rewarding as generously and effusively as required the child's accomplishments and positive behavior.

After school hours the parent surrogate is constantly available to his two children. He stays with them through the dinner period and settles them in bed for the evening. His or her shift starts at 3:00 P.M. and ends at 11:30 P.M. by which time the children have been in bed and sleeping for one or two hours.

Children in the age group we are describing (4 or 5 to 13 years) need the structure provided by a meaningful adult in their life. The younger they are the more this is true. They need clear, consistent, fair, predictable, and age-appropriate limits. They need the positive rewards, admiration, affection, and narcissistic supplies that their meaningful adults (usually the parents) must supply. They need adults to help master the struggle with their own impulses and to keep their behavior within the boundaries of such limits, when they are unable to do so by themselves. Yet, for all this to happen as ideally as possible it is absolutely fundamental that the adult object available to the child (the primary caretaker) to be a constant one, daily and through the weeks and months of the treatment. The more objects that share the care of the child, the less consistent and intimate the relationship to the one adult is, the more we are departing from those ideal conditions necessary to ensure not only the therapeutic climate, but also the type of relationship and environment in which children's development thrives.

The more the role of the primary caretaker is diluted and distributed among several members of the staff, the less effective the system becomes. Unfortunately it is not only that the system becomes *less effective*—it can in fact become detrimental to the welfare of the child and his best developmental interests. Systems that do not take the above as one of the basic rules for inpatient services for children are not effective and may well be very damaging.

Briefly then, the emotional growth, character development, and general well-being of a child up to the end of the latency stage require a satisfactory interaction with a meaningful, constant adult—one that the child admires, values, and preferably loves. That person is in fact the catalyst that sustains not only growth but the development of those controls that are necessary for living in an organized society. He is also one of the essential motivational sources of the behavior of the child. For example, the child will tend not to follow the pleasure principle as blindly as he would for much of the time only because his meaningful adult will be distressed if he does. In return the child expects affection, support, admiration, and genuine concern. Fortunately, the meaningful adult's influence on the child grows so large in the emotional feeling tone of the child that the latter is more than willing to accept limits, renounce gratifications or postpone them, accept deprivations, etc. for the sake of the valued object. In short, human beings are educable because in the competition between instincts and objects, objects end up by gaining the upper hand—but only if they are valued, if they become significant to the child.

It follows then that the primary caretaker system relies heavily on these characteristics and developmental needs of children. It relies too on the fact that in the absence of his primary objects, the child is willing to accept a substitute, a parent surrogate.

Clearly then the primary caretaker's essential task is to make himself or herself, valuable and meaningful to the child. This implies that the primary caretaker must elicit as many as possible of the positive transferential elements of which the child is capable. The process is very much facilitated in an inpatient setting by the fact that the child is away from his parents or other figures in his life. And if there were none we are in the privileged position of providing them for the first time, thus fulfilling some of the most basic rights and needs of the child.

In this respect the objection is raised that we are giving such children a temporary haven from which they will have to return to a devastating home situation. At least in some cases, this is certainly true. Nevertheless, we should not forget that the child is right in the middle of his or her development. For this reason a period of time in an environment that promotes their personality growth along the right paths may be invaluable to the child's future. The corrective emotional experiences he will be exposed to may well show him alternatives that he may one day take. This could be so if the total experience was a treasured one that led to growth in some important areas.

Children come into this relationship like an organic chemical compound with an open valence. As such chemicals do, the child will strongly link himself with the right compound, the right person, since this in fact is a developmental imperative for him. The linkage will not happen automatically, just because the child has the need. The primary caretaker must earn the attachment through his attitude toward the child and his interactions with him.

Beyond a general positive attitude toward children, there are other things favoring the establishment of a meaningful relationship: the ability to "come down" to their level, to be sensitive to their needs; the ability to be flexible and yet firm; the capacity to become genuinely interested in the child's activities; the capacity to play with him; the capacity to love him without becoming seductive; the ability to be flexible and fair, the ability to see the child as a person in his own right, and the ability to respect the child's idiosyncrasies within reasonable limits.

Since the primary caretaker is given the most influential role in the child's life, he can use this position to great advantage. He or she can gratify or deny the wishes of the child, and negotiate on his behalf with other staff (including the therapist). He is the child's advocate in relation to things and situations that are of interest to the child. In addition, the primary caretaker takes the child out into the community after school hours for activities and functions that are highly desirable and pleasurable for him. As far as possible, this should be done as a family, and not in large groups. On occasion, of course, two or three families can go together, as happens in real life, to the movies, roller skating, bicycling, to a park, a museum, to a shop, etc. This helps further enhance the importance and value of the primary caretaker in the child's eyes. As such it helps to develop and cement their relationship. Other devices used for this purpose are, for example, a weekly allowance. The child receives it from his primary caretaker. He can spend it on toys, candies, or in any other way he likes as long as he has the approval and cooperation of his parent surrogate.

Like in any sensible family, all the above pleasurable activities and privileges are in some measure related to the child's behavior and accomplishments. They are extra rewards for his positive behaviors and achievements and consequently tend to be positive reinforcers of positive behaviors and interactions. By the same token these activities can be restricted, limited, or regulated in constructive ways by the parent surrogate as part of the educational and therapeutic approach to the child.

As the relationship between the child and the parent surrogate develops the latter becomes more and more capable of stopping or aborting negative behavior by means of a glance, by calling the child's name, or by a simple look of concern, displeasure, or disappointment. The stronger the positive ties between the child and the primary caretaker the easier it becomes to set appropriate limits in the behavior of the child without massive restrictive (and quite negative) interventions.

It will be obvious that since the child spends most of his time in the "milieu", the nature and quality of his experiences are a vital and integral part of his developmental and therapeutic progress as well as of his therapeutic plan.

Most of the children are in one or another form of "uncovering psychotherapy" two, three, and occasionally more times a week. Psychotherapy aims at dealing with the conflicts and psychopathological structures acquired up to that point in the child's life. It aims at the resolution of fixation points, at the undoing of regressions, at the interpretive analysis of maladaptive defenses, etc. The effectiveness and value of this effort may be undermined if the child's support structures fail to meet developmental requirements—if they keep the child in a continuous anxiety state because of lack of appropriate controls over the conditions of life in the ward, exposing the child to negative interactions and traumas.

In such a setting psychotherapy aimed at resolving the child's problems is not more capable of success than it could be in a chaotic, disorganized, and unpredictable family environment. Yet, as we all know, unless maxium care is exercised an inpatient ward can become nightmarish, unsettled, dehumanized, and chaotic. When that occurs many among the children and some among the senior staff may be living in constant fear of what might happen next. In some more extreme cases many of the children and some of the staff may be living in a state that approaches a permanent panic. Constant questions are being asked as to who is going to explode next, or to become aggressive, abusive, or destructive, or what is going to be destroyed, or who is going to get hurt and how badly, etc. Frequent trips to the emergency rooms at such times testify to the reality of such fears, at least before we changed over to the primary caretaker system.

Against that background psychotherapy is, in my view, next to impossible. The same is true of any form of treatment.

No less important in all these considerations is the fact that children (and more especially so the younger ones) who come to us for a variety of conflicts and reasons, have not as yet finished their developmental processes. Quite the contrary, they are very actively engaged in this process. They are still structuring their character and personalities, making constant identifications, learning new adaptive techniques, new ego skills, establishing ego and superego ideals, more adaptive defenses, etc. But for this development to continue to take place as ideally as possible, certain minimal conditions must be present. The "milieu," the ward and the parent surrogates must provide the right climate, the necessary holding environment, the right structure. In short, they must meet the child's developmental needs and rights efficiently. At the same time they must remove as quickly and as completely as possible all those factors and negative influences that are potentially serious obstacles to the adequate unfolding of the different developmental paths that must remain open to the child.

It is clear that the child's development will continue to take place on the ward whether we want it or not. The conditions in the artificial holding environment constituted by the ward and the quality of the experience with the human objects (and especially the primary caretaker) will determine if that development is going to follow desirable and favorable routes or undesirable and unfavorable ones. It is in this very fact that one of the great strengths of the inpatient treatment of children lies. It can remove a child from an unfavorable (in the developmental sense) environmental situation and place him in a more favorable one. Thus, the dangers implicit in separating a child from his objects can be turned into a valuable asset.

The Ward Liaison vis-a-vis the Primary Caretaker

I will not attempt to define or describe in detail other inpatient systems, but only mention a few of their salient aspects. In any case, it is not a simple task to describe social systems; they evolve through many years partly as the result of planning (based on certain legitimate assumptions and theoretical tenets), and partly in an unplanned manner through the actual experiences on the service, through apathy, dissatisfactions in the staff, and the thousand and one other factors that determine changes in any social system.

(I am aware that the following descriptions may be somewhat biased because of my own theoretical orientation. That I do not consider other systems to be good enough goes without saying, since I have changed ours and reorganized it as speedily as I could. I should add that no particular criticism is implied of any other systems for running inpatient wards for children. It is indeed quite conceivable that a few years hence another psychiatrist will be looking, perhaps not in very favorable terms, at the primary caretaker approach, for which I must assume full responsibility.)

In other systems the emphasis is, on the surface, but frequently only on the surface, not all that different from the primary caretaker approach. The children are assigned to therapists for the formal treatment of their presenting disturbance at the same time that somebody on the ward is assigned as the child's staff person. This person is generally called the ward liaison of the child. The main and most significant difference from the primary caretaker system is that the relationship between the ward liaison and the child is from the start extremely loose (or can easily become so) and is not based on a careful consideration of the developmental needs of children. In actual practice this staff person may not be available to the child consistently and for most of the needed time. The ward liaison person is assigned to a variety of tasks on the ward which clearly prevent him or her from interacting with the child regularly and consistently on a day-to-day basis. This excludes the degree of closeness that is essential in the primary caretaker system in order to meet the developmental needs of children and to accomplish the many other aims described earlier. The ward liaison is frequently loosely defined as somebody the child could go to, but not a parent surrogate having the responsibility for the life of the child in every detail while on the unit.

The Therapeutic Milieu and Group Care

There is in other systems a strong emphasis on the effect of the whole milieu on the child. The therapeutic milieu is expected to effect a significant influence on the child and to help bring about the desired changes in him. There can be no question as to the essential therapeutic role played by the milieu in the life of the child. Indeed, as we will see, the primary caretaker system relies heavily on its "curative" value. What has to be clearly understood is that an assembly of professional people, however well intentioned, does not by itself constitute a therapeutic milieu. They most certainly constitute a milieu but one that in spite of its good will may in actual fact be detrimental to the children. For a milieu to be truly therapeutic it must have a certain structure that is itself finely tuned to the developmental rights and needs of children.

Each one of its members' roles must be strictly defined in terms of interactional function with specific children, with the whole group of children on the ward, and with the other members of the staff. Unless constant and special care is exercised the milieu becomes a theoretical myth, under which can hide the fact that the situation may have degenerated into some form of loosely structured group care for the children. In that case the system may have partly or wholly lost the ability to care for the individual needs of each of the children.

I must emphasize that group care for children, which tends to deprive them of a very close, consistent, and sustaining relationship with a meaningful adult is highly detrimental for the child. In my view such an approach should not be considered a second best, as is frequently done, except in the most extraordinary circumstances. We only need to remind ourselves, for example, of the devastating effects that orphanages, where such conditions attained, had on children.

The Group Approach, The Phenomenon of Gang
Formation, and its Consequences

The group approach gives little or no positive help in the control of the children's behavior. Since individual members of the group of caretakers seldom have deep relationships with any child, the staff is forced to rely on the use of punitive measures to control behavior. Even in those cases where someone in the staff group has managed to establish a special contact with one child or another, it will be found that his influence is limited. The child will tend to side with his peer group as war is declared between the two groups. This, as we know, can become a daily happening. This is not surprising since the process is much facilitated by a group approach to the children.

In an enclosed environment such as a ward, the constitution of one group with common interests which affect the other members of the milieu naturally forces them into a similar group organization, with interests and aims generally quite contrary to those of the first group. Though this specific type of group formation is quite deleterious, various forms of group organizations in a children's ward are not only unavoidable, but even desirable. It is, nevertheless, essential that such groups serve positive and constructive functions; that they be based on positive feelings and experiences rather than in negative ones. The latter is one of the very many undesirable contributions an inpatient setting can make to the welfare of the children and staff. It should be noted that negative groupings such as this are a very sensitive barometer as to how healthy or unhealthy the ward climate is.

None of the above is by any means uncommon in any inpatient setting, but on occasion the situation may reach such a climax that a quasi-permanent state of war exists between the staff as a group and the children as a group. This can be facilitated by the presence of two or three highly disturbed and aggressive children that quickly take control of the group. Soon enough they may organize other children for the performance of highly violent and destructive acts. The staff as a group has at this point little effective influence on this behavior. They may be afraid of being hurt (quite rightly) and of the violence of the frequent outbursts. Understandable as this is, this situation will leave many children with no alternative but to join in this disruptive behavior. Some will do so for fear of reprisals by the leaders and other members of the gang. Others will join in because such behavior is highly exciting. Such participation is seductive for children who feel neglected, unwanted, and emotionally deprived and at the same time either lack the necessary controls by themselves or do not find in the environment the much needed adult support.

As we know, a frightened person becomes highly punitive and even violent, though that violence may be well disguised and somewhat controlled. For the staff, massive, though controlled retaliation can become the rule. Then, children are restricted physically; two or three staff being required to overwhelm the most aggressive. In the process someone on the staff or a child often gets hurt. Trips to the emergency room can become common. Indeed, three to four a week may be the norm at such times.

Under these circumstances children are frequently placed in the so-called quiet rooms. They may be left in isolation for prolonged periods of time. Indeed, in one case I know, a child was forgotten in a quiet room for several hours. The assumption is that the rages and violence should exhaust themselves so that the child could not harm anybody or anything. However, violence only engenders more violence. The quiet rooms themselves may soon look as if a tornado had gone through. They may be set on fire on occasion, requiring calls to the fire brigade. I have seen quiet room doors so badly burned that it was miraculous that the child who set it on fire was not hurt.

Once the situation is this far out of hand the conditions of the wards in general cannot be expected to be much better. Ceilings, furniture, equipment, toys, etc. may be in absolute shambles. New objects may have an expected life of no more than a few days, sometimes just a few hours. Children can no longer have any toys or possessions since they get stolen, destroyed, or simply taken away by one bully or another. Such things as plants and pictures on the walls are simply impossible to keep for the same reason. Damage to property and incidents of stealing are not necessarily restricted to the wards. Other areas of the hospital or the institution may be vandalized. Nothing can be considered safe since the children may have managed to acquire master keys.

I have in one occasion seen a ward where the staff had grown so apathetic and hopeless that the evening I visited I was unable to walk into the children's rooms safely. They were littered with upturned chairs, tables, pillows, and general rubbish. The bed sheets were strewn on the floor while many of the children were sleeping on their bare mattresses. And yet I should strongly emphasize that the staff responsible for this ward was constituted not of calloused human beings, but of a rather fine group of professionals and their ancillaries. But, they had been driven to despair.

Incidents of children running away can become a common occurrence. Visitors to the wards may be received in a verbally assaultive manner. "Fucker," "get the hell out of here," "who is this son of a bitch," may become not uncommon greetings. And that is perhaps better than being hit at the door, or somewhere along the hall, by a fist, a flying book, or even a piece of furniture.

In short, it can become not only unpleasant, but unsafe to visit such wards.

As you would expect, under such circumstances not only are the children and the staff in constant terror, but the turnover of the staff becomes absolutely incredible. Such staff will honestly state how they dreaded coming on duty, and leaving the ward after a shift of duty was felt as an enormous relief. Many of them felt confused, and at a loss as to what to do or how to do it. Self-esteem runs low. They can describe too the apathy that can overtake the system during such periods. Whenever ugly conflicts arise, the whole staff may hang back, waiting for somebody else to intervene first. No one feels any particular responsibility for the children creating the uproar and no one wants to get hurt. Naturally, this can lead to unnecessary escalation of all kinds of minor incidents among the children. By the time the staff can no longer avoid intervening, they will have a major crisis on their hands.

It is my opinion that for most of this type of deterioration the real culprit is the fact that the staff slides back gradually into a group approach under the misguided impression that the "milieu" will do the required job. In fact, direct links between the children and individual staff members are weakened. Thus, there is no longer a healthy balance between the peer culture group (of whatever quality it happens to be) and the necessary sustaining and ordering attachment of the children to the senior staff. In the deprivational conditions in which the children feel left, all hell is bound to break loose, and it generally does.

Yet, all that I have described so far is in no way unique to any particular setting. I have no doubt that much of it, if not most of it is easily recognizable by those with experience in the inpatient treatment of children. They are the potential operative negative forces always present in different degrees in such services. They simply wait for the right opportunity to materialize.

Conflicting opinions among the psychiatrists responsible for the various methods of care delivery and their merits are to be expected. As I see it, that is an unavoidable difficulty. Therefore I will try to introduce later on a number of what I consider to be more "objective" and quantifiable criteria in order to assess the benefits derived from the changes associated with the primary caretaker system in our setting.

ADVANTAGES OF THE PRIMARY CARETAKER FROM THE POINT OF VIEW OF THE CHILDREN

1. It provides them with one immediately recognizable, constant, sympathetic, and willing parent substitute from the very instant they join the unit. The child is initially free to regulate how much or how little use he will want to make of the primary caretaker according to age, stage of development, type of psychopathology, special needs and/or situations that led to the child's referral to the inpatient unit. In the long run it is absolutely essential that the primary caretaker works his or her way into as positive and meaningful a relationship as can be developed.

2. The very specific relationship to the same person (primary caretaker), rather than to a large number of different individuals facilitates the child's finding out the expectations of the system. They quickly learn what behaviors are acceptable or unacceptable, since all of this is mediated by his primary caretaker. This helps to make such limits consistent, constant, and predictable, since the same person sets them. Further, since all of his attention is concentrated on the welfare of his two charges, he can enforce them evenly if and when necessary. Even more important, he can negotiate and explain to the specific child the reasons for the limits, indeed the desirability of such limits and the necessity to respect them not only for the sake of other, but in terms of one's own best interests.

3. The primary caretaker, given his constant relationship to the child, can offer positive, pleasurable, and constructive interactional models for effectively relating to other children and adults. His manners, his concern for others, his respect for others, his problem-solving attitudes, all constitute effective models for ego-building identifications for the child. In our experience this is particularly valuable for children who lacked such opportunities in their own environment or who lived in a highly negative one.

We should note that identifications of this type tend to take place surprisingly quickly and effectively once a strong, positive tie has been developed between the child and his parent surrogate.

4. Through this relationship the child has a permanent, eager, and sympathetic adult object in whom he can confide, go to with his problems, and go to for comfort and affection when comfort and affection are required. In contrast to a group situation, he does not have to wait his turn or compete for attention and affection. In group situations many children are not able to compete with the more outgoing and aggressive ones for the favors of any willing staff. Under such circumstances many tend to withdraw, become depressed, and act-out negatively in order to get the attention from another human being to which they are entitled. In the primary caretaker program they have their own special person always readily available to them. Furthermore, this person has "special value" since much effort was put into developing a meaningful relationship between the child and the parent surrogate. Thus, the child does not have to compete excessively or inappropriately with large numbers of children to have his developmental rights and needs met appropriately.

5. The child's therapist can relate consistently to one person in the child's milieu—the very person who has the most responsibility for his patient in the ward. He can relay to the primary caretaker his specific recommendations for the management of the child's problems. It is pretty well impossible to expect a whole staff of twenty or more people to be consistent in the handling, for example, of certain behaviors of the child, let alone to remain aware of the specific recommendations made for each one in a group of eighteen children.

6. The child is under constant benign supervision. This is particularly useful for children with certain types of problems. But more important, the child has freedom to organize his free time and activities constructively under this benign supervision. If he does not know how his free time can be structured for him by the primary caretaker (as a parent would for his child) in a form that is not only enjoyable for the patient, but constructive in ways that promote ego growth. He can of course choose to play with his

parent surrogate, or they can go together to interesting places in the community if they so choose.

This helps to avoid the negative possibilities, even traumatic situations, that easily develop in large and loosely supervised groups of children in institutions. It is not that we ban or do not expect to see some negative behaviors or highly aggressive interactions. Yet, we expect them to take place in reasonably well controlled situations where the possibility of escalation to experiences of traumatic proportions, physical harm, or destruction can be controlled in time, without a massive uproar on the ward and/ or retaliatory interventions on the part of the staff. Otherwise, these may become necessary in order to ensure everyone's safety.

7. The close and carefully developed relationship between the primary caretaker and his two charges tends to avoid the common and frequently highly destructive phenomenon of group interaction known as gang formation. Gang formation is one of the most negative and destructive situations possible in an inpatient unit. A loose group milieu situation very much favors this outcome. Children without close ties to meaningful adult objects in the ward will group together (as they do in real life when family ties and organization are meaningless in terms of the needs of the child) in a highly aggressive and destructive gang. Usually it declares war on the staff and the institution and spends much of its time in devising new and ever more destructive means of acting-out and provocation. Soon there are two camps, the staff camp and the children's camp, on the way to an ever escalating war with each other. Both camps are frightened, the adults because of the natural horror of that much unleashed and uncontrollable aggression (with a similar fear of their own reactions to it) as well as the fear of getting hurt, maimed, or even killed. The children, caught in the middle of a hostile and destructive orgy over which they lose control, end up being traumatized by the overwhelming strength of their aggressive drive, by the guilt experienced in relation to their behavior, by the fear of not being able to control themselves, and by the failure of the adult world to control them. Frequent repetition of this situation is extremely detrimental to the welfare of the children for all the above reasons; but more importantly, in

some ways it acts as a habit-forming drug with heights of excitement that must be periodically reexperienced. When such situations repeat themselves at periodic intervals, one has to conclude that the ward has lost its helping, curative capacities and has become the training ground for psychopathic, asocial, and criminal behavior.

If we take into account that most inpatient settings will have several children with overt psychopathic or sociopathic inclinations, serious problems with the control of their aggression, or children that have declared war on society, we can see how easy it is for such phenomena to develop. Further, if we understand group psychology, the contagion phenomenon, and the readiness with which chaotic groups (including those of children) will follow the behavior of the most psychopathic or destructive of its leaders, we can readily understand the potential danger always looming in an inpatient ward organization.

THE PROCESS OF CHANGE AND ITS RESULTS

In spite of a consensus among the ward staff, teachers, activity therapists, social workers, psychologists, and psychiatrists that the wards were not running as efficiently as they could at that point, there was still enormous resistance to any change. Established social systems are well known to be very resistive to change.

A brief look at some of the objections to the proposed change to the primary caretaker system may be of interest.

Since the new system is based on the establishment of a strong positive relationship between the parent surrogate and the children and by extension of the whole of the human elements in what ought to be a truly therapeutic milieu for the children, I made the decision to get rid of the quiet rooms on the wards. This created something close to a panic situation among the staff. Most did not think that the wards could be run without them, and feared for their own safety as well as that of the children. We held discussions about the dehumanizing aspects of quiet rooms (actually isolation cells as in mental hospitals), the multiple negative messages conveyed to the children at conscious and unconscious levels (such as: you are dangerous and cannot be controlled, that is why we have quiet rooms and place you there); about their undermining effect in terms of learning to develop more adaptive and positive means of negotiating conflictual situations with the children; about its closing effect on possible attempts to help them express their anger by more socially acceptable methods, since at the drop of a hat and without much discussion the quiet room was the automatic solution to many behavioral problems, especially those of an aggressive nature; and even about the fact that some occasional staff members ventilated their sadism by confining children in the quiet rooms. However, closing the quiet rooms led, in combination with other factors, to various staff members' spontaneous resignations from the system. Later on, some of those who remained as the changes took place mentioned that former staff members were quite incredulous about the fact that we could do without the quiet rooms. They asked, "But how can you possibly run the wards without them?" The current staff answered that as the new system developed the incidents of violence became rare and the quiet rooms are nowadays unnecessary. The wards were never safer than they are now. This was met with similar incredulity and astonishment.

The children themselves were no less disturbed than the staff at the idea that the "quiet rooms" were to disappear and were not to be used. Since they knew I was responsible for the decision many approached me in disbelief with various inquiries. Some of the children were simultaneously pleased and frightened. A few showed clearly that they had been fully trained by the procedure into thinking that they were like dangerous animals, incapable of controlling their behavior and as such had to be managed by brutal force and placed in the quiet room. Two or three of the children asked me, with obvious terror in their voices and faces, "How will I be controlled when I have my hairies?" They shook their heads in disbelief, thinking I was making a big mistake when I answered that I did not think their hairies—the children's lingo for "seemingly" uncontrollable aggressive outbursts and destructive behavior—were the only way of expressing anger. There were better ways that they would learn if we did not have the quiet rooms. I was sure that they could control themselves and did not really need either the hairies or the quiet rooms. Indeed they do not. Such behavior is rarely observed nowadays on the wards under the primary caretaker system. There are, of course, occasional aggressive outbursts, but they rarely acquire frightening proportions. The primary caretaker influence on the children is such that a word, a glance, calling a child's name, a small talk, or some "room time," manages to prevent escalation into major incidents.

Previously, in the course of a week, any one of the wards would send to my office fifteen to twenty-five reports concerning the use of the quiet room, but I do not get any such reports today. By the same token, the number of trips to the emergency room that in the past averaged between three to five in any given week, is now essentially nil. An occasional trip tends to represent the sort of incident one would expect in a place where there are thirty-six very active young children in a relatively confined space. I mean such things as tripping, taking a fall from a bike or roller skates, etc.

A more unexpected source of objections among a few of the ward staff was based on an extraordinary reluctance to accept full responsibility for two children only. They preferred the earlier, more indiscriminate group approach to the children. It seemed that a few feared the degree of emotional commitment that the change would imply. The new system offered little buffering for the inordinate demands that children, especially disturbed and emotionally neglected children, can place on an available adult. In the group approach one could keep the interactions to one's level of tolerance, or even avoid them altogether by keeping busy with other more neutralized activities.It was my impression that in some cases that level was so low that one or two of the staff members were unsuitable for work with children.

The new system clearly delineated the primary caretaker functions and responsibilities. This was generally regarded as an advantage since there was much dissatisfaction with the unclear perimeters of duties and functions in the group situation. Many, on the other hand, were not pleased with the aloofness of the group approach and were very anxious for closer contact and responsibilities in regard to specific children. The arguments for and against continued to rage for a while. It was clear too that the primary caretaker would be more exposed. One's performance would be more visible to everybody, and more open to criticisms and evaluation.

Some staff members objected that one could not really play the role of a parent for the child. They argued that even if it could be done, it was undesirable since we should not compete in this area with the real parents. But they were not asked to play the role of the parent for the child, but only that of a surrogate. Indeed, no competition with the parents is intended by the system. The only intention was to substitute temporarily as a reliable, meaningful, and constant adult in the life of children whose placement in our service separated from their real objects. Staff was asked only to fill the gap, to provide the support and structure that had been artificially removed from the children's lives and to provide it only in that measure that the children required.

Perhaps one of the most dreaded implications of the new system was the fear of the repeated losses the staff would be exposed to. Anybody working closely with children is well aware of the enormous countertransference feelings that arise, of the intensity of the attachments that may develop. This is even more so for some adults, with certain character structures, needs, and life experiences. The new system encouraged the development of close relationships, with the concomitant feelings that are bound to grow. Yet, at one point or another the relationship would have to be terminated. When that happens the relationship and the feelings do not go away with the child. They cause pain and lead to mourning. The staff will hardly be able to recover from the experience or complete their mourning when another child will arrive. The whole enjoyable and painful cycle repeats itself. Of course, all human beings are shy of pain, but if this type of work with children is going to be effective and humane the price must be paid.

Some among the staff can establish a healthy balance between their general professional aims of helping children in distress, and attachment to one specific child. Thus for them any child is one among the many they hope to help; though this does not avoid the pain, loss and mourning, it acts as a balancing wheel. Others in spite of a clear awareness of their professional aims get lost in the pain, at least for a while.[1]

PRACTICAL CONSIDERATIONS AND DIFFICULTIES IN IMPLEMENTATION

The staff shifts are of eight continuous hours starting at 3:00 P.M. and ending at 11:30 P.M. We decided to organize the primary caretaker system around this period of time because this represented the nonstructured time in the life of the children. In this way we tried to maximize the hours of close contact between the primary staff and the child. The children go to school from 8:30 A.M. to 3:30 P.M. During this period the school staff is responsible for them, as in ordinary life. The school staff is responsible for the lunch hour as well.

The primary staff works five days a week and takes two days off. This poses no significant difficulty with many of the patients since we like as many of them as possible to spend the weekend at home with their families. Yet, there are a number of children that for clinical or other reasons cannot go home. Sometimes they are not wanted there by their parents. For these children, who are the ones in most need, the continuity of the relationship with their primary staff breaks down. This is unavoidable. The primary staff have their own private lives, their families, friends, or even their studies to pursue since many of them are students. In any case, they need this break to recover from an extraordinarily demanding and at times an exhausting job. They need it too to restore distance, emotional feeling tone and so on.

Furthermore, no one can avoid a cold, flu, an accident, or an illness. At such times the continuity of the relationship breaks. In

---

1. Because of the dyanamics involved it would seem salutary that once in a while the primary staff be given a backup role for a time. Those in a backup role can in turn move to primary staffing. This might help to distribute the burden.

order to cope with these unavoidable breaks, a backup system was devised. Thus, as in an extended family, there is a second person in the staff that substitutes in the case of absences of the primary staff. That person is clearly identified for the child as another member of his or her family, like a benevolent, friendly and reliable aunt or uncle that comes to take care of things when the parents must be absent. Like an uncle or aunt, though he is of great importance to the child in the absence of the primary staff, he must not assume the role of the parent surrogate. He must not overstep his limits. He is there to fill the gap and meet the child's need without competing with the primary staff for that privileged position. To do so would tend to dilute the intensity and quality of the relationship between the primary staff and his children. That would be a step in the wrong direction, back toward group care.

Another problem in the continuity of the relationship through the course of a day between the child and the primary staff takes place during the waking time period. It proved impossible to have the primary staff come early in the morning for an hour and a half to deal with the waking time period (desirable as this obviously is) and then return for their afternoon shift. This of course would be ideal. This period is of enormous importance in the shape that the rest of the day will take for the child. The same is true of the feeling tone the child will carry with him. One must realize that every awakening takes place in a strange environment and in the absence of the actual parents. One must realize too that the child's ego shortly after waking up is not at its best, but in fact is frequently regressed. During this time many negative things can happen, all of them with the tendency to escalate beyond reasonable proportions because of the temporarily altered ego state.

It is for this reason that we considered it important to have large numbers of staff with the children during this period. An attempt at constancy is introduced by having the same person handle the waking up of children. They are called "morning care assistants" and are mostly well selected students who need a couple of hours of work a day. They provide constancy and structure, help the children to get ready for school, and try to avoid negative interactions among them. In this way the children are off to a good start.

Not much more is expected of the morning care assistant than a brief, pleasant interaction and a structuring role for the activities of which they are in charge. Here again, any dilution of the intensity of the relationship to the primary staff is avoided.

SOME RESULTS OF THE CHANGE

I mentioned the difficulties of being objective in the evaluation of the results brought about by the change of system. The ones listed below seem to me to introduce at least some measure of objectivity.

1. The dramatic decrease in the use of the quiet room as a "resource" to control behavior. As already explained, they no longer exist on the wards and more important, the staff does not feel that they are needed. As an added bonus, the staff has developed more sophisticated skills for the humane management of conflicts, disruptive behaviors, aggressive outbursts, etc.

2. The wards have a pleasant, humane atmosphere. it is not that there are no incidents. Of course there are, but they are of a different quality, they are modulated differently. Aggressive outbursts do occur, but once again, they are of a different quality, not as primitive and uncontrollable as in other systems. As the result of the above neither the children or the staff get hurt. Trips to the emergency room are essentially nil. As explained earlier, when one is required, it is usually the result of a bona fide accident. The fact that neither the staff nor the children have gotten hurt for a period of over twenty months—coinciding with the implementation of the new system—seems to me an objective measure of the positive significance of the changes.

3. Similarly the unrelenting destruction of the physical plant of the ward, furniture, and other objects has essentially stopped. There may be the occasional incident, but not the systematic and constant damage that is a way of life in many inpatient settings. The remnants of such damage are still visible in some areas where repair has not been possible. They stand there as silent witness,

much as the wounds of a city devastated by war testify to the earlier violence. Such an area is, for example, the ceilings of the wards. They are built of a special metallic tile that could not be replaced. In many rooms there was hardly any left intact. I referred earlier too to the short life expectancy of any new object brought onto the ward.

Today, after significant repairs such as painting, adding new furniture, drapes, carpets, and pictures as well as notice and display boards, plants, toys, etc. the wards look quite different. The senseless damage has come to an end. These different new improvements made at great expense have stood the test of time. They are still unharmed.

I can remember, for example, that the locksmith had to be called two and three times a week to repair the lock of the entrance door to one of the wards. The children's favorite pastime was to damage it, as was the case with anything else. After weeks of constant calls to the locksmith, the maintenance department sent a memo refusing to repair them again! The same door has not required the services of the locksmith for a period of over twenty months.

4. I cannot recall a single incident of children running away from the service for well over a period of a year though the wards are open at all times. In contrast several runaways a week were not unusual under the previous system.

5. Children can now have their toys and other personal possessions in their rooms. They are very rarely destroyed or stolen. In the old system, personal toys were simply out of the question since they were destroyed or stolen almost immediately. The same was true for other objects such as plants, pictures, and so on. These things find themselves in a relatively safe environment today.

6. Newcomers to the patient population were frequently received with a flood of information as to how to fight the staff, and quite effective lessons in the arts of aggression and destruction. In sharp contrast staff members describe how newcomers are welcomed now into the "family" by the other children. They include constructive suggestions as to how to behave and explanations of limits. The implication here is that they expect the newcomers to adhere to the rules.

7. The turnover of staff is now enormously reduced, and is now commensurate with the staff population. In the past, large numbers left out of fear of being hurt, general disatisfactions with their roles, despair about their usefulness, and the general unpleasantness of the milieu situation.

8. Practically everyone on the ward staff, including nurses, psychiatric care workers, teachers, psychiatrists, psychologists, and social workers recognizes the enormous positive changes brought about through the primary caretaker system. But more important, they are reasonably happy and contented about their jobs. It is not that there are no tensions and dissatisfactions. There are. But they do not interfere with their basic, positive feelings toward their professional activities in the wards. Furthermore, the immediate ward staff gets much gratification because the results of their efforts are visible in the significant improvements in many of the children.

The degree of consensus among the staff as to the benefits derived from the change is quite remarkable, especially for a psychiatric setting. Many among the ward staff have many years of experience. They have operated under various approaches. Yet, they tend to verbalize a marked preference for the primary caretaker approach.

INDEX